Statistical Methods
in Epidemiology

Monographs in Epidemiology and Biostatistics
edited by Brian MacMahon

Monographs in Epidemiology and Biostatistics
Volume 12

Statistical Methods in Epidemiology

HAROLD A. KAHN

CHRISTOPHER T. SEMPOS

New York   Oxford
OXFORD UNIVERSITY PRESS
1989

Oxford University Press

Oxford   New York   Toronto
Delhi   Bombay   Calcutta   Madras   Karachi
Petaling Jaya   Singapore   Hong Kong   Tokyo
Nairobi   Dar es Salaam   Cape Town
Melbourne   Auckland

and associated companies in
Berlin   Ibadan

Library of Congress Cataloging-in-Publication Data
Kahn, Harold A.
Statistical methods in epidemiology.
(Monographs in epidemiology and biostatistics; v. 12)
Rev. ed. of: An introduction to epidemiologic
methods/Harold A. Kahn.   1983.
Includes bibliographies and index.
1. Epidemiology—Statistical methods.
I. Sempos, Christopher T.   II. Kahn, Harold A.
Introduction to epidemiologic methods.
III. Title.   IV. Series.   [DNLM: 1. Epidemiologic Methods.
W1 M0567LT v.12 / WA 950 K61i]
RA652.2.M3K34   1989   614.4'072   88-22380
ISBN 0-19-505751-1
ISBN 0-19-505049-5 (pbk.)

9 8 7

Printed in the United States of America
on acid-free paper

For LENORA and JUDITH

Preface

This book is a major revision of H. A. Kahn's *An Introduction to Epidemiologic Methods* [Oxford University Press 1983]. New topics include Cox regression, Kaplan–Meier life tables, adjusted relative risk using person-year data, confidence limits for relative risk by methods analogous to Woolf's method for odds ratios, adjustment for confounding variables that are related only to the disease of interest but not to the risk factor being investigated, additional methods for estimating confidence limits on the standardized mortality (morbidity) ratio (SMR), the Mantel–Fleiss prescription for evaluating the validity of the Mantel–Haenszel summary χ^2, and comparing life tables with adjustment for confounding variables using the Mantel–Haenszel procedure.

We have incorporated an Appendix of Framingham (Massachusetts) Heart Study data to serve two objectives. First, it permits us to apply the various analytical methods described to an *identical data set* so that results may be compared. It is our opinion that a comparison of results between a complex procedure that many students think of as a "black box" and a simpler procedure that they can completely comprehend and calculate personally will be extremely helpful. The Appendix also provides a source of real data for the student exercises that are now included. These exercises in which students are asked to assemble data from the listing (and tabulations) in the Appendix are always based on small samples. This is done deliberately to avoid an overload of clerical work. The statistics computed for such exercises can be expected to have wide confidence limits and may at times seem to contradict our teaching that different methods will usually reflect similar results. The contradiction is apparent rather than real because large numeric differences often exist in combination with substantive agreement. For example, confidence limits for an odds ratio that range from 0.4 to 5.2 are not substantively different from limits of 0.6 to 7.9. In addition, our teaching emphasizes that agreement can usually be expected among various methods only if the data are based on a reasonably adequate sample size.

The original objective, to write a book about statistical methods for chronic disease epidemiology that could be read and understood by nonstatisticians, has been maintained. In addition, wherever reconsideration has suggested to us that the original text was obscure or ambiguous, we have tried to make improvements. This book would be appropriate for an Epidemiologic Methods class where the prerequisites were Principles of Epidemiology and at least one course in statistics.

At the suggestion of Martha Linet, and to encourage proper perspective, we have added a chapter on data collection. This is in keeping with our view that the accuracy and completeness of the data collection process usually have more effect on a study's ability to answer the questions posed than does the choice among alternative methods of analysis.

We wish to thank again George Comstock, Sidney Cutler, Fred Ederer, Uri Goldbourt, Lawrence Gould, the late Abraham Lilienfeld, Eric Peretz, Lenora Kahn, Nathan Mantel, Jack Medalie, Paolo Pasquini, James Schlesselman and Stanley Schor who helped with *An Introduction to Epidemiologic Methods,* the precursor to the present volume. We are also grateful to James Tonascia for permission to reprint unpublished data on sample size and to the literary executor of the late Sir Ronald A. Fisher, F.R.S.; to Frank Yates, F.R.S.; and to Longman Group, London, for permission to reprint random numbers from their book *Statistical Tables for Biological, Agricultural and Medical Research* [6th ed., 1974].

George Comstock, Nathan Mantel, and James Schlesselman read an early draft of this book and provided us with many helpful comments and suggestions that we wish to acknowledge with gratitude. We also wish to thank the National Heart, Lung, and Blood Institute, NIH, DHHS for providing us with Framingham Heart Study data; Anne Looker for her helpful comments; Yvonne Jones, Roy Milton, Joel Novak, Warren Pendleton, and Paul Sorlie for assistance with computer operations; and Stephen Kraft for the artwork. Of course, the views expressed in this book are those of the authors and do not necessarily reflect the views of those who have assisted us.

Silver Spring, Maryland   H. A. K.
July 1988   C. T. S.

Contents

Abbreviations

AR	Attributable risk
CHD	Coronary heart disease
CL	Confidence limits
DBP	Diastolic blood pressure
DSR	Direct standardized rate
FRW	Framingham relative weight
ISR	Indirect standardized rate
M–H	Mantel–Haenszel
MP	Matched pairs
OR	Odds ratio
RF	Risk factor
RR	Relative risk
SBP	Systolic blood pressure
SMR	Standardized morbidity (or mortality) ratio

Statistical Methods
in Epidemiology

1
Review of Selected Elementary Statistics

Although almost all readers of this book will have completed one or more introductory statistics courses, our experience tells us that many students will benefit from a brief review of vocabulary, notation, elementary algebra, mean and variance formulas, and related topics. The items included in this review are needed to understand many of the epidemiologic methods to be discussed in later chapters. This section is *not* a capsule review of an introductory statistics course and is not intended to be used as such.

VOCABULARY

A *population,* or *universe,* which should always be well defined by the investigator, can often be effectively described by certain summary constants called *parameters.* As an example we might cite the mean and standard deviation of systolic blood pressure values for all persons selected for service in the United States armed forces during the period 1942–1945. The complete set of blood pressure values for this group during 1942–1945 constitutes a population, and the mean and standard deviation of these values are parameters that, if known, can be used to describe this particular population. In this case, since the population values are almost certainly not normally distributed, the mean and standard deviation would not perfectly describe the population distribution of blood pressure values.

A random *sample* of blood pressure values could be taken from selective service records for 1942–1945 and the mean and standard deviation of the sample values calculated. These two summary values are called *statistics* and are generally used in estimating the corresponding *parameters.*

Systolic blood pressure is a variable reported in *discrete* values, such as 140, 126, 138. This variable is, however, at least in concept, a *continuous variable* and can assume any value within its range, such as 126.359021 . . . .

A special type of variable that we shall refer to frequently is *dichotomous*—sick or well, male or female, inducted into service or not inducted into service, etc. Dichotomous variables are usually assigned a value of 1 if the attribute is present and a value of 0 if it is not. The average value of the variable will then be between 0 and 1 and equal to the probability that the attribute is present.

A *null hypothesis* (H_0) states that the statistics (such as sample means) being compared are the result of random sampling from the same population and thus any difference between them is due to chance. A test of a null hypothesis is subject to two types of errors. *Type I error* is the result of rejecting the null hypothesis when it is in fact true. *Type II error* is the result of failing to reject the null hypothesis when it is in fact false. However, if the null hypothesis is true, type II error is nonexistent and irrelevant. Similarly, if the null hypothesis is false, type I error has no meaning. Because we do not know the actual facts of the populations from which our samples are derived (i.e., whether or not the null hypothesis is true), we invariably want studies that are designed to limit both types of errors. Thus, *if* the null hypothesis is true, we want to limit the type I error to a value α, which is usually specified to be .01 or .05. If the null hypothesis is false and some alternative hypothesis (H_a) is true, we want to limit the type II error to a value β, commonly specified to be about .10. The *power* of a test to reject H_0 when H_a is true is equal to $1 - \beta$.

NOTATION AND ELEMENTARY ALGEBRA
The letters

$$X_1, X_2, \ldots, X_j, \ldots, X_N$$

represent values of a variable for the 1st, 2nd, . . . , *j*th, . . . , and *N*th individuals in a *population* of size *N*.

The letters

$$x_1, x_2, \ldots, x_j, \ldots, x_n$$

represent values of a variable for the 1st, 2nd, . . . , *j*th, . . . , and *n*th individuals in a *sample* of size *n*.

The notation

$$\sum_{j=1}^{N} X_j$$

represents the sum of all values of X_j from X_1 through and including X_N. Note: where the meaning is clear, we shall use ΣX_j or even ΣX to represent the sum of all values of X in place of the more complete notation.

The following are other common notations used in statistical analysis:

$|x|$ the absolute value of x, i.e., $|7|$ or $|-7| = 7$

$E(X)$ the expected value of X; equals each value of X multiplied by the probability of that value, summed over all values; the mean value of X

$\cong$ approximately equal to

$>$ greater than ($a > b$ indicates that a is greater than b)

$\geqslant$ greater than or equal to

$<$ less than ($a < b$ indicates that a is less than b)

$\leqslant$ less than or equal to

Note: students having difficulty remembering whether *less than* is represented by $<$ or by $>$ should note that the point of the wedge is next to the smaller quantity: $7 < 10$ and $5 > 2$.

If a quadratic equation is in the standard form

$$ax^2 + bx + c = 0$$

then

$$x = \frac{-b \pm \sqrt{b^2 - 4ac}}{2a}$$

If $10^x = y$, then x is the logarithm of y, using base 10.

If $e^x = y$, then x is the logarithm of y and y is the antilogarithm of x, both using base e.

The letter e represents the base used in natural logarithms and can be defined as the limiting value of the expression $(1 + \frac{1}{x})^x$ as x increases in size indefinitely. To illustrate: if $x = 2$, then $(1 + \frac{1}{2})^2 = (1.50)^2 = 2.250$; if $x = 100$, then $(1 + \frac{1}{100})^{100} = (1.01)^{100} = 2.705$. To three decimal places, $e = 2.718$. That is, even if $x = 1\,000\,000$ or more, $(1 + \frac{1}{x})^x$ will be less than 2.719. Hereafter, we shall refer only to logarithms using base e.

Also,

$$\ln y = \text{logarithm of } y, \text{ using base } e$$

$$\ln(xy) = \ln x + \ln y$$

$$\ln(a^x) = x(\ln a)$$

$$\ln(x/y) = \ln x - \ln y$$

$$e^0 = e^{x-x} = e^x e^{-x} = 1$$

$$e^{-x} = 1/e^x$$

$$x^{1/2} = \sqrt{x}$$

MEAN AND VARIANCE FORMULAS

The equations given below and the ideas corresponding to them occur frequently in epidemiologic analysis, and the reader should therefore be familiar with them.

$$\sum_{j=1}^{N} X_j/N = \mu \tag{1-1}$$

where μ represents the mean of the population.

$$\sum_{j=1}^{N} (X_j - \mu)^2/N = \text{var}(X) \tag{1-2}$$

where $\text{var}(X)$ represents the population variance.

$$\sum_{j=1}^{n} x_j/n = \bar{x} \tag{1-3}$$

where $\bar{x}$ represents the mean of the sample. If the sample is picked at random, the expected value of $\bar{x}$, that is, its average value over all possible sample selections, is μ. In symbols,

$$E(\bar{x}) = \mu \tag{1-4}$$

$$\sum_{j=1}^{n} (x_j - \bar{x})^2/(n-1) = \hat{\text{var}}(X) \tag{1-5}$$

where $\hat{\text{var}}(X)$ is an estimate of $\text{var}(X)$ based on sample data. Note: when we are discussing both sample statistics and parameters or whenever necessary for clarity, we shall use a circumflex (ˆ) to indicate the sample statistic and the absence of any such mark to indicate a parameter. Since parameters do not have variances, we can dispense with the circumflex over the statistic in expressions for the variance or the standard error of a statistic. We make two exceptions to these conventions. The first is for the parameter and statistic of a binomial distribution. Instead of P and $\hat{P}$ for the proportion with the characteristic under study, we shall use P and p for the *parameter* and *statistic*, respectively. The second exception is for the number of cases in each cell of a table. Here, too, the population values will be designated by capital letters—A, B, C, ... —and the sample values by lower case letters—a, b, c, ...

$$\text{var}(\bar{x}) = \frac{\text{var}(X)}{n} \frac{(N-n)}{(N-1)} \tag{1-6}$$

$$\text{SE}(\bar{x}) = \left[\frac{\text{var}(X)}{n} \frac{(N-n)}{(N-1)} \right]^{1/2} \tag{1-7}$$

$SE(\bar{x})$ is the standard error of the sample mean. It is usually estimated by $\left[\dfrac{\hat{var}(X)}{n}\dfrac{(N-n)}{(N-1)}\right]^{1/2}$ in which case we write $\hat{SE}(\bar{x})$. Whenever the sample size is less than 10 percent of the population size, the term $(N-n)/(N-1)$, known as the finite sampling factor or finite multiplier, has little effect and can be omitted from the equation. The variability of the sample mean, or any other sample statistic derived from a sample of size n, relates to the dispersion of an imaginary distribution of the sample statistic *in all possible samples* of size n from the population being sampled. The standard error of the sample statistic is, in fact, the standard deviation of this imaginary distribution.

VARIANCE FORMULAS FOR FUNCTIONS OF VARIABLES

The following formulas for the variance of simple functions are very useful.

$$\text{var}(X + Y) = \text{var}(X) + \text{var}(Y), \text{ if } X \text{ and } Y \text{ are independent} \qquad (1\text{-}8)$$

$$\text{var}(X - Y) = \text{var}(X) + \text{var}(Y), \text{ if } X \text{ and } Y \text{ are independent} \qquad (1\text{-}9)$$

$$\text{var}(KX) = K^2 \text{var}(X), \text{ where } K \text{ is a constant not subject to sampling variation} \qquad (1\text{-}10)$$

MEAN AND VARIANCE FORMULAS FOR GROUPED DATA

Data are often summarized in groups, such as blood pressure classes 120–129, 130–139, ... The following definitions are used:

X_i = value assigned to each member of the ith class; usually taken as the midpoint of the ith class interval

f_i = number (frequency) of individuals in the ith class

m = number of classes

Then

$$\sum_{i=1}^{m} f_i X_i \bigg/ \sum_{i=1}^{m} f_i \cong \mu \qquad (1\text{-}11)$$

The approximation may be better or worse depending on the distribution of the actual values within each group.

Similarly,

$$\dfrac{\sum\limits_{i=1}^{m} f_i X_i^2}{\sum\limits_{i=1}^{m} f_i} - \left(\dfrac{\sum\limits_{i=1}^{m} f_i X_i}{\sum\limits_{i=1}^{m} f_i}\right)^2 \cong \text{var}(X) \qquad (1\text{-}12)$$

MEAN AND VARIANCE FORMULAS FOR ATTRIBUTE DATA

In a population where all values of X_i are either 1 or 0 (usually signifying the presence or absence of disease or some other attribute), let the proportion of the N values that are 1 be P. Then the frequency of 1's and 0's is NP and $N(1-P)$, respectively, and from Equations 1-11 and 1-12

$$\mu = \frac{NP(1) + N(1-P)(0)}{NP + N(1-P)} = P \tag{1-13}$$

$$\mathrm{var}(X) = \frac{(NP)(1^2) + N(1-P)(0^2)}{NP + N(1-P)}$$

$$- \left[\frac{NP(1) + N(1-P)(0)}{NP + N(1-P)}\right]^2$$

$$\mathrm{var}(X) = \frac{NP}{N} - \left(\frac{NP}{N}\right)^2 = P - P^2 = P(1-P) \tag{1-14}$$

In this case, the formulas for grouped data give exactly correct results because the two values are perfectly represented by the two X_i values. Thus P is the mean and $P(1-P)$ is the variance of a population of 1's and 0's. If we take a sample of size n, the variance of the sample mean using Equation 1-6 without the finite multiplier is

$$\mathrm{var}(\bar{x}) \cong \frac{\mathrm{var}(X)}{n} = \frac{P(1-P)}{n} \tag{1-15}$$

For attribute data, it is usual for p to be used in place of $\bar{x}$ for the sample mean, and thus we can write the above

$$\mathrm{var}(p) \cong \frac{P(1-P)}{n} \tag{1-16}$$

We rarely know P and usually estimate it with p. This leads to the usual formula

$$\widehat{\mathrm{var}}(p) \cong \frac{p(1-p)}{n} \tag{1-17}$$

Sometimes, interest is focused not on the sample mean from an attribute population but on the number of 1's in the sample. In this case, the sample statistic to be considered is not p but np, which is the total number of individuals with the characteristic in the sample. Using Equation 1-17 for $\widehat{\mathrm{var}}(p)$ and Equation 1-10 on the variance of a variable multiplied by constant, we have

$$\text{vâr}(np) \cong \frac{n^2 p(1-p)}{n} = np(1-p) \tag{1-18}$$

It is very common for $(1-P)$ and $(1-p)$ to be written Q and q, respectively.

MEAN AND VARIANCE OF THE POISSON DISTRIBUTION

The Poisson distribution reflects the probability of a certain number of events when the number of trials is extremely large but the chance of an event occurring in any one trial is small. It is somewhat similar to a binomial distribution for large n and small p. We shall use the fact that the mean and the variance of the Poisson distribution are equal and the distribution has only one parameter. The number of events observed estimates this Poisson parameter without the need for any supplementary information such as sample size. If 20 events were observed in binomial trials, we could not estimate P without information as to the number of trials (n). If 20 events are observed for a Poisson variable, no further information is needed. We can estimate the Poisson parameter as 20.

CONFIDENCE LIMITS

When a standard error of a sample mean has been calculated and the sample size is large or the population being sampled approximates a normal distribution, confidence limits (CL) for the population mean can be calculated as follows:

$$95\% \text{ CL} = \bar{x} \pm 1.96 \, \hat{\text{SE}}(\bar{x}) \tag{1-19}$$

$$99\% \text{ CL} = \bar{x} \pm 2.58 \, \hat{\text{SE}}(\bar{x}) \tag{1-20}$$

Note: as given, Equations 1-19 and 1-20 are not correct, even for large samples from a normal distribution. To make them exactly correct, we should substitute $\text{SE}(\bar{x})$ for $\hat{\text{SE}}(\bar{x})$. However, for large samples the distinction is slight. For small samples from a normal universe the values 1.96 and 2.58 should be changed in accordance with tables of Student's t values [Armitage 1971]. For small samples from a nonnormal universe, it may be advisable to consult with a statistician.

The justifications for using the confidence limits given above are that (a) the distribution of sample means in all possible samples from a normally distributed population is normal and (b) the distribution of all possible sample means based on large samples is approximately normal, whether or not the variable is normally distributed in the population being sampled. Our estimated standard error of the sample mean is an estimate of the standard deviation of the imaginary normal distribution of all possible sample means. In a normal distribution, only 5 percent of the values are more than ±1.96 standard deviations away from the expected value. Since $E(\bar{x}) = \mu$, we can say that only 5 percent of the possible sample mean values are more than ±1.96 $SE(\bar{x})$ distant from μ. We do not know $SE(\bar{x})$ but use instead $\hat{SE}(\bar{x})$, derived from sample data. For large samples, this is entirely satisfactory.

Assuming adequate sample size or normality of the population, we can add and subtract 1.96 $\hat{SE}(\bar{x})$ to $\bar{x}$ and consider the resultant range to include μ. Only if our value of $\bar{x}$ is one of the 5 percent that is more than ±1.96 $\hat{SE}(\bar{x})$ distant from μ will our range of values fail to include μ. Thus $\bar{x} \pm 1.96$ $\hat{SE}(\bar{x})$ is a 95 percent confidence interval for μ. The identical argument applies to 99 percent confidence intervals using $\bar{x} \pm 2.58$ $\hat{SE}(\bar{x})$.

CHI-SQUARE FORMULAS

Most students of epidemiology are familiar with the formula relating χ^2 (chi square) to the quotient (observed frequency − expected frequency)^2 divided by expected frequency, summed over all the frequencies in a correlated set:

$$\chi^2 = \sum \frac{(f_{obs} - f_{exp})^2}{f_{exp}}$$

Correlated frequencies are not all free to vary since if some observed frequencies are larger than expected, others will have to be smaller than expected. However, some students do not know that the above formula is a special instance of the basic formula for χ^2, which in the case of a single variable from a normal distribution expressed as a deviation from its expected value is

$$\chi_1^2 = \frac{[x - E(x)]^2}{\text{var}(x)} \tag{1-21}$$

where the subscript 1 refers to one degree of freedom. In the case of K variables that are constrained to add to a fixed sum,

$$\chi_{(K-1)}^2 = \sum_{i=1}^{K} \frac{(x_i - \bar{x})^2}{\text{var}(x)} \tag{1-22}$$

STANDARDIZED NORMAL DEVIATE

By taking the square root of each side of Equation 1-21 we get

$$[\chi^2]^{1/2} = \frac{x - E(x)}{\text{standard deviation of } (x)} = z \qquad (1\text{-}23)$$

If x is derived by a random process from a normally distributed population with mean equal to $E(x)$ and standard deviation as specified, z is a standardized normal deviate. In that case the probability of a value of z as large or larger than that observed can be read from tables of the normal distribution. If this probability is small the hypothesis that x is a random sample from a population with mean and standard deviation equal to the values specified in Equation 1-23 is rejected. Note that the "x" in Equations 1-23 or 1-21 can be a single observation or a complex statistic. For example, if "x" were a sample value of a particular multiple logistic regression coefficient, β_i (see Chapter 6), then a standardized normal deviate could be calculated as

$$z = \frac{\beta_i - E(\beta_i)}{\text{SE}(\beta_i)} \qquad (1\text{-}24)$$

Squaring both sides leads to

$$z^2 = \frac{[\beta_i - E(\beta_i)]^2}{\text{var}(\beta_i)}$$

which should be recognizable as Equation 1-21 with z^2 written for χ^2.

2
Random Sampling

This book treats only samples that include a random element in the selection process. Nonrandom samples based on volunteers or on the judgment of the sampler as to the desirability or nondesirability of including a particular individual in the sample may be excellent or terrible as estimators of population parameters, but there is no objective way of judging which adjective applies. Statements such as "we are 95 percent confident that the mean percentage of cholesterol contained in high-density lipoproteins is between 17 and 19" can be made only for random samples.

SIMPLE RANDOM SAMPLING

Simple random sampling is simple in theory [Remington and Schork 1970] but less so in practice. In theory, one has a list of N elements (usually individuals), a number is assigned in sequence from 1 to N to each element in sequence, and then a table of random numbers is used to select n individuals out of the N who are in the sample. For those unfamiliar with random number tables [The Rand Corporation 1954, Snedecor and Cochran 1980], a sample page of such a table is shown in Table 2-1 [Fisher and Yates 1974]. The mechanics of using the table are simple. Suppose, for example, that the population to be sampled has 8059 elements and a sample of 300 is to be selected. Consider the random number table in any arrangement that will produce a sequence of four-digit numbers. One way is to use columns of four digits. In Table 2-1, starting at the upper left corner of the page, this would result in 0347, 9774, 1676, etc. On reaching the bottom of the page, continue with the next column of four digits: 4373, 2467, etc. An alternative way of

Table 2-1. Random Sampling Numbers

03	47	43	73	86	36	96	47	36	61	46	98	63	71	62
97	74	24	67	62	42	81	14	57	20	42	53	32	37	32
16	76	62	27	66	56	50	26	71	07	32	90	79	78	53
12	56	85	99	26	96	96	68	27	31	05	03	72	93	15
55	59	56	35	64	38	54	82	46	22	31	62	43	09	90
16	22	77	94	39	49	54	43	54	82	17	37	93	23	78
84	42	17	53	31	57	24	55	06	88	77	04	74	47	67
63	01	63	78	59	16	95	55	67	19	98	10	50	71	75
33	21	12	34	29	78	64	56	07	82	52	42	07	44	38
57	60	86	32	44	09	47	27	96	54	49	17	46	09	62
18	18	07	92	46	44	17	16	58	09	79	83	86	19	62
26	62	38	97	75	84	16	07	44	99	83	11	46	32	24
23	42	40	64	74	82	97	77	77	81	07	45	32	14	08
52	36	28	19	95	50	92	26	11	97	00	56	76	31	38
37	85	94	35	12	83	39	50	08	30	42	34	07	96	88
70	29	17	12	13	40	33	20	38	26	13	89	51	03	74
56	62	18	37	35	96	83	50	87	75	97	12	25	93	47
99	49	57	22	77	88	42	95	45	72	16	64	36	16	00
16	08	15	04	72	33	27	14	34	09	45	59	34	68	49
31	16	93	32	43	50	27	89	87	19	20	15	37	00	49
68	34	30	13	70	55	74	30	77	40	44	22	78	84	26
74	57	25	65	76	59	29	97	68	60	71	91	38	67	54
27	42	37	86	53	48	55	90	65	72	96	57	69	36	10
00	39	68	29	61	66	37	32	20	30	77	84	57	03	29
29	94	98	94	24	68	49	69	10	82	53	75	91	93	30

Source: Fisher and Yates 1974 (by permission).

using the table is to select four-digit numbers from a single-digit vertical column. Using this procedure 0911, 5186, and 3512 would be the first three numbers in Table 2-1.

To avoid choosing the same sample each time, a method to vary the starting point is desirable. This method need not be elaborate. For example, perhaps opening a book to a "random" page shows pages 270 and 271. Use the first two digits of these pages as a starting point and begin with the twenty-seventh four-digit number in your random number table. In Table 2-1, using four-digit columns, this is 2467. Alternatively, the 27 could be used to begin with the seventh four-digit number on page 2 of the random number collection. Have some simple rule in mind and carry it through to produce a variable starting point. If more than one or two samples are to be selected, the method described below, although usable, is not the most efficient. The mechanics for allocation of a total population into K random samples, or subgroups, is described in [Mantel 1969].

We return now to the details of selecting 300 individuals from a population of 8059. In some way, perhaps using existing reference numbers (such as patients' clinic numbers or student identification card numbers), assign to each individual in the population one, and only one, four-digit number from 0001 to 8059. Using the numbers shown in Table 2-1 in the format of four-digit columns and using the twenty-seventh four-digit number as a starting point, the first 10 random numbers are 2467, 6227, 8599, 5635, 7794, 1753, 6378, 1234, 8632, and 0792. Numbers 8599 and 8632 are not assigned to anyone in the population being sampled and thus have no relevance for this example of sample selection. If a number had been repeated we would ignore the later selection.

Thus, from the first 10 random numbers, 8 individuals are selected for the sample. Continue selecting individuals corresponding to the random numbers in the table until 300 sample individuals have been identified. This is the simple part of simple random sampling.

STRATIFIED RANDOM SAMPLING

Sometimes it is possible to identify separate sections of the population, which we call *strata,* and to take advantage of them in our sampling plan so as to reduce the sampling error below that for a simple random sample. Examples of variables that are often used for stratification are sex, race, age, and socioeconomic status. The fundamental aspect of stratified sampling is that the strata are sampled separately and the results then appropriately combined in the analysis. If much of the variability in what we are measuring is between strata, we can use stratification to reduce sampling variance. By sampling within strata and then combining the results appropriately, our results are completely free of the variability between strata, however great that might be.

An extreme (unrealistic) example illustrates this idea. A sample study is proposed to estimate the average length of postoperative hospital stay for a certain disease. Separate lists exist (or information is available that allows us to make such lists) for hospitals having fewer than 25 beds, those having 25 to 99 beds, and those having 100 beds or more. Suppose further that all hospitals with fewer than 25 beds keep such patients exactly nine days, all hospitals of 25 to 99 beds keep such patients exactly seven days, and hospitals of 100 beds or larger keep these patients exactly five days. By simple sampling of a combined list that includes all sizes of hospitals, it would be possible to get samples with averages as low as five days and as high as nine days. With stratified sampling, however, the estimate for hospitals with fewer than 25 beds would always be nine days, no matter which hospitals of this group were selected. Similarly, the possible samples for the other strata could yield only the sample means of five days and seven days, regardless of which hospitals were selected within each stratum. In this extreme case, all of the variance in length of

stay are between strata. *Within each stratum there is no variance at all.*
Using stratified sampling (and suitable combination of the results of each
stratum's sample into an overall average), there would be no sampling
variance. All possible samples would yield the same results.

One other artificial example illustrates the potential benefits of
stratification. Imagine a population, or universe, consisting of just eight
elements as follows: 0_a 0_b 0_c 0_d 1_a 1_b 1_c 1_d, with subscripts used to permit
identification of individual elements. Our purpose in introducing this
miniuniverse is to permit students to hold in their hand, so to speak,
some of the elements of sampling theory. For any real example, we can
appeal only to concepts, but through the device of this miniuniverse,
students can get a feel for what is meant by "all possible samples,"
"standard error of the mean," etc. The superficial point of the illustration
is to show how sample design (simple or stratified random) affects
sampling variance. The deeper purpose is to give students clearer insight
into the fundamentals of sampling theory without the necessity of
working through that theory.

For this population, $P = 0.5$ is the mean and $P(1 - P) = 0.25$ is the
variance. A simple random sample of size 2 might result in any one of the
28 possible samples listed in Table 2-2. Summarizing these and ignoring
the individual identification, we get:

Sample	Sample mean	Frequency
0–0	0	6
0–1	0.5	16
1–1	1.0	6
All		28*

To calculate the mean and variance of this distribution of all possible
sample means of size 2, we use Equations 1-11 and 1-12 on the following

Table 2-2. All Possible Samples of Size 2 in Simple
Random Sampling from a Population Consisting of
$0_a 0_b 0_c 0_d 1_a 1_b 1_c 1_d$

$0_a 0_b$	$0_b 0_c$	$0_c 1_a$	$0_d 1_d$
$0_a 0_c$	$0_b 0_d$	$0_c 1_b$	$1_a 1_b$
$0_a 0_d$	$0_b 1_a$	$0_c 1_c$	$1_a 1_c$
$0_a 1_a$	$0_b 1_b$	$0_c 1_d$	$1_a 1_d$
$0_a 1_b$	$0_b 1_c$	$0_d 1_a$	$1_b 1_c$
$0_a 1_c$	$0_b 1_d$	$0_d 1_b$	$1_b 1_d$
$0_a 1_d$	$0_c 0_d$	$0_d 1_c$	$1_c 1_d$

data:

$\bar{x}$	f	$f\bar{x}$	$f\bar{x}^2$
0	6	0	0
0.5	16	8.0	4.0
1.0	6	6.0	6.0
	28	14.0	10.0

The mean of all possible sample means is

$$\frac{\Sigma f\bar{x}}{\Sigma f} = \frac{14}{28} = 0.5 = P$$

Note that the mean of all possible sample means equals P, the mean of the universe from which we are sampling. Thus, our sample means are unbiased estimates of the population mean. The standard error of the sample mean is the standard deviation of the *distribution of all possible sample means,* which equals

$$\left[\frac{\Sigma f\bar{x}^2}{\Sigma f} - \left(\frac{\Sigma f\bar{x}}{\Sigma f}\right)^2\right]^{1/2} = \left[\frac{10.0}{28.0} - (.5)^2\right]^{1/2} = \left(\frac{3}{28}\right)^{1/2}$$

In real sampling applications, the number of all possible samples becomes enormous and the distribution of all possible sample means is only a concept and not an actual enumerated distribution. In the example cited earlier of a sample of 300 from a population of 8059, there are over 10^{554} different samples possible. Obviously, the standard error of the sample mean applicable to real samples needs to be determined by methods other than the direct calculation of the standard deviation of all possible means. It is, of course, calculated by formula. The formula for simple sampling appropriate for either binomial or continuous variables, as previously stated in Equation 1-7, is

$$\text{SE}(\bar{x}) = \left[\frac{\text{var}(X)}{n}\left(\frac{N-n}{N-1}\right)\right]^{1/2} \tag{2-1}$$

The term $(N-n)/(N-1)$, called the *finite sampling factor,* is useful whenever the sample represents 10 percent or more of the total population; otherwise it may be omitted.

In practical sampling problems, $\text{var}(X)$ is usually unknown and $\hat{\text{var}}(X)$ is used as an estimate. In the artificial example we are investigating, var(X) is known and its use in Equation 2-1 results in

$$[\text{var}(\bar{x})]^{1/2} = \left[\frac{.5(.5)}{2}\left(\frac{8-2}{8-1}\right)\right]^{1/2} = \left[\frac{1}{8}\left(\frac{6}{7}\right)\right]^{1/2} = \left(\frac{3}{28}\right)^{1/2}$$

exactly as calculated by direct enumeration.

If by the use of supplementary information, such as sex, area, or age, for example, we were able to divide the population into two strata that tended to include the 1's in one stratum and the 0's in the other, we might have

$$\text{Stratum 1} \qquad 0_d 1_a 1_b 1_c$$

$$\text{Stratum 2} \qquad 1_d 0_a 0_b 0_c$$

We can now select a stratified random sample of size 2 by taking one element at random from stratum 1 and one clement at random from stratum 2. Under these conditions the possible sample selections are

From stratum 1	From stratum 2
0_d	1_d
0_d	0_a
0_d	0_b
0_d	0_c
1_a	1_d
1_a	0_a
1_a	0_b
1_a	0_c
1_b	1_d
1_b	0_a
1_b	0_b
1_b	0_c
1_c	1_d
1_c	0_a
1_c	0_b
1_c	0_c

Combining samples of similar composition by ignoring identification of individual elements results in

Sample	Sample mean	Frequency
0–0	0	3
0–1	0.5	10
1–1	1.0	3
All		16[†]

The reduction in total number of possible samples from 28 to 16 is characteristic of stratified sampling. This can easily be understood by recognizing that some of the samples possible under simple sampling are no longer possible when a stratified sampling procedure is used. For example, selection of 1_a and 1_b from stratum 1 is not possible under the stratified plan of selecting one from each stratum; however, the combination of 1_a and 1_b is one of the possibilities in simple sampling.

We now calculate the mean and variance of the 16 possible sample means of size 2 from the stratified sample:

$\bar{x}$	f	$f\bar{x}$	$f\bar{x}^2$
0	3	0	0
0.5	10	5.0	2.50
1.0	3	3.0	3.00
	16	8.0	5.50

The mean of all possible sample means is

$$\frac{\Sigma f\bar{x}}{\Sigma f} = \frac{8.0}{16.0} = .5 = P$$

In this illustration of stratified sampling, our results show that the mean of all possible sample means is the mean of the universe. When this is the case, the sample mean is said to be *unbiased*.

The variance of all possible sample means is

$$\frac{\Sigma f\bar{x}^2}{\Sigma f} - \left(\frac{\Sigma f\bar{x}}{\Sigma f}\right)^2 = \frac{5.50}{16} - (.5)^2 = \frac{3}{32}$$

and the standard deviation of all possible sample means is $(3/32)^{1/2}$. Equation 2-2 is appropriate for estimating the overall population mean using data from a stratified sample:

$$\bar{x}(\text{strat}) = \sum_{i=1}^{r} \frac{N_i}{N} \bar{x}_i \tag{2-2}$$

where $\bar{x}_i$ is the sample mean and N_i is the population size of the ith stratum, r equals the number of strata, and N equals the total population size $(i = 1, 2, \ldots, r)$.

Weighting the sample mean of the ith stratum $(\bar{x}_i)$ by the proportion that the ith stratum size is of the total population size provides an unbiased estimate of the overall mean. Note that the weighting factors relate to population sizes $(N_i$ and $N)$ and not to sample sizes $(n_i$ and $n)$. If stratified sampling allocation of n_i is not proportional to stratum size N_i, n_i/n will not equal N_i/N, and it is N_i/N that must be used as the proper weighting factor. The variance of an overall stratified sample mean derived by weighting the sample means for individual strata as in Equation 2-2 is

$$\text{var}(\bar{x}) \text{ strat} = \sum_{i=1}^{r} \left(\frac{N_i}{N}\right)^2 \frac{\text{var}_i(x)}{n_i} \left(\frac{N_i - n_i}{N_i - 1}\right) \tag{2-3}$$

where $\text{var}_i(x)$ is the variance of x within the ith stratum.

Applying Equation 2-3 to our artificial example of sample size 2, we obtain

$$\text{var}(\bar{x}) \text{ strat} = \left(\frac{4}{8}\right)^2 \frac{.75(.25)}{1} \left(\frac{4-1}{4-1}\right) + \left(\frac{4}{8}\right)^2 \frac{.25(.75)}{1} \left(\frac{4-1}{4-1}\right)$$

$$= \frac{1}{4} \left(\frac{3}{4}\right)\left(\frac{1}{4}\right) + \frac{1}{4} \left(\frac{1}{4}\right)\left(\frac{3}{4}\right) = \frac{6}{64} = \frac{3}{32}$$

as the variance of the distribution of all possible stratified means of size 2. The square root of this, $(3/32)^{1/2}$, is the standard deviation of this distribution and is the standard error of $\bar{x}$ (strat). The value $(3/32)^{1/2}$ is exactly equal to what we obtained earlier as the standard deviation of all possible stratified samples of size 2.

Recalling that the standard error of $\bar{x}$ (simple) was $(3/28)^{1/2}$, we see, in this artificial example, that stratification may result in reduction of sampling error. If the allocation of sample n_i to the several strata is proportional to stratum size (N_i), then the variance of $\bar{x}$ (strat) will be the same as or less than the variance of $\bar{x}$ (simple) for samples of the same size. The reduced variance for stratified sampling depends on the differences between strata for the variable of interest. The more stratum means differ from each other, and the more strata are alike within themselves, i.e., the smaller the variance within strata, the more potential benefit there is in stratified sampling.

If the investigator has a reasonably good basis for estimating $[\text{var}_i(x)]^{1/2}$—for the binomial this is equivalent to estimating P_i since $(P_iQ_i)^{1/2} = [\text{var}_i(x)]^{1/2}$—for the several strata and believes they differ appreciably, consideration should be given to allocating n_i proportional to

$$\frac{N_i[\text{var}_i(x)]^{1/2}}{\sum_i N_i[\text{var}_i(x)]^{1/2}}$$

This is called *optimum allocation* and provides the smallest possible sampling variance obtainable with stratified sampling, provided the estimates of $[\text{var}_i(x)]^{1/2}$ are not far from the truth. Although the sample size in each stratum may be determined by optimum allocation as just described, by proportional allocation, or otherwise, Equation 2-2 provides the correct estimate of the overall mean. If optimum allocation is attempted on the basis of poor estimates of $[\text{var}_i(x)]^{1/2}$, it is possible that the resultant sampling variance will be larger than for simple random sampling.

To summarize, allocate stratified sample size proportional to N_i unless you have good reason to do otherwise.

SYSTEMATIC SAMPLING

Systematic sampling is a common type of sampling based on selecting every rth individual from a list or file after choosing a random number from 1 to r as a starting point. Going back to the example used for simple random sampling, choosing 300 from a population of 8059, we now obtain a systematic sample by calculating the ratio $N/n = 8059/300 = 26.9$ and selecting every twenty-sixth (or twenty-seventh) individual in the file beginning with a random start between 1 and 26 (or 27). Note that using $r = 26$ results in a sample size of 309 and $r = 27$ results in a sample size of 298. It is typical of systematic sampling procedures that they yield sample sizes approximately, rather than exactly, equal to the targeted sample size.

Systematic sampling is based on a fixed nonrandom rule and is not limited to selection from an actual file. Thus, selection of all those born on the (randomly chosen) fifth day of any month or of everyone whose social security number ends in (the randomly chosen digits) 12, 65, or 87 is similar to systematic sampling procedures yielding approximately 3 percent samples. Of course, the choice of the sampling scheme has to be relevant to the population being sampled. A population that is not completely covered by social security would be unsuitable for sampling by means of social security numbers. A primitive population that did not record and remember birthdays could not be sampled using date of birth.

The reason for the popularity of systematic sampling is its simplicity and, in many instances, its superiority over simple sampling. The simplicity is obvious, the potential superiority less so. We shall consider this aspect in terms of an example. Suppose we want to systematically sample a chronological list of all hospital admissions for one year. If the sampling objective is to estimate the proportion of all hospital admissions during the year that are due to infectious diseases, it is quite probable that a systematic sample of admissions is preferable to a simple random sample. Consider that admissions for infectious diseases may have seasonal peaks and that by systematic sampling from a chronological list we are sure to obtain $(1/r)$th of the admissions in each season. In simple random sampling, however, some of the possible samples would include admissions only from a particular season and thereby improperly reflect the proportion of annual admissions for infectious disease. As in the foregoing example, if the list is ordered in a manner related to the study objective, systematic sampling is in some respects analogous to stratified sampling. If the list is in random order, systematic sampling is analogous to simple random sampling.

If however, the list is in cyclical order so that every rth element is in some way special, then systematic sampling can be disastrous. Investigators must be on guard with regard to this last situation, but it rarely occurs. An example commonly cited relates to choosing a sample of homes. In such a situation, it is possible that if the random start provides a corner house, every rth house thereafter might also be a corner house. If corner houses are related to above-average economic status or above-average family size or some other aspect of relevance to the study, systematic sampling might provide misleading data. As stated earlier, such a constellation of events is not very probable, but be sure to give it some thought.

How should the sampling variance of means derived from systematic sampling be estimated? Whereas the number of possible simple random samples of 300 from 8059 is more than 10^{554}, the number of possible samples of 300 using systematic sampling from a list of 8059 is *only* 26. There are 26 possible starting points on the list in accordance with the random number chosen and thus only 26 possible different systematic samples. Clearly the distribution of all possible sample means and consequently the formulas for calculating the sampling error for simple samples (and also within strata for stratified samples) do not apply to systematic sampling. There are formulas that depend on the serial correlation coefficient [Madow and Madow 1944] and split sample methods, but they are clumsy to apply [Deming 1950]. However, our recommendation is to use Equation 1-6 for simple random sampling and to consider the results as approximately correct if the list being used is ordered at random or not ordered in any way known to be relevant to the variable of interest. The formulas applicable to simple random sampling can be considered as overstating the sampling variability if the ordering of the list is relevant to the variable under study.

For systematic samples not derived from a real list, such as the example given of choosing all those born on the fifth of any month, we must first be able to assume that the day of the month is unrelated to our study objectives. Without this qualification, we would not have a random element in our sample. Next, we must recognize that such a sample, which in this case is made up of all those born on the fifth of the month, lacks the characteristics of a systematic sample drawn from a list whose order is in some way relevant to study interests. We have no guarantee that using birth date we will get about one-thirtieth of those of every age, one-thirtieth of those living in every geographic section, one-thirtieth of the men, one-thirtieth of the women, etc., but instead we have an excellent approximation to the size and kind of sample we would have obtained by sampling every thirtieth from a list arranged at random.

The selection of every rth person from a list ordered by age is an excellent approximation to stratified sampling with proportional allocation. If the list ordering is relevant to what we want to measure—and age is relevant to practically everything the epidemiologist is interested in measuring—the sections of the list may be thought of as strata that differ as to strata means. This is the feature of list ordering that provides the basis for reduction in sampling variance.

The increased efficiency of systematic sampling can be substantial, but it is altogether dependent on the degree to which the variable of interest is associated with the order of population elements on the list. Although systematic sampling can be equivalent to a type of stratified sampling, there is no practical way to use the standard error formulas appropriate to stratified sampling.

CLUSTER SAMPLING

The individuals in the population we wish to sample are often grouped into clusters, e.g., families, villages, or hospital wards. Although it is often convenient or administratively desirable to first sample clusters and then investigate the individuals in the chosen clusters rather than to sample individuals directly from the population, the effect on sample results needs to be understood. There is an important distinction, for example, between picking a sample of 1000 from a population of 100 000 by direct random selection and picking 1000 individuals from 250 randomly selected nuclear families.

To illustrate the problem, we consider estimating the proportion of 1981 hospitalized patients diagnosed as having myocardial infarction (MI) who report having taken a specified amount, or more, of aspirin during the week prior to diagnosis. Depending upon study objectives, the investigator may wish to compare the proportion of myocardial infarction patients positive for aspirin with suitable controls. However, for the purpose of discussing and explaining cluster sampling, reference to the hospitalized patients only will be sufficient.

Assume that, in the study area, there are 17 hospitals treating myocardial infarction patients, that during 1981 they discharged about 1000 such patients and that we need about 250 cases for the precision desired. Further assume that the hospitals are generally similar with respect to patient populations, accuracy in diagnosis, etc.

We might, of course, proceed by simple random, stratified random, or systematic random methods to select 250 of the 1000 patients for inclusion in the study. However, to carry out such a study we would have to assign a part-time interviewer to each hospital and the expense would be much greater than if the study could be limited to a few hospitals. Each hospital represents a cluster of patients, and to use cluster sampling, we first pick several hospitals at random. In the present example, perhaps 6 of the 17 would be selected and then only the MI patients or a sample of the MI patients in these six hospitals would be included in the study.

The greater ease and convenience of carrying out a study in 6 rather than 17 hospitals is evident. What then is the drawback? Why are not all sample studies initiated by selection of convenient clusters? The answer to both questions is that sampling variance is likely to be increased. Although likely, it is not a certainty that cluster sampling variance will be larger than simple random sampling variance, and there is even some chance that cluster sampling variance will be smaller [Cochran 1963].

We use an extreme example to explain how selecting clusters affects sampling variance. Suppose a population consists of three clusters, A, B, and C. For the variable of interest, each cluster is composed of perfectly homogeneous elements, i.e., every individual in a cluster is like every other individual in that cluster. Assume that our variable is the presence of rheumatoid arthritis and that each cluster is made up of only one type of individual. In cluster A all are negative, in cluster B all are positive, and in cluster C all are doubtful with respect to rheumatoid arthritis. We now pick one cluster at random and then study all or a sample of all the individuals therein with respect to rheumatoid arthritis. No matter how large our sample size is, it is clear that we cannot learn anything more about the cluster than could have been learned by a sample of one from the same cluster. Furthermore, we have no indication that the individuals in the two clusters not selected are completely different from the individuals in our sample. Of course, this is an extreme example, but it illustrates the fact that if the characteristic of interest is *positively correlated within clusters,* as is very often the case ("birds of a feather flock together"), *n* sample observations will produce fewer than *n* independent units of information. In addition, if clusters vary greatly from one to another so that at least some of them must deviate substantially from population parameters, the clusters selected may not provide good estimates of the proportion of the total population having the characteristic being studied.

If clusters are random assemblages of individuals, then cluster sampling has no greater sampling variance than simple random sampling. In this case it is wise to take advantage of the practical benefits of cluster sampling. However, if clusters are positively correlated within themselves, i.e., more homogeneity than would result from chance association, cluster sampling variance will be larger than simple random sampling variance. If clusters are negatively correlated within themselves, however, i.e., more heterogeneity than would result from chance association, cluster sampling benefits the investigator both by reduced variance for fixed sample size and by reduced costs. Calculation of cluster sampling variance depends on the intraclass correlation coefficient [Deming 1950], which epidemiologists are unlikely to know. However, only if clusters are formed at random or reflect negative correlation within themselves for the variable of interest will the variance obtained from the simple random sampling formula equal or overestimate the real sampling variance of cluster sampling.

Since simple random sampling variance can grossly underestimate the true cluster sampling variance we do not recommend using it for that purpose. Cluster sampling variance can be many times larger than the variance calculated by assuming a simple random sample [Abraham 1986]. Such differences can lead to qualitatively different conclusions about the significance of the study findings. We suggest obtaining statistical advice whenever attempting to analyze data from surveys based on cluster sampling design such as the National Health and Nutrition Examination Surveys [Landis et al 1982].

SAMPLE SIZE

"How large a sample do I need?" is a frequent question, applicable to all types of epidemiologic studies. We shall first consider it from the viewpoint of simple random sampling and then indicate how sample size is affected by stratified, systematic, and cluster sampling methods.

We consider two types of sample size calculations and, for ease of exposition, start with estimates of binomial variables. First we will calculate the sample size needed to estimate a single parameter, then the sample size needed to estimate whether or not two parameters differ by a specified amount.

Sample Size for Single Binomial Parameter

Suppose we wish to estimate the proportion (P) of regular current cigarette smokers in the freshman class entering a large university and we would like our estimate (p) to have a high probability of being within $\pm\Delta$ of the true value (P), where Δ signifies a specific difference (such as .03 or .05) between our estimate and the true value.

Before calculating the sample size needed in order to estimate the proportion of freshmen who smoke cigarettes, we must take what seems to be a ridiculous step: we must estimate what that proportion is. The basic reason for this is that sample size depends on the standard error of the variable to be estimated, and, as was shown earlier, the standard error of p equals

$$\left[\frac{P(1-P)}{n}\right]^{1/2}$$

If we judge the proportion of cigarette smoking among freshmen to be .30 and specify Δ as .04, then

$$1.96\,\text{SE}(p) = 1.96\left[\frac{P(1-P)}{n}\right]^{1/2} = .04$$

$$= 1.96\left[\frac{(.30)(.70)}{n}\right]^{1/2} = .04 \tag{2-4}$$

expresses the prior opinion that we would like 1.96 standard errors of our estimate to equal .04. If $1.96\,\text{SE}\,(p) = .04$, then our sample estimate has about a 95 percent chance of being within four percentage points of the truth. This assumes that n is large enough to make the distribution of all possible sample p values approximately normal. For epidemiologic studies this is usually the case. We can now solve for n. Doing this, we get $n = 504$. Thus, if the true value is in fact .30, the mean of a sample of size 504 will be within $\pm.04$ of .30, or from .26 to .34, 95 percent of the time. We now repeat these calculations assuming $P = .10, .20, .40,$ and .50:

$$1.96\left[\frac{(.10)(.90)}{n}\right]^{1/2} = .04 \qquad n = 216$$

$$1.96\left[\frac{(.20)(.80)}{n}\right]^{1/2} = .04 \qquad n = 384$$

$$1.96\left[\frac{(.40)(.60)}{n}\right]^{1/2} = .04 \qquad n = 576$$

$$1.96\left[\frac{(.50)(.50)}{n}\right]^{1/2} = .04 \qquad n = 600$$

The corresponding ranges within which 95 percent of sample p values fall are given in Table 2-3.

Table 2-3. Sample Size Required for Selected Values of P with .95 Confidence Limits Fixed at $\pm.04$

P	Sample size	95% of sample p's will be between
.10	216	.06 and .14
.20	384	.16 and .24
.30	504	.26 and .34
.40	576	.36 and .44
.50	600	.46 and .54

What happens if our estimate of P is a poor one? Suppose we estimate $P = .20$ and calculate a sample size of 384, but in fact P is .40. With $P = .40$, the true variance of all possible sample means of size 384 is $(.4)(.6)/384 = .000625$, with standard error of the sample mean equal to $(.000625)^{1/2}$, or .025. Two standard errors would equal .05, and 95 percent of the sample p's based on a sample size of 384 would be between .35 and .45. If we observe a p of .35 in our sample and use it to estimate $SE(p)$, we would estimate the true mean as between .30 and .40 with .95 confidence. Of course, we are not going to take all possible samples, only one, and it may happen that the p for the sample we select is extremely low. In that case we might continue to think that the true value is about .20. However, it is much more likely that the sample result will contribute to changing our prior opinion about the prevalence of cigarette smoking among freshmen. This illustration of results following a poor estimate of P indicates that useful findings may not be critically dependent on good preliminary estimates of P.

Let us examine this same question of the sample size needed to estimate a single parameter with a specified precision from a slightly different viewpoint. Suppose instead of specifying precision as within four precentage points, we specify precision as a proportion of P. If we want $1.96\ SE(p)$ to equal $P/5$, this would be equivalent to $\pm.05$ if $P = .25$ and to $\pm.02$ if $P = .10$. Often this is the better way to describe desired precision. For example, the specification $\pm.05$ is not too useful if $P = .01$. To set up the equation in this form, with $1.96\ SE(p) = P/K$, we have

$$1.96\ SE(p) = 1.96\left[\frac{P(1-P)}{n}\right]^{1/2} = \frac{P}{K} \tag{2-5}$$

If K is specified as 5, we need only insert our preliminary estimate of P and then solve for n.

For $P = .01$, the specification that 95 percent of samples should fall between .008 and .012 requires an n of 9508 according to Equation 2-5. This rather large sample size could exceed the total size of the freshmen class, which would certainly remind us to use the finite sampling factor, $[(N-n)/(N-1)]$, as part of the variance equation. If the total freshmen class at our hypothetical large university were 5000, the equation to solve for n with $P = .01$ and approximately 95 percent assurance of $\pm P/5$ is

$$1.96\left[\frac{.01(.99)}{n}\left(\frac{N-n}{N}\right)\right]^{1/2} = \frac{.01}{5}$$

$$1.96\left[\frac{.01(.99)}{n}\left(\frac{5000-n}{5000}\right)\right]^{1/2} = .002 \qquad n \approx 3300$$

Note that to simplify the arithmetic we use N instead of $N-1$ in the denominator of the finite sampling factor. For $N = 5000$, this is an inconsequential change.

Difference Between Binomial Parameters

Often the epidemiologist's interest is not in estimating a single parameter but in comparing two parameters. Sample size calculations are most commonly applied to this situation. The sample size needed for a randomized, controlled clinical trial is an example. Suppose it is proposed to conduct a trial of some type of medication or diet to study its effect on reducing the incidence of myocardial infarction. Setting aside the many practical problems of conductng such a trial [Ederer 1975], we direct our attention to estimating the sample size needed.

In order to estimate the sample size needed for a study capable of detecting a change in incidence rate, it is necessary to have a preliminary estimate of what that incidence rate is. Suppose we are planning a three-year study and have data suggesting that the population we intend to study, taking into account age, sex, etc., has an incidence rate of new cases of myocardial infarction of 1 percent per year, or about 3 percent for the three-year study period. In addition to estimating the existing incidence rate, it is necessary to stipulate what degree of change (associated with the treatment being investigated) the study is supposed to detect with a high probability. The difference to be detected (i.e., if it exists, we shall have a high probability of not missing it) is determined by a blend of subject matter considerations and the investigator's judgment. Determining whether a proposed program might reduce the annual incidence of myocardial infarction from .030 to .029 seems inappropriate. Conceivably circumstances may exist in which detection of this change is desirable, but in general it is unwise to try and identify such a small difference. A program causing a slight reduction is very likely to be superseded before long by some improved alternative. Thus, a difficult, expensive, and time-consuming study might come to the conclusion that program A does seem to reduce annual incidence by .001, only to be overtaken by the emergence of program B, which is thought to lower incidence by .005.

If the true control group incidence rate is 3 percent per three-year study period and the treatment reduces this to 2.9 percent, the sample size needed to detect this slight difference will necessarily be larger than the sample size needed to detect a reduction from 3 percent to 1 percent. In general, the larger the difference to be detected, the smaller the sample size required. (Using the word *detect* is a form of shorthand because what we are actually referring to is the detection of a statistically significant difference between the two groups.) If the control and treatment incidence rates are as stipulated, the four factors we must know for calculating the sample size needed in order to have a stated probability of detecting a significant difference are

P_c true incidence rate in the control group
P_e true incidence rate in the experimental group, usually derived as a
       proportional reduction from P_c
α probability of type I error in performing the test of significance, i.e.,
       concluding that there is a difference between P_c and P_e when in fact
       the sample data regarding each are only random variations arising
       from the same parameter, P_c
β probability of type II error in performing the test of significance,
       i.e., failing to reject the null hypothesis when in fact P_c and P_e differ
       as stipulated

Before putting these components together in a way that will enable the various formulas for sample size calculation to make sense, we remind readers about the variance of the difference between *independent variables* as previously stated in Equation 1-9:

$$\text{var}(x - y) = \text{var}(x) + \text{var}(y)$$

Independence can be illustrated with the following examples. Height and weight are not independent, as knowledge of height permits an improved estimate of weight. Obviously the improved estimate is far from perfect, but it is nevertheless better than the estimate possible in the absence of any information. For adults, height and social security number are probably independent, as knowledge of either for any individual is not likely to improve your estimate of the other.

At present we are interested in the variance of the difference between p_c and p_e (sample estimates of P_c and P_e, respectively). In a properly conducted trial, knowledge of the sample result for p_e, e.g., that it was above or below the true value of P_e, would not provide any basis for knowing that in the same trial p_c was above or below the true value of P_c. Thus, the sample data p_e and p_c are independent and

$$\text{var}(p_c - p_e) = \text{var}(p_c) + \text{var}(p_e)$$

We now consider a specific example. What is the sample size needed, with equal numbers of subjects in control and experimental groups, to detect a significant difference between p_e and p_c with a two-sided type I error of .05 (i.e., reject the null hypothesis if the difference between p_e and p_c is large and positive *or* large and negative) and a type II error of .10, if P_c really is .03 and P_e really is .02. Figure 2-1 presents these concepts in nonquantitative form.

Our explanation of sample size calculations rests upon Figures 2-1 through 2-6. If you understand what has been added or changed from

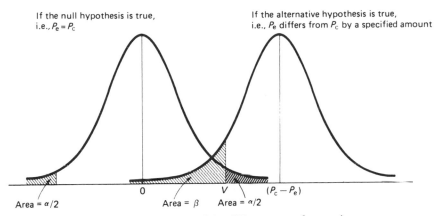

If the null hypothesis is true, i.e., $P_e = P_c$

If the alternative hypothesis is true, i.e., P_e differs from P_c by a specified amount

Area = $\alpha/2$ Area = β Area = $\alpha/2$

$(P_c - P_e)$

Figure 2-1. Distribution of all possible differences of sample means.

each figure to the next, you should have a clear conception of the ideas involved. In Figures 2-1 through 2-6 the total area under each sampling distribution is standardized at unity. Thus, if a labeled area is shown as equal to .025, it can be read as meaning that the *probability* of a sample difference being in that specific area of the distribution is .025.

For our specific example, we need to calculate $\text{var}(p_c - p_e)$ if the null hypothesis is true. Recognizing that in this instance both p_c and p_e represent sample estimates of a parameter of .03 (i.e., P_e is *not* different from P_c, which equals .03), we have

$$\text{var}(d): H_0 = \frac{.03(.97)}{n} + \frac{.03(.97)}{n}$$

where $d = p_c - p_e$ and $\text{var}(d): H_0$ is the variance of the difference under the null hypothesis.

The standard error of the difference $p_c - p_e$ if the null hypothesis is true is the square root of the above:

$$\text{SE}(d): H_0 = \left[\frac{.03(.97)}{n} + \frac{.03(.97)}{n} \right]^{1/2}$$

This formulation is the same as that used to calculate n on the basis of specified confidence limits. However, in order to bring into the calculations the power of our sample size to reject the null hypothesis when a specified alternative is true, we are now considering sample size calculations from the viewpoint of hypothesis testing. Of course, after the data have been collected, presenting results in terms of confidence limits on the unknown difference between the two parameters is always more informative than simply rejecting or not rejecting the null hypothesis.

Recalling that in our test of the null hypothesis we have a two-sided type I error of .05, we can identify the critical value as the point marked "V" in Figure 2-1. This point is $1.96\,\text{SE}(d): H_0$ above the mean value of zero difference, given that the null hypothesis is true. If this is not immediately obvious, consider the following argument. We are investigating two possible states. Either both control and experimental groups have $P = .03$, which is the null hypothesis state, or $P_c = .03$ but $P_e = .02$, which is the alternative hypothesis state. A type I error of size α specifies the proportion of times we will reject the null hypothesis *when it is true.* If the null hypothesis is true, any sample difference falling in the two areas marked $\alpha/2$ will result in falsely rejecting the null hypothesis; for these two symmetric areas to have a total probability of .05, they must each be $1.96\,\text{SE}(d): H_0$ from the mean.

Here again we are making use of characteristics of the normal distribution. For the sample sizes appropriate to epidemiologic studies, the normality assumption is almost always justified.

In Figure 2-2 we repeat Figure 2-1 with some simplifications and an indication that V is $1.96\,\text{SE}(d): H_0$ from the mean (zero) of the distribution of all possible sample differences under the null hypothesis.

Suppose the true state is that of the alternative hypothesis. In that case some of the possible sample differences will fall in the region to the left of the point V. Keep in mind that in real sampling, as opposed to that discussed in a textbook illustration, you would not know that the sample came from the population specified by the alternative hypothesis. You would know only that the sample difference is not large enough to fall in the upper rejection region ($\alpha/2$) for the null hypothesis. As a consequence you fail to reject the null hypothesis when the alternative is true. This is the type II error (of size β), and in this particular example we have set β equal to .10. Thus, 10 percent of all possible sample differences observed when the *alternative hypothesis is true* will result in a failure to reject the null hypothesis when it is, in fact, false.

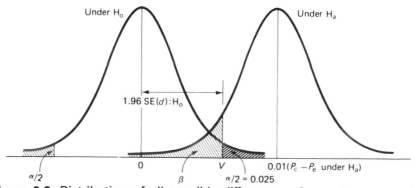

Figure 2-2. Distribution of all possible differences of sample means with type I error (α) set equal to .05.

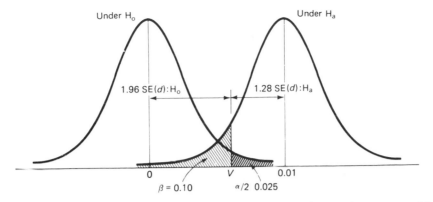

Figure 2-3. Distribution of all possible differences of sample means with type I error (α) set equal to .05 and type II error (β) set equal to .10.

Perhaps a better way of thinking about type II error is to state the probability desired for rejecting H_0 when the alternative is true, which is $(1 - \beta)$. The quantity $(1 - \beta)$ is referred to as the "power" of the test. If we want this to be .90, then $(1 - \beta) = .90$ and $\beta = .10$.

Again making use of the characteristics of the normal distribution, we know that 10 percent of the tail area on one side of the mean is located beyond 1.28 standard deviations from the mean. In this example the standard deviation of the distribution of all possible sample differences under the alternative hypothesis is

$$\text{SE}(d): H_a = \left[\frac{.03(.97)}{n} + \frac{.02(.98)}{n} \right]^{1/2}$$

and we can add to the diagram that V is 1.28 SE(d): H_a from the mean of the distribution of all possible sample differences under the alternative hypothesis. This is shown in Figure 2-3, which can be used to derive a formula for calculating n. Note that 1.96 SE(d): $H_0 + 1.28$ SE(d): H_a equals exactly the distance between the means of the two sampling distributions. Thus, we have 1.96 SE(d): $H_0 + 1.28$ SE(d): $H_a = .01$, from which we can calculate n:

$$1.96 \left[\frac{.03(.97)}{n} + \frac{.03(.97)}{n} \right]^{1/2} + 1.28 \left[\frac{.03(.97)}{n} + \frac{.02(.98)}{n} \right]^{1/2} = .01$$

$$1.96 \left(\frac{.2412}{\sqrt{n}} \right) + 1.28 \left(\frac{.2207}{\sqrt{n}} \right) = .01$$

$$\sqrt{n} = 75.52$$

$$n = 5703$$

The sample size of 5703 is required for each group (control and experimental). This huge sample size is needed because we are attempting to discover if a small difference (between .02 and .03) exists. In reviewing the components of the sample size equation immediately above, we observe that 1.96 was used for $Z_{\alpha/2}$, the standardized normal deviate appropriate to a one-sided area of $\alpha/2$ (two-sided error $= \alpha$). If the two-sided α is set equal to .01, we use 2.58 instead of 1.96. The value of var(d): H_0 represents the variance of the difference between two sample means, both drawn from a binomial universe with $P = P_c$, which in this case is .03. The value 1.28 represents the Z_β that is appropriate to the standardized normal deviate beyond which in one direction the proportion β of the distribution lies. If the type II error had been set at .05 instead of .10, Z_β would be 1.64 instead of 1.28. The value used for var(d): H_a represent the variance of the difference of two binomial means, one drawn from a population with $P = .03$ and the other from a population with $P = .02$. We now restate, in general terms, the equation to be solved for sample size n, using Q to represent $1 - P$:

$$Z_{\alpha/2}\left(\frac{2P_cQ_c}{n}\right)^{1/2} + Z_\beta\left(\frac{P_cQ_c}{n} + \frac{P_eQ_e}{n}\right)^{1/2} = P_c - P_e\ddagger \tag{2-6}$$

Most texts, references, and experts [Halperin et al 1958, Fleiss 1981] would argue that the above equation is wrong and that $2P_cQ_c$ should be replaced by $2\bar{P}\bar{Q}$, where $\bar{P} = (P_c + P_e)/2$. While not agreeing with the majority on this point, we want to present their view. In simplest terms, the disagreement arises because the actual significance test performed *after* data have been collected tests whether the two observed values p_c and p_e could both represent samples from a population whose parameter is $(p_c + p_e)/2$, or $\bar{p}$. We would perform the same test, but our view is that the null hypothesis (to use the arithmetic values from the preceding illustration) states that both parameters are .03 (value of P_c), not that both are .025 $[(P_c + P_e)/2]$. The sampling variance under the null hypothesis follows from the null hypothesis. The sample size calculated from Equation 2-6 is exactly the sample size appropriate to the question "If the true control proportion is P_c and the true experimental proportion P_e, what sample size is needed to be $1 - \beta$ sure of detecting a significant difference at the α level between control and experimental means?" Having computed the sample size appropriate to this question, we shall use the data actually collected to answer a different question: Are p_c and p_e random samples from a binomial universe with $(p_c + p_c)/2$ as mean?

As a practical matter, it is useful to note that this difference of opinion has only a moderate effect on the calculated value of n.

Unrelated to the previous discussion of the correct formula is an approximation to Equation 2-6 that substitutes $\bar{P} = (P_c + P_e)/2$ for both P_c

and P_e. Using Δ to represent $P_c - P_e$, this short form becomes

$$Z_{\alpha/2}\left(\frac{2\bar{P}\bar{Q}}{n}\right)^{1/2} + Z_\beta\left(\frac{2\bar{P}\bar{Q}}{n}\right)^{1/2} = \Delta$$

$$(Z_{\alpha/2} + Z_\beta)\left(\frac{2\bar{P}\bar{Q}}{n}\right)^{1/2} = \Delta$$

$$(Z_{\alpha/2} + Z_\beta)^2\left(\frac{2\bar{P}\bar{Q}}{n}\right) = \Delta^2$$

$$n = \frac{(Z_{\alpha/2}Z_\beta)^2(2\bar{P}\bar{Q})}{\Delta^2} \qquad (2\text{-}7)$$

Unequal Sample Size in Groups to Be Compared

Unlike Equation 2-6, Equation 2-7 requires an equal number of subjects in both groups. Equation 2-6 is simple to solve for n even if written so that there are n subjects in one group and $2n$ or $3n$ in the other (e.g., for study designs with two or three controls for each case). If you are investigating a possible difference between cases and controls (see Chapter 3 for the source of P_c and P_e values in sample size calculations related to case-control studies) and few cases are available for study but controls are plentiful, you might decide to choose three controls per case. In that event Equation 2-6 becomes

$$Z_{\alpha/2}\left(\frac{P_cQ_c}{3n} + \frac{P_cQ_c}{n}\right)^{1/2} + Z_\beta\left(\frac{P_cQ_c}{3n} + \frac{P_cQ_c}{n}\right)^{1/2} = P_c - P_e^{\ddagger} \qquad (2\text{-}6a)$$

Equation 2-6a indicates that the variance of the sample mean under the null hypothesis is $P_cQ_c/3n$ for the control group and P_cQ_c/n for the cases. The divisors of $3n$ and n reflect the different sample sizes for the two groups. Equation 2-6a also indicates that the variance of the sample mean for the control group remains $P_cQ_c/3n$ under the alternative hypothesis but the variance of the case group changes to P_eQ_e/n.

Choosing Between Alternative Parameters Using One Sample

The preceding sections on the sample size needed to estimate whether two parameters differ have been written with respect to *two independent samples*. With one small simplification, exactly the same logic and computations are applicable to the situation in which only *one sample* is used to choose between alternative parameters.

Return to the example on the extent of smoking in the freshman class cited in the section Sample Size for Single Binomial Parameter. We now modify that example in the following way. Past experience has shown that freshman classes include about 25 percent who are cigarette smokers. We hypothesize that is true for the current entering class as well *but we want to be 90 percent confident that if the new class includes 33 percent smokers or more, we will reject the hypothesis of 25 percent.* The specification of a hypothesis (H_0) that $P = .25$ *and an alternative* (H_a) *that* $P = .33$ leads to sample size calculations that are almost identical to those explained in Figures 2-1 through 2-3. In the case of the two independent samples, the two distributions diagrammed in these figures are distributions of *differences* between sample means drawn from two populations. In the case of the single sample, the distributions diagrammed are distributions of *sample means* drawn from two populations. We will designate P_0 and P_a for the alternative parameters in the instance of a single sample. Then the equation to be solved for n, analogous to that given for two samples in Equation 2-6, is

$$Z_{\alpha/2}(P_0 Q_0/n)^{1/2} + Z_\beta (P_a Q_a/n)^{1/2} = P_a - P_0{}^\ddagger \qquad (2\text{-}8)$$

The only changes from Equation 2-6 are the expressions in the parentheses. In Equation 2-6 these are the variances of the *differences in sample means* under the two hypotheses. In Equation 2-8, these are just the variances of *sample means* under the two hypotheses.

Sample size calculations presented herein relate to simple random sampling. If the same equations are used with stratified, systematic, or cluster sampling, it should be with full recognition that good stratification or relevant ordering of a list from which a systematic sample is taken will increase precision (reduce sampling variance) from that specified and, with few exceptions, cluster sampling will reduce precision (increase sampling variance) from that specified.

Continuous Variables

All the preceding examples of sample size calculations relate to binomial variables. Exactly the same principles apply to continuous variables (e.g., blood pressure or weight) with $\text{var}(X)$ substituted for $P(1 - P)$ and μ for P. Equation 2-4 rewritten for a continuous variable becomes

$$1.96\,\text{SE}(\bar{x}) = 1.96\left[\frac{\text{var}(X)}{n}\right]^{1/2} = \Delta \qquad (2\text{-}9)$$

where Δ equals the difference between estimate and parameter that we are willing to tolerate. Equation 2-5 rewritten for a continuous variable becomes

$$1.96\,\text{SE}(\bar{x}) = 1.96\left[\frac{\text{var}(X)}{n}\right]^{1/2} = \frac{\mu}{K} \qquad (2\text{-}10)$$

Equation 2-6 rewritten for a comparison of continuous variables, with X representing the result of standard treatment and Y the result of experimental treatment, becomes

$$Z_{\alpha/2}\left[\frac{2\,\text{var}(X)}{n}\right]^{1/2} + Z_{\beta}\left[\frac{\text{var}(X)}{n} + \frac{\text{var}(Y)}{n}\right]^{1/2} = \mu_x - \mu_y^{\S} \quad (2\text{-}11)$$

For binomial variables, if means differ so must the variances as they are directly related (P and PQ). Continuous variables, however, can have var(X) equal to var(Y) even though $\mu_z \neq \mu_y$. If var$(X) = $ var(Y), Equation 2-11 can be simplified to

$$Z_{\alpha/2}\left[\frac{2\,\text{var}(X)}{n}\right]^{1/2} + Z_{\beta}\left[\frac{2\,\text{var}(X)}{n}\right]^{1/2} = \mu_x - \mu_y^{\S}$$

Using Δ to represent $\mu_x - \mu_y$

$$(Z_{\alpha/2} + Z_{\beta})\left[\frac{2\,\text{var}(X)}{n}\right]^{1/2} = \Delta$$

$$(Z_{\alpha/2} + Z_{\beta})^2\left[\frac{2\,\text{var}(X)}{n}\right] = \Delta^2$$

$$\frac{(Z_{\alpha/2} + Z_{\beta})^2[2\,\text{var}(X)]}{\Delta^2} = n \quad (2\text{-}12)$$

This is exactly equivalent to Equation 2-7 for binomial variables when the variance under both the null and alternative hypotheses is approximated by $\bar{P}\bar{Q}$.

Estimates of the variances required for calculating sample size appropriate for the study of continuous variables must depend on prior data and on the investigator's informed judgment.

Summary

It may be helpful for students to consider the effect of different sizes of n on the distribution of all possible sample differences, as shown in Figures 2-1 to 2-3. First let us imagine how the distributions might look if n were very large, thus reducing the size of both SE(d): H_0 and SE(d): H_a, but without changing the location of V. This is shown in Figure 2-4, wherein both $\alpha/2$ and β are smaller than in Figures 2-1 to 2-3.

Suppose (as is traditional) that, despite the larger sample size, α is kept constant at .05 and $\alpha/2$ at .025. Then the distributions for very large n would look like Figure 2-5, in which V' is the critical value above which we make a type I error if the null hypothesis is true and below which we make a type II error if the alternative hypothesis is true. The cross-

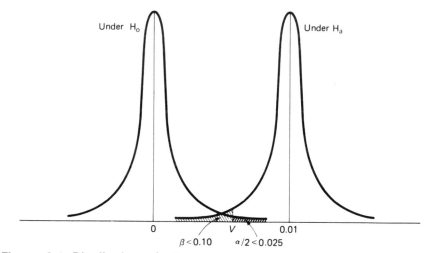

Figure 2-4. Distribution of all possible differences of sample means if sample size is very large.

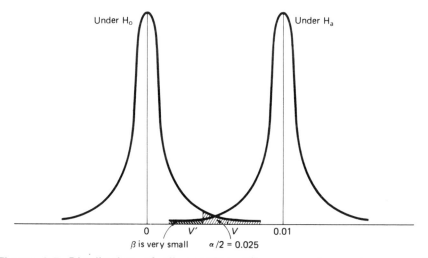

Figure 2-5. Distribution of all possible differences of sample means if sample size is very large but type I error (α) is kept equal to .05.

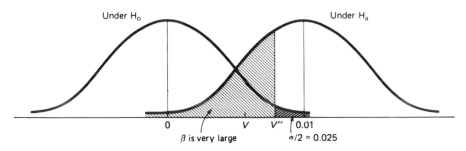

Figure 2-6. Distribution of all possible differences of sample means if sample size is *not* large and type I error (α) is kept equal to .05.

hatched area immediately to the right of V' represents $\alpha/2 = .025$ of the total area under the distribution, given H_0. Note how much *farther V' is from the mean of the distribution under the alternative hypothesis* relative to our original critical value, V. As a consequence, the probability of a type II error has been drastically reduced. If in fact the alternative hypothesis is true, we have very little chance of accepting the null hypothesis ($\beta < .01$, estimated from Figure 2-5).

Next look at Figure 2-6, in which we consider the effect on the two distributions of a small n (but still large enough to justify our use of the normal curve for the distribution of all possible sample differences). Again the two-sided α is fixed at .05.

Now V'' is the critical value above which we make a type I error if the null hypothesis is true. This error is again fixed at .05 (two-sided), but observe how large β has become. Since for values of $p_c - p_e$ below (to the left of) V'' we do not reject the null hypothesis, Figure 2-6 shows that we shall be doing this about 25 percent of the time that samples are actually taken from the universe specified by the alternative hypothesis.

To review, Figures 2-4, 2-5, and 2-6 show that for a fixed type I error, the probability of failing to reject the null hypothesis when the alternative is true (β) will be small for large samples and large for small samples.

A final note about sample size. Sample size calculations are needed to ensure that the study design is adequate for at least some question of interest. As a practical matter, there are always subsidiary questions of importance related to differences between subgroups. Furthermore, some individuals assigned to a treatment will refuse, and others may not adhere to the schedule of treatment or be lost to follow-up . All these factors reduce the effect that can be observed. Experienced investigators know that sample size, however calculated, is invariably inadequate for some purposes. Some methods of analysis, such as matching or multiple adjustment, tend to reduce the variance of sample statistics and thus to reduce the sample size needed to a value lower than that obtained by using Equations 2-4 to 2-12. Unfortunately, this favorable influence is more than balanced by the increased sample size necessary for subgroup comparisons. We advise the use of Equations 2-4 to 2-12, modified when necessary by inclusion of the finite sampling factor, together with an appreciation that the resultant sample size usually reflects minimum needs.

APPLICATION TO FRAMINGHAM HEART STUDY DATA

The Appendix data from the Framingham Heart Study are included in this book to help show the extent to which alternative methods of analysis lead to different results. Although it would not be necessary to list the detailed data to demonstrate these comparisons, we want to encourage students to use the Appendix data to calculate some of the simpler methods themselves. Simple and complex methods will often be in general agreement and students who have personally computed the simpler ones should then find the complex ones less mysterious.

Since sampling procedures are common to all methods for analyzing data, applications for this chapter do not relate to the goal stated above. However, there is a benefit to the student in using Appendix data to demonstrate sampling calculations and suitable examples are included below. From another viewpoint, the Appendix data are definitely related to this chapter on sampling through the question "How was the Framingham population sampled?" Because results from the Framingham Heart Study are so well known around the world, we briefly outline its "sampling origins."

Originally thought of as a 20-year study, the population under age 30 was excluded because the investigators estimated that too few would develop arteriosclerotic or hypertensive heart disease before the study's end. By contrast those over 59 were excluded because too many may already have cardiovascular disease at the study's start. A sample size of 6000 was feasible and estimated to be sufficient for 2000 new cases of cardiovascular disease to develop by the end of the twentieth year. This number of new cases would be "large enough to insure statistically reliable findings" [Dawber et al 1951]. Since 6000 was considerably smaller than the town population in the target ages, a random sampling plan to avoid the unknown bias of self-selection was adopted.

Sampling was based on the annual publication by the Town of Framingham of a list of all residents age 20 or over. The list was stratified by family size and by precinct of residence. Within strata the list was arranged by address. So as not to break up families, e.g., include a husband in the sample but exclude his wife, sampling selection was of families not individuals. Within each stratum, a systematic sample of two families was selected from each successive group of three families on the list. Everyone aged 30–59 inclusive in the selected families was considered to be in the sample. The prediction was that about 90 percent of the selected individuals could be examined. In fact, the acceptance rate was 69 percent. When this lower acceptance rate became known it was decided to accept additional study subjects who were volunteers so as to have an adequate number under study. The final study population consisted of 4469 sample respondents and 740 volunteers. In early publications from the study these two groups were shown separately, with little important distinction ever noted between them insofar as incidence findings are concerned. Not much attention has ever been given to Framingham prevalence findings and as stated in Chapter 10, the opportunity for biased selection when studying prevalence is considerable. The possibility of bias is much reduced if the study relates to associations with the future occurrence of disease.

The Appendix list represents a further selection of the Framingham Heart Study data (sample respondents and volunteers combined). When the first examinations were made in 1948, serum cholesterol was not recognized as a potential risk factor. Very many of the first examinations had been completed before cholesterol measurements began. Excluded from the Appendix are all persons without a serum cholesterol value on exam 1 and also all those under age 45 at examination 1. We have selected only 13 (including coronary heart disease incidence and mortality by cause through examination 10) from the 394 variables on the tape provided by the National Heart Lung and Blood Institute to provide the desired material for comparison of methods and for student exercises. Of course, the Appendix is not a random sample of the Framingham data for the first 10 examinations (examinations were every two years and we have 18 years of follow-up), nevertheless it is useful for our specific objectives. A description of the 13 variables appears at the beginning of the Appendix.

For more complete information on the Framingham sample, see [Dawber et al 1951, Gordon and Kannel 1968, Dawber 1980].

If in a large population you plan to study, the risk of developing coronary heart disease (CHD) over an 18-year period is thought to be .144 for women (as in the Appendix data), what sample size is needed to be 90 percent confident of detecting a significant difference at the .05 level between the risk for men and women, if the risk for men is, in fact, .255 (as in the Appendix data)?

$$P_c = .144 \qquad \alpha = .05, \qquad Z_{\alpha/2} = 1.96$$
$$P_e = .255 \qquad \beta = .10, \qquad Z_\beta = 1.28$$

Using Equation 2-6 we have

$$1.96 \left[\frac{2(.144)(.856)}{n} \right]^{1/2}$$

$$+ 1.28 \left[\frac{(.144)(.856)}{n} + \frac{(.255)(.745)}{n} \right]^{1/2} = .255 - .144$$

$$1.96 \left(\frac{.2465}{n} \right)^{1/2} + 1.28 \left(\frac{.1233}{n} + \frac{.1900}{n} \right)^{1/2} = .111$$

$$\frac{.9731}{\sqrt{n}} + \frac{.7165}{\sqrt{n}} = .111$$

$$\frac{1.6896}{.111} = \sqrt{n}$$

$$n = 232 \text{ (each sex)}$$

You estimate that in a large population, 18-year risks of coronary heart disease are .18 for those with cholesterol values under 260 (as in the Appendix data). What sample size is needed to be $1 - \beta$ confident of detecting a significant difference at the α level, between the risks for those with cholesterol < 260 and those with levels ≥ 260, if the risk is actually .24 for the higher cholesterol group? For the following levels of α and β shown below calculate, for yourself, the estimated sample size using Equations 2-6 and 2-7, and compare your results to those shown in the table that follows.

$$P_c = .18 \qquad P_e = .24$$

$\alpha = .05$ and $\beta = .05,$ $\quad \alpha = .05$ and $\beta = .10,$ $\quad \alpha = .05$ and $\beta = .20$
$\alpha = .01$ and $\beta = .05,$ $\quad \alpha = .01$ and $\beta = .10,$ $\quad \alpha = .01$ and $\beta = .20$

Values of Z corresponding to two-sided tail areas for α of .05 and .01 are 1.96 and 2.58, respectively. Values of Z corresponding to one-sided tail areas for β of .05, .10, and .20 are 1.65, 1.28, and .84, respectively.

		Estimated sample size needed in each group	
α	β	Using Equation 2-6	Using simplified Equation 2-7
.05	.05	1125	1201
.05	.10	900	968
.05	.20	665	723
.01	.05	1534	1649
.01	.10	1269	1373
.01	.20	986	1078

You are asked to investigate whether the reported equality of mean systolic blood pressure between men and women in city C is correct. You presume that the standard deviation of individual systolic blood pressure values given in the Appendix for men and women combined is applicable to city C. What sample size is needed to be 90 percent confident that if mean female systolic pressure is 5 mm Hg higher than that for males you will find a significant difference at the .05 level in your sample?

The Appendix data show an overall standard deviation for systolic blood pressure on examination 1 of 28.0. The variance is the square of the standard deviation or 784. Using Equation 2-6 with 784 in place of all the variance symbols (which are PQ for binomial variables) we have

$$1.96\left[\frac{2(784)}{n}\right]^{1/2} + 1.28\left[\frac{2(784)}{n}\right]^{1/2} = 5$$

$$\frac{77.6}{\sqrt{n}} + \frac{50.7}{\sqrt{n}} = 5$$

$$\frac{128.3}{5} = \sqrt{n}$$

$$n = 658 \text{ (each sex)}$$

EXERCISES

(Note: Unless otherwise indicated, exercise calculations in this and later chapters relate to the complete Appendix listing.)

Ex. 2-1. From the listing of men aged 45–49 select a random sample of 30 and estimate (a) the proportion with serum cholesterol values of 260 or more and (b) the standard error of this estimate. Since the sample size is more than 10 percent of the population size (30/212) it is helpful to use the finite multiplier in calculating the standard error. Does the sample proportion ±1.65 estimated standard errors include the population proportion (.175)?

The above work is to be carried out independently by each student. The resulting sample estimates can then be assembled into a frequency distribution. Find the standard deviation of this frequency distribution and compare it to (a) the theoretical standard error using the known population variance and (b) standard errors estimated by individual samples. What fraction of the samples included the population value within estimated 90 percent confidence limits?

Suppose the class has 15 students and you assume (correctly) that the best estimate of the population proportion would be derived from combining the results of all 15 samples. This single sample of 450 will necessarily have to include some individuals more than once and represents a different kind of sample than we have considered to this point. Previously we have sampled without replacement and had ignored all later appearances of a random number already selected. By combining separate samples that may result in the same individual being selected more than once, we are sampling with replacement (of previously selected individuals). Because this is, in a way, equivalent to sampling from an infinite population, and our sample is surely less than 10 percent of infinity, the finite sampling factor is not applicable and should not be used. Do the 90 percent confidence limits on the combined estimate include the parameter (.175)?

Ex. 2-2. From the entire Appendix listing, select a simple random sample of 50 and estimate the proportion of those at risk (CHD $\neq$ 1) who developed coronary heart disease during 18 years follow-up (CHD $>$ 1). Calculate 90 percent confidence limits and observe whether the limits include the true value (.197). Note: It is not wrong to use the finite sampling factor in this exercise but it would make little difference since

$$(N - n)/(N - 1) = (1363 - 50)/1362 = 0.964.$$

Ex. 2-3. Use the age–sex groupings in the Appendix data as strata and select, from those at risk, a stratified random sample of 50, proportional to stratum size. After rounding the stratum sample sizes to the nearest

integer, the sample size will turn out to be 49 rather than 50. Add one to
the stratum for which the rounding reduction was closest to 1/2. Estimate
the proportion of those at risk who developed coronary heart disease
under observation. Calculate 90 percent confidence limits for your
estimate. Do they include the true value (.197)? How does this estimate
compare with that from Exercise 2-2? Is an estimate from a stratified
random sample always closer to the truth than that from a simple random
sample of the same population? Are the confidence limits always
narrower for a stratified sample? What is the general relationship
between a simple random sample and a stratified random sample of the
same population?

Ex. 2-4. The Appendix list is sorted by age sex groups, within groups
by CHD status, and within CHD status by systolic blood pressure on
examination 1.

a. Pick a systematic sample of 50 and estimate mean Framingham
   relative weight. Note: $N/n = 28.12$. If you choose a random number
   from 1 to 28, select that individual and every twenty-eighth thereafter,
   you will have a sample of exactly 50 only if your starting number was 7
   to 28 inclusive. If your starting number was 1 to 6, the sample size will
   be 51 when the end of the list is reached.
b. Pick a random sample of 50 and estimate mean Framingham relative
   weight. How do the systematic and random samples compare?
c. Use the systematic sample of 50 to estimate the proportion of those at
   risk who did develop coronary heart disease in the 18-year follow-up.
   With the Appendix list ordered as it is, would you expect this to be a
   poor, adequate, or excellent estimate? How close is your estimate to
   the true value (.197)?

Ex. 2-5. Select a stratified random sample of 50 men age 55 or over
from the two strata 55–59 and 60–62. Choose the sample size within each
stratum proportional to stratum size. Estimate the overall average
systolic blood pressure on examination 1 within this specific population.
Each student should do this work independently and then the class can
assemble these independent estimates into a frequency distribution. Note
whether this frequency distribution resembles a normal distribution.
Calculate the standard deviation of this set of independent estimates.
How does it compare to the theoretical calculation of the standard error
of the mean blood pressure for this method of sampling from this specific
population. Using the known population values and the square root of

Equation 2-3, this is

$$\text{SE(SBP}_{\text{strat}}) = \left[\left(\frac{184}{246}\right)^2 \left(\frac{712.89}{37}\right)\left(\frac{184-37}{184-1}\right) \right.$$
$$\left. + \left(\frac{62}{246}\right)^2 \left(\frac{745.29}{13}\right)\left(\frac{62-13}{62-1}\right) \right]^{1/2}$$
$$= 3.40$$

Ex. 2-6. Given that the true proportion of individuals with diastolic blood pressure greater than or equal to 115 mm Hg is $(82/1406) = .058$, what sample size is needed to estimate this proportion with 95% confidence that the estimate will be:

a. Within 2 percentage points (± 0.02) of the truth?
b. Differ from the truth by not more than 20 percent of the true proportion?

Ex. 2-7. Given that the true variance of diastolic blood pressure values is 201.64, what sample size is needed to estimate the population mean for this variable with 95 percent confidence that your estimate will be:

a. Within 5 mm Hg of the true mean ($=90.2$)?
b Differ from the true mean by not more than 5 percent of the true mean?

Ex. 2-8. Given that the 18-year incidence of coronary heart disease among those with systolic blood pressure of less than 165 mm Hg on examination 1 is .162, what size sample is needed to be 90 percent confident ($\beta = .10$) of finding a significant ($\alpha = .05$) difference in risk between those with SBP < 165 and those with SBP $\geqslant 165$, if the latter's risk were actually .321?

NOTES

* To check that no possibilities have been omitted, we can calculate the number of combinations of eight elements taken two at a time. The first element selected could be any one of the eight, and for each of these there are seven possible ways of picking the second selection. Thus, there are 56 different possibilities for selecting two from eight, but these include permutations, such 0_a0_b and 0_b0_a. Since in either case exactly the same two elements make up the sample, the order in which they were chosen is unimportant to us and they are alike for our purpose. To reduce the 56 permutations to combinations that involve different elements, we need only divide by the possible number of permutations of two things, which is 2. Thus $56 \div 2 = 28$ different samples of two, in agreement with the direct count.

[†] There are only 16 possible different stratified samples of size 2, as compared to 28 for simple sampling. The total of 16 can be checked as follows. If we pick from stratum 1 four choices are possible and for *each* of these four choices are possible from stratum 2, the total is 16. Picking first from stratum 2 only introduces permutations of the 16 samples already cited. Since we are interested in different samples and not in the order of choosing sample elements, these permutations can be ignored.

[‡] Depending on the direction of the change expected from the experimental treatment, this should be written $P_c - P_e$ or $P_e - P_c$, whichever shows a positive difference.

[§] This should be written $\mu_x - \mu_y$ or $\mu_y - \mu_x$, whichever reflects a positive difference.

3
Relative Risk and Odds Ratio

Since Cornfield showed that under suitable conditions retrospective (case-control) studies* can provide estimates of relative risk [Cornfield 1951], this statistic (as well as the odds ratio, which is closely related to it) has been used extensively in epidemiologic investigations as a measure of strength of association between a disease and a risk factor. Although, for reasons to be discussed later, we prefer the odds ratio, for historical reasons the discussion begins with relative risk.

RELATIVE RISK
Definition

In a prospective study participants are selected without reference to the presence or absence of disease. After excluding prevalence cases present at baseline, the population is then followed over time. The number of new cases occurring during a specified time period divided by the population at risk is the incidence rate.[†] Consider a population followed prospectively as described in Table 3-1. The risk of disease developing among those with the risk factor is $A/(A + B)$. Similarly, the risk of disease developing among those without the risk factor is $C/(C + D)$. The risk for those with the risk factor relative to those without the risk factor is the ratio of the two risks, $[A/(A + B)] \div [C/(C + D)]$.

Thus, in a prospective study relative risk can be defined as the ratio of incidence rates (or of risks) [see Chapter 8 for the difference between rates and risks (probabilities)] and

$$\text{relative risk} = \frac{\text{Incidence rate of disease in exposed group}}{\text{Incidence rate of disease in unexposed group}}$$

Table 3-1. Classification of a Population by Risk Factor Status and Disease Development in an Incidence Study

Risk factor classification	Disease incidence +	Disease incidence −	Total at risk
+ (present)	A	B	$A + B$
− (absent)	C	D	$C + D$
Total	$A + C$	$B + D$	T

Before we proceed with an example, we define RR as the symbol for relative risk in the population and $\widehat{RR}$ as the symbol for an estimate of RR based on sample data. The same convention will also be applied to OR and $\widehat{OR}$ as symbols for odds ratios.

Table 3-1A illustrates the calculation of relative risk using prospective data from the Honolulu Heart Program [Abbott et al 1986]. It shows the 12-year risk of stroke as $171/3435 = .0498$ for smokers and $117/4437 = .0264$ for nonsmokers. The ratio of these two risks or the risk of becoming a stroke victim during the next 12 years for smokers, *relative* to this risk for nonsmokers, is

$$\frac{171/3435}{117/4437} = \frac{.0498}{.0264} = 1.89$$

These data estimate that smokers are 1.89 times as likely to have a stroke over the next twelve years as nonsmokers. The relative risk (1.89) is certainly useful but knowledge of the separate risks for smokers (.0498) and nonsmokers (.0264) is even more valuable. A relative risk of 2 can derive from risks of .20 and .10 or from risks of .002 and .001. In general, these separate risks are not available from retrospective studies.

Table 3-1A. Twelve-Year Risk of Stroke among Male Smokers and Nonsmokers

Smoker	Stroke Yes	Stroke No	Total
Yes	171	3264	3435
No	117	4320	4437
Total	288	7584	7872

$$RR = \frac{171/3435}{117/4437} = 1.89$$

Source: Abbott et al 1986.

In cross-sectional data, although presence of disease and exposure to risk factors are both measured at the same time, both specific group risks and relative risk can be estimated from such data. In this case, $A/(A + B)$ and $C/(C + D)$ relate to prevalence. Their ratio estimates the relative risk of being a case. Such a relative risk estimate may or may not differ substantially from a relative risk estimate based on incidence data. In particular, if disease duration is unrelated to the risk factor, they will be in agreement.

For retrospective studies, however, direct assessment of risk for specific groups is often impossible and the estimation of relative risk (using $\widehat{OR}$) is the most that can be accomplished. Before proceeding to the mechanics of relative risk estimation in retrospective studies, we shall briefly review the logical foundation for obtaining relative risk from such studies.

From Case-Control Studies for Rare Diseases

In a retrospective study the objective is to compare cases and controls with respect to the presence of a reported risk factor. Exposure to the risk factor is often measured at the time of the study. Sometimes exposure data are obtained from preexisting records or from biological specimens collected in the past, e.g., frozen sera. However, whether data are measured at the time of the retrospective study or earlier, the most basic requirement for obtaining relative risk estimates from retrospective studies is that the cases in the study be representative of all the cases in the population under consideration and that the controls in the study be representative of all the noncases in the same population. The word *representative* refers to representativeness *with respect to the risk factors being evaluated*.

Suppose that both cases and controls are taken from a private hospital principally used by patients in high socioeconomic categories. If the intent is to study the disease-risk factor association in this upper-class subpopulation, restricting cases and controls to such a hospital can be defended. If the intent is to study the risk-disease association in the total population, the restriction to private hospital data may be challenged. Evidence may exist establishing that risk does not vary by social class, but more likely the applicability to the total population of findings based on a particular subpopulation would be unknown. As a practical matter, it will often be true that the disease-risk factor association found for a subpopulation will apply fairly well to the total population. Although sampling error makes it unlikely that the study cases and controls include the identical proportion with the risk factor as all cases and all noncases, respectively, strong bias must be absent. Sampling error, although always present, is not a fundamental difficulty because it is controllable with adequate sample size. However, if cases are selected so that the method of selection produces important differences from all cases—and similarly for controls relative to all noncases—then it is quite possible that the proportion with the risk factor among *cases in the study* will differ by much more than sampling error from the proportion with the risk factor among *all relevant cases*. Details regarding selection of cases and controls are discussed in many texts on epidemiology [Breslow and Day 1980; Kelsey et al 1986; Lilienfeld and Lilienfeld 1980; Schlesselman 1982] but the essential requirement is the one stated above.

Although prospective studies can estimate the relative risk with respect to becoming sick (incident cases), retrospective, i.e., case-control studies can usually estimate only the relative risk with respect to being sick (prevalent cases). The practical importance of this distinction ranges from trivial to enormous. The retrospective study that compares *existing* cases with noncases (controls) on one or more potential risk factors cannot, in principle, relate to *all cases* occurring (incident) during the past *n* years because some of these incident cases may no longer be alive. The prospective study can, in principle, relate to all incident cases, whether early deaths or not, because risk factor status is measured at the onset of observation. For a disease such as myocardial infarction, in which a large fraction die promptly upon the very first clinical manifestation of the disease, relative risks derived from case-control studies *may* be quite different from those obtained in prospective studies. *If* early myocardial infarction deaths are unrepresentative of the myocardial infarction prevalent cases with respect to the risk factor being investigated, the difference can be great. In other words, if duration of disease is related to the risk factor, results from a retrospective study can be biased compared to a prospective study. Furthermore, a retrospective study tends to identify factors related to improved survival as risk factors for being sick. On the other hand, relative risk for a disease such as senile cataract, which is not associated with increased mortality risk, is, in principle, equally estimable in prospective and case-control studies.

A second major qualification for retrospective studies to be able to provide estimates of relative risk equivalent to those from a prospective study relates to when risk factor information is collected. In prospective studies, these data are collected prior to the development of disease and thus cannot be influenced or biased by disease status. (The possibility that ascertainment of disease in a prospective study may be biased by knowledge of risk factor status is a separate problem to be guarded against in study procedures.) In retrospective studies, risk factor data are collected after disease status is known and are subject to potential bias for that reason. Similar to differences arising from the use of incident or prevalent cases, the practical consequences of this potential problem vary greatly depending on the specific disease and risk factor under consideration. To illustrate, Table 3-2 lists several specific risk factors, in relation to myocardial infarction, showing a range of potential measurement bias from nonexistent to major.

Table 3-2. Illustration of Bias Potential in Retrospective Study Measurement of Risk Factors for Myocardial Infarction

Risk factor	Potential measurement bias due to measuring *after* disease status is known
Age began smoking	It is possible that those with the disease may try harder than controls to recall correctly an event of many years past.
Current smoking	Obvious major bias since myocardial infarction patients are almost always forbidden to smoke by attending physician. Current smoking probably does not reflect the risk factor intended for study. This is typically avoided by changing the risk factor from "current smoking" to smoking habits of "a month ago," "a year ago," "prior to your illness," etc.
Years of education completed	It is possible that those with the disease may be more (or less) given to exaggeration about a variable of social importance. However, for this variable the possibility exists of locating official records, thereby completely eliminating measurement bias.
Blood type	Bias is nonexistent for any objectively measurable genetic trait.

Investigators conducting retrospective studies must be aware of these (and other) potential biases. The final logical requirement for a successful retrospective study is that data collection methods for risk factors be similar for cases and controls. If risk factor data for cases come from relatives of cases, so should data for controls. If risk factor data for cases come from records, so should data for controls. If risk factor data are obtained by interviewers, the same interviewers should contact both cases and controls, without knowledge as to which is which, insofar as this is possible.

Assuming that we have conducted a retrospective study and chosen study cases and controls so as to represent all cases and all noncases in the population being investigated, have avoided measurement bias due to differences in data collection methods between cases and controls, have minimized bias due to risk factor measurement after disease has developed, and have been able to rule out important differences in risk factor frequency between incident cases and prevalent cases, we can summarize study results as in Table 3-3.

Table 3-3. Association of Risk Factors and Disease in a Retrospective Study Sample

Risk factor classification	Cases	Controls	Total
+ (present)	a	b	m_1
− (absent)	c	d	m_2
Total	$a + c = n_1$	$b + d = n_2$	$m_1 + m_2 = t$

Table 3-4. Association of Risk Factor and Disease
in a Population Cross Section

Risk factor classification	Cases	Noncases	Total
+ (present)	A	B	M_1
− (absent)	C	D	M_2
Total	$A + C = N_1$	$B + D = N_2$	$M_1 + M_2 = T$

Frequently, $b + d$ is chosen to equal $a + c$, that is, the total number of controls equals the total number of cases. Since the number of cases and the number of controls are usually determined *without knowledge* of how many cases and how many noncases actually exist in the population of interest, it is impossible to use any ratio of cases to controls to reflect the risk for a specific group. The ratio $a/(a + b)$, for example, does *not* estimate the risk of disease for those with the risk factor. This ratio is in fact useless by itself.

The key to understanding how the data in Table 3-3 can be used to estimate relative risk is in recognizing that $a + c$ is a sample of total cases and $b + d$ is a separate sample of noncases. Thus, although the relationship of a to b or a to $a + b$ promises no meaningful data (since it reflects in part decisions such as having one or two controls per case), the relationship of a to c provides an estimate of how all cases are divided into those with and without the risk factor. Similarly, whereas the ratios c/d and $c/(c + d)$ are usually uninterpretable, the ratio b/d estimates the distribution of the risk factor among all noncases.

Table 3-4 cross-classifies the total population from which the cases and controls in Table 3-3 were selected, and a/c and b/d in Table 3-3 can be interpreted as estimates of A/C and B/D in Table 3-4. Thus, although we cannot estimate the risk of disease for those with and without the risk factor, we can estimate how the risk factor is distributed among those with and without disease.

We now use Table 3-4 to explain how the retrospective study data a/c and b/d can be used to estimate relative risk. Analogous to what has been stated for incidence, the relative risk of having disease for those with compared with those without the risk factor is $[A/(A + B)]/[C/(C + D)]$. This ratio referred to Table 3-1 definitions is the relative risk of *becoming* sick; with reference to Table 3-4 definitions, it is the relative risk of *being* sick. For diseases that are uncommon, and happily for humanity many diseases fit this requirement, $A + B$ can usually be satisfactorily approximated by B. Similarly, $C + D$ can usually be approximated by D. Making these substitutions, we have

$$\frac{A/(A + B)}{C/(C + D)} \simeq \frac{A/B}{C/D} = \frac{AD}{BC} \tag{3-1}$$

To repeat, if the disease is rare *in the population* (how common or rare it is in the sample studied depends on how many controls were selected per case), the relative risk is closely approximated by AD/BC, commonly called the *odds ratio*. Thus we can use $(a/c) \div (b/d) = ad/bc$ to estimate AD/BC, which in turn is an estimator of relative risk for rare diseases. The odds ratio can also be defined directly, rather than as something approximately equal to the relative risk under certain conditions, and we will soon do so.

From Case-Control Studies for Any Disease

It is sometimes claimed that retrospective studies can estimate relative risk only for rare diseases because it is only for rare diseases that the population relative risk is approximated by the population odds ratio. Although this is frequently true as a practical consequence of how retrospective studies are conducted, exceptions are possible. We shall use the notation of Tables 3-3 and 3-4 to make this point.

If, as is rarely done, controls are selected not to represent noncases but to represent the *total population* (for example, selecting an area sample for controls), the relative risk can be estimated without regard to disease rarity. The study data in this instance, a/c, estimates A/C and b/d estimates $(A + B)/(C + D)$. The ratio $(a/c) \div (b/d)$ would then estimate $[A/(A + B)]/[C/(C + D)]$ whether or not the disease is rare. Since controls are rarely samples of the total population, the usual rule that retrospective studies can estimate relative risk only for rare diseases is correct. If, however, controls do represent the total population rather than just noncases, this need not be. Again, we emphasize that whether or not the disease is rare, $(a/c) \div (b/d)$, where $b + d$ is a sample of noncases, is an appropriate estimator of AD/BC, the odds ratio in the population.

ODDS RATIO
Definition

The distinction between risk and odds can be illustrated using the notation of Table 3-4, where $A/(A + B)$ is the *risk* of disease among those with the risk factor and A/B is the *odds* of disease to nondisease among those with the risk factor. The application of odds that might be familiar to most readers relates to gambling. Odds of 2 to 1 are equivalent to a probability of 2 out of 3. Odds of 5 to 2 are equivalent to a probability of 5 out of 7. Odds thus have the same numerators as probabilities, but the denominators count only those events not counted in the numerator. The denominator of a probability is always a count of all relevant events, including those counted in the numerator. If in Table 3-4 A has the value 1 and B the value 99, the risk of disease for those with the risk factor would be 1/100 and the odds of disease to nondisease for those with the risk factor would be 1/99.

Again referring to Table 3-4, the odds ratio relating the *odds of being a case to not being a case* for those with the risk factor (A/B) to these same odds for those without the risk factor (C/D) is $(A/B)/(C/D)$, which has just been shown to be a good approximation to the relative risk for uncommon diseases. Interestingly, the other odds ratio obtainable from Table 3-4, i.e., relating the *odds of having or not having the risk factor* for those who are cases (A/C) to these same odds for those who are not cases (B/D) also equals $(A/B)/(C/D)$. This is easy to see:

$$\frac{A/C}{B/D} = \frac{A}{C}\left(\frac{D}{B}\right) = \frac{A}{B}\left(\frac{D}{C}\right) = \frac{A/B}{C/D} \tag{3-2}$$

The odds ratio is usually reported in its simplest form, which is AD/BC. However, the algebraic equivalents of AD/BC, $(A/C)/(B/D)$, or $(A/B)/(C/D)$ express the odds in the numerator and denominator of the ratio more clearly than does AD/BC.

If instead of population data in Table 3-4, we make use of sample data in Table 3-3 to calculate odds ratios, as we previously explained, we are not able to use a/b or c/d as estimates of the odds for disease to nondisease in the population. However, we can and do use a/c and b/d as estimates of the population odds for having, relative to not having, the risk factor. As shown in Equation 3-2, however, the ratios $(A/C)/(B/D)$ and $(A/B)/(C/D)$ are identically equal to AD/BC, the population odds ratio.

Arrangement of 2 × 2 Tables

At this point, a brief digression concerning the ordering of rows and columns in 2×2 tables may be helpful. Note that both Tables 3-3 and 3-4 are arranged so that data for those *with* the risk factor is in the first row and data for cases is in the first column. Often, locating data for those with the risk factor in the first row is contrary to natural numeric ordering. For example, the first row might contain data for those with higher blood pressure and the second row data for those with lower blood pressure. This is done deliberately. Consider the symbolic sample data arrangement in Table 3-3. Under the proper conditions of sampling and measurement, ad/bc estimates the ratio in the population of the odds of being a case for those with the factor present, to the odds of being a case for those with the factor absent. This particular odds ratio is no more correct than the other odds ratio that can be estimated from these data; it is just customary and convenient for the odds ratio to be in this form. In Table 3-4, AD/BC is the odds of being a case for those with the factor present (A/B) divided by the odds of being a case for those with the factor absent (C/D). In sample data arranged the same way, ad/bc provides an estimate of AD/BC.

If both the population and the sample data in Tables 3-3 and 3-4 had been arranged so that the first row of the table was "risk factor absent" and the second row was "risk factor present" but with the A-B-C-D and a-b-c-d labeling for the four cells unchanged, then AD/BC would represent the odds of being a case for those *with factor absent (A/B)* divided by the odds of being a case for those *with factor present (C/D)*. Thus, with this changed ordering of the data, calculating ad/bc from the sample estimates a population odds ratio different from the one estimated from an identical sample 2×2 table but with row data reversed. If presence of the factor raises the risk of disease, then AD/BC from Table 3-4 will have a value greater than unity and AD/BC from a table similar to Table 3-4 but with row data reversed will have a value less than unity. There are only two odds ratios definable from a 2×2 table, and each is the reciprocal of the other. Returning to Table 3-4 notation, the possibility for calculating odds in terms of *disease* are A/B and C/D *or* B/A and D/C. The odds ratios possible are odds for those with factor present divided by odds for those with factor absent and odds for those with factor absent divided by odds for those with factor present. The possibilities for calculating odds in terms of *risk factors* are A/C and B/D or C/A and D/B. In this instance, the odds ratio could relate odds for those with disease to odds for those without disease or odds for those without disease to odds for those with disease. Using all possible combinations, we get

$$\frac{A/B}{C/D} = \frac{A/C}{B/D} = \frac{D/C}{B/A} = \frac{D/B}{C/A} = \frac{AD}{BC}$$

$$\frac{C/A}{D/B} = \frac{B/A}{D/C} = \frac{C/D}{A/B} = \frac{B/D}{A/C} = \frac{BC}{AD}$$

To better visualize the effect on the odds ratio of changes in the order of rows or columns, Table 3-4A restates the essential data of Table 3-1A and then repeats the data but with row and column changes. In Table 3-4A all computations of the estimated odds ratio are made using ad/bc. However, with various row and column reordering it should be clear that the ad/bc calculation does not always estimate the same odds ratio.

It is always essential to know what you are doing with respect to summarization of data, but it is still convenient to be able to use the routine calculation of a cross-product ratio, ad/bc, in obtaining an estimate of the odds ratio of interest. Recognizing that reversing the two rows (or the two columns) of the table leads to estimating the reciprocal odds ratio often helps identify any instances when the table is arranged in

Table 3-4A. Effect on the Odds Ratio Calculation Using *ad/bc* of Changes in the Ordering of Rows and Columns

		Stroke	
	Smoker	Yes	No
A. *Rows and columns as in Table* 3-1A	Yes	171	3264
	No	117	4320

$OR = ad/bc = 1.93$, indicating that smoking increases the odds of having a stroke.

		Stroke	
	Smoker	Yes	No
B. *Rows reversed from Table* 3-1A	No	117	4320
	Yes	171	3264

$OR = ad/bc = .52$ (=1/1.93), indicating that not smoking is protective against a stroke

		Stroke	
	Smoker	No	Yes
C. *Columns reversed from Table* 3-1A	Yes	3264	171
	No	4320	117

$OR = ad/bc = .52$ (=1/1.93), indicating that smoking *reduces* the odds of *not* having a stroke.

		Stroke	
	Smoker	No	Yes
D. *Rows and columns reversed from Table* 3-1A	No	4320	117
	Yes	3264	171

$OR = ad/bc = 1.93$ (=1/.52), indicating that the odds of *not* having a stroke are increased for nonsmokers.

a manner other than intended. (Reversing both rows *and* columns of the table leads to inverting an inverted ratio, which leaves it unchanged.)

A final comment on row and column ordering. The cross-product ratio *ad/bc* is affected by which of the two rows is on top and which of the two columns is on the left. Having fixed these, whether the disease–nondisease data are in rows and the risk factor data in columns or vice versa does not affect the cross-product ratio.

From Case-Control Studies

To recapitulate, a properly designed and conducted case control study:

1. Provides no data on disease odds separately for risk factor groups.

2. Does provide estimates of risk factor odds separately for cases and noncases. For Table 3-3, this is a/c and b/d.
3. Provides an estimate, ad/bc, of the population odds ratio, AD/BC, which for rare diseases (perhaps prevalence less than .05) is a good approximation of the population relative risk $[A/(A + B)]/[C/(C + D)]$.

One aspect of using retrospective study data to estimate relative risk that seems inadequately understood is that the sample data, ad/bc, are *always* usable as an estimator of the population odds ratio, AD/BC, whether or not the disease is rare in the population. When the disease is rare, AD/BC is sufficiently close to $[A/(A + B)]/[C/(C + D)]$ to make ad/bc an estimate of relative risk as well as the odds ratio. Since odds are not as much a part of ordinary usage as chance or probability or risk, many people find the concept of an odds ratio less meaningful than a relative risk. We think this is a matter of custom rather than of basic superiority of one method over the other and that odds and odds ratios will be increasingly used by epidemiologists in the future.

An Odds Ratio Advantage

One aspect of the odds ratio that is superior to the relative risk is the former's insensitivity to whether a study stresses death or survival. This point is illustrated by Table 3-5. Using Table 3-5 data to compare community A with community B, the relative risk of dying is $(2/100) \div (1/100) = 2$. The same comparison of odds leads to the odds ratio $(2/98) \div (1/99) \cong 2$. Thus, both measures indicate double or about double the risk of dying in community A relative to community B.

We now use Table 3-5 data to compare the two communities, but this time with respect to *surviving* instead of dying. The relative "risk" for surviving is $(98/100) \div (99/100) \cong 1$. The odds ratio for surviving is $(98/2) \div (99/1) \cong 1/2$. The use of relative risk leads to different results depending on whether the study is summarized with respect to death or to survival. Using the odds ratio, however, it does not really matter. Community A has about twice the odds of community B with respect to dying and about half the odds of community B with respect to surviving.

Table 3-5. Comparison of Mortality Experience in Two Communities

Community	Number dying	Number surviving	Total
A	2	98	100
B	1	99	100
Total	3	197	200

This indifference as to whether stress is placed on counting the events or the nonevents is obviously a desirable property of a summary statistic. The odds ratio has this property, the relative risk does not.

INTERPRETATION OF RELATIVE RISK AND ODDS RATIO ESTIMATES

Estimates of RR and OR are both used to measure the strength of the association between exposure and disease. Both ratios can take on values between 0 and infinity with the same general interpretation. Possible categories for RR and OR are greater than 1, zero, and less than 1, but never less than zero. A value greater than 1 indicates that risk or odds of disease is greater when exposed to the specified risk factor (positive association). A value of 0 indicates no association between exposure and disease. A value less than 1 indicates reduced risk or odds of disease with exposure to the risk factor (negative association). There may be differences in the numerical values for RR and OR (with OR always further from unity than RR) but they always point in the same direction.

CONFIDENCE LIMITS
Woolf's Method for Odds Ratios

We shall use OR as a symbol for AD/BC in the population and $\widehat{OR}$ as a symbol for an estimate of OR based on sample data. For data as in Table 3-3, the odds ratio, for odds of being a case comparing those with risk factor positive to those with risk factor negative, is estimated as $\widehat{OR} = ad/bc$. To obtain 95 percent confidence limits on OR using Woolf's method [Woolf 1955], we calculate $\ln \widehat{OR}$ and its estimated standard error:

$$\text{SE}(\ln \widehat{OR}) = \left(\frac{1}{a} + \frac{1}{b} + \frac{1}{c} + \frac{1}{d}\right)^{1/2} \tag{3-3}$$

Then 95 percent confidence limits on $\ln OR$ are

$$\ln \widehat{OR} \pm 1.96\left(\frac{1}{a} + \frac{1}{b} + \frac{1}{c} + \frac{1}{d}\right)^{1/2}$$

For 99 percent confidence limits, substitute 2.58 for 1.96. When confidence limits on $\ln OR$ have been obtained, confidence limits on OR are derived by taking antilogs. If $\ln OR_U$ and $\ln OR_L$ are the upper and lower confidence limits for $\ln OR$, then $e^{\ln OR_U}$ and $e^{\ln OR_L}$ are the upper and lower confidence limits for OR.

Some authors advocate the addition of 1/2 to each of the cell frequencies a, b, c, and d before calculation of $\widehat{OR}$ or of SE $\ln \widehat{OR}$

Table 3-6. Relationship of Cataract and Diabetes in a Case-Control Study, Age 50 to 69

Diabetes	Cataract cases	Fracture patients (controls)
+ (present)	55	84
− (absent)	552	1927

Source: Hiller and Kahn 1976.

[Haldane 1956; Fleiss 1979]. Others do not use the 1/2 adjustment or have reservations concerning it [Mantel 1977; Miettinen 1979]. We make no recommendation about this except to emphasize two points. First, if any cell frequency is zero, it may be impossible to carry out the calculations outlined in this and later chapters unless the 1/2 is added. Second, epidemiologic studies summarized into 2×2 tables with cell totals of zero or with cell totals so small that adding 1/2 will substantially affect the summary calculations are rarely of adequate precision to contribute anything of importance to our knowledge.

To illustrate the use of Woolf's method in calculating 95 percent confidence limits on OR, we apply the method to the data in Table 3-6, taken from a case-control study on the relationship of cataract to diabetes [Hiller and Kahn 1976].

$$\widehat{OR} = \frac{55(1927)}{84(552)} = 2.29$$

$$\ln \widehat{OR} = .8286$$

$$SE(\ln \widehat{OR}) = \left(\frac{1}{55} + \frac{1}{1927} + \frac{1}{84} + \frac{1}{552}\right)^{1/2} = .1800$$

$$\ln \widehat{OR} \pm 1.96 SE(\ln \widehat{OR}) = .8286 \pm .3528$$

95 percent CL on $\ln OR = .4758$ and 1.1814

95 percent CL on $OR = e^{.4758}$ and $e^{1.1814} = 1.6$ and 3.3

These same data were used to calculate confidence limits on the odds ratio using Cornfield's method as reported by Gart [1971]. That method, which requires an iterative procedure, is not as convenient as Woolf's method but is generally acknowledged to be more accurate. In this instance, however, the more accurate method makes no difference. The 95 percent confidence limits derived from the above data using Cornfield's method are also 1.6 and 3.3. In order to compare the two methods when the 2×2 table has cells of much smaller size, we make use of additional data reported by Hiller and Kahn [1976] for subgroups. The

Table 3-7. Comparison of 95% Confidence Limits on Odds Ratio Relating Cataract and Diabetes for Various Race and Control Groups, Age 50 to 69

Race	Control diagnoses[a]	$\widehat{OR}$	Cornfield (Gart [1971])	Woolf [1955]	Cell	Row or column total
			95% CL on *OR*		In 2 × 2 table, size of smallest	
All races	Hemorrhoids	2.1	1.1–4.2	1.1–4.0	12	67
All races	Varicose veins	3.6	1.8–7.4	1.9–6.9	11	66
White	Fractures	2.0	0.9–4.5	1.0–4.2	9	61
Nonwhite	Fractures	2.2	1.1–4.7	1.1–4.4	13	45

[a] Presumably reflecting the nondiabetic population.
Source: Hiller and Kahn 1976.

resultant confidence limits are shown in Table 3-7. Although the size of the smallest cell is smaller in Table 3-7 than in Table 3-6, differences between the two methods are not large, and Woolf's method can be properly said to provide results very similar to those from the more precise method. As shown in Chapter 5, the methods outlined in this book for calculating confidence limits on odds ratios differ to an important extent only when the data do not support a clear inference. However, for those desiring the greater precision of Cornfield's method, see Gart [1971].

Poisson Variable Assumption for Relative Risk

Odds ratios are now more commonly encountered in published reports than direct estimates of relative risk. However, if the individual risks are low enough for the observed events to be treated as Possion variables, then the number of observed events contains all the relevant information and approximate confidence limits can be computed without great difficulty [Ederer and Mantel 1974]. The approach outlined below should be reasonably satisfactory for risks less than .10. Let

o_1 represent observed events in sample group 1
o_2 represent observed events in sample group 2
n_1 represent the population size or person-years of observation in sample group 1
n_2 represent the population size or person-years of observation in sample group 2

Then

$$\widehat{RR} = \frac{o_1/n_1}{o_2/n_2} = \left(\frac{o_1}{o_2}\right)\left(\frac{n_2}{n_1}\right) \tag{3-4}$$

The confidence limits we shall derive relate only to samples of size n_1 and n_2 with *the sum of the actually observed events* equal to $o_1 + o_2$. The reasons for this can be clarified by imagining the distribution of all possible sample values of o_1 and o_2 arising from all possible samples of size n_1 and n_2. Of all the possible sample outcomes, our attention is restricted to those in which the sum of observed events equals the $o_1 + o_2$ sum in our actual sample. This amounts to taking a slice of the set of all possible samples, but it is a slice that permits inclusion of very large or very small observed values of relative risk. Restricting interest to this set of results enormously simplifies the calculation of the sampling error. We first place confidence limits on the parameter P, which represents the true proportion of the events that are in group 1. Then we use the confidence limits on P to derive confidence limits on the parameter RR, which is our objective.

Sample data can be summarized in the binomial variable

$$p = \frac{o_1}{o_1 + o_2} \qquad (3\text{-}5)$$

As a binomial variable based on a fixed number of trials (remember that $o_1 + o_2$ is constant over all samples under consideration) and using Equation 1-16, the sampling variance of p can be written

$$\text{var}(p) = \frac{P(1 - P)}{o_1 + o_2}$$

If our data set is large enough to justify using the normal approximation (see [Ederer and Mantel 1974] if it is not), our sample result of p will be within $1.96[P(1 - P)/n]^{1/2}$ of P 95 percent of the time. In fact, the lowest value of P for which *the observed data would not be unusual* (at the .025 level) is

$$P_L = p - 1.96 \left[\frac{P_L(1 - P_L)}{o_1 + o_2} \right]^{1/2} \qquad (3\text{-}6)$$

We denote this lower 95 percent confidence limit for P by the symbol P_L.

Another way of stating the relationship shown in Equation 3-6 is that p will not be greater than $P + 1.96 \, [SE(p)]$ unless p happens to be one of those unusually large sample values that occur in only 2.5 percent of all possible samples under consideration. Similar reasoning with respect to unusually small sample values of p, which occur in only 2.5 percent of all possible samples under consideration, leads to

$$P_U = p + 1.96 \left[\frac{P_U(1 - P_U)}{o_1 + o_2} \right]^{1/2} \qquad (3\text{-}7)$$

where P_U is the upper 95 percent confidence limit for P. Since we have found parameter values compatible with p being unusually large or unusually small at the .025 level, solving Equations 3-6 and 3-7 results in 95 percent confidence limits for P. Note that in both Equations the standard error of p is given in terms of P (not p) so that in solving for the upper confidence limit the standard error is based on P_U and in solving for the lower confidence limit the standard error is based on P_L.

We now divide numerator and denominator of Equation 3-4 by $(o_1 + o_2)$ and define the estimated relative risk in terms of the observed binomial proportion p from Equation 3-5:

$$\widehat{RR} = \frac{o_1}{o_2}\left(\frac{n_2}{n_1}\right) = \frac{o_1/(o_1 + o_2)}{o_2/(o_1 + o_2)}\left(\frac{n_2}{n_1}\right) = \frac{p}{1 - p}\left(\frac{n_2}{n_1}\right) \tag{3-8}$$

If we substitute $P/(1 - P)$ for $p/(1 - p)$, we have the true relative risk:

$$RR = \frac{P}{1 - P}\left(\frac{n_2}{n_1}\right) \tag{3-9}$$

The confidence limits on P relate to confidence limits on RR in the following way. If P is at its .025 lower limit P_L, then $1 - P_L$ is at its .025 upper limit and $P_L/(1 - P_L)$ *will be at its* .025 *lower limit*. Also, if P is at its .025 upper limit P_U, then $(1 - P_U)$ will be at its .025 lower limit and $P_U/(1 - P_U)$ *will be at its* .025 *upper limit*. Thus, the limits we have identified for P permit us to calculate confidence limits for RR as well:

$$RR_L = \frac{P_L}{1 - P_L}\left(\frac{n_2}{n_1}\right) \tag{3-10}$$

$$RR_U = \frac{P_U}{1 - P_U}\left(\frac{n_2}{n_1}\right) \tag{3-11}$$

All that remains is to solve Equations 3-6 and 3-7. Since these are quadratic equations, they need to be put into the standard form, $ax^2 + bx + c = 0$ and then solved for x using the formula

$$x = \frac{-b \pm \sqrt{b^2 - 4ac}}{2a}$$

We shall use the data on the 16-year incidence of myocardial infarction in Framingham by serum cholesterol level [Shurtleff 1970], shown in Table 3-8, to illustrate these computations, first for P_L and then for P_U.

Table 3-8. Development of Myocardial Infarction in Framingham after 16 Years, Men Age 35 to 44, by Level of Serum Cholesterol

Serum cholesterol (mg%)	Developed MI	Did not develop MI	Total
>250	10	125	135
≤250	21	449	470

Source: Shurtleff 1970.

Substituting Table 3-8 data into Equation 3-6, we have

$$P_L = \frac{10}{10 + 21} - 1.96 \sqrt{\frac{P_L(1 - P_L)}{10 + 21}}$$

$$P_L - .323 = -1.96 \sqrt{\frac{P_L(1 - P_l)}{31}} \qquad (3\text{-}12)$$

Squaring both sides of the equation, we get

$$P_L^2 \quad .646P_L + .104 = 3.842 \left[\frac{P_L(1 - P_L)}{31} \right]$$

which in standard form is

$$34.842P_L^2 - 23.868P_L + 3.224 = 0$$

The coefficients of this standard quadratic equation are

$$a = 34.842$$

$$b = -23.868$$

$$c = 3.224$$

so that

$$P_L = \frac{23.868 \pm \sqrt{569.681 - 4(34.842)(3.224)}}{69.684}$$

$$P_L = \frac{34.839}{69.684} \text{ or } \frac{12.897}{69.684} = .500 \text{ or } .185$$

as the two solutions to our quadratic equation. Clearly our choice for the lower limit is .185. However, the .500 is also of interest to us, as we shall soon see.

To solve for the upper limit, we substitute Table 3-8 data into Equation 3-7:

$$P_U = \frac{10}{10 + 21} + 1.96 \sqrt{\frac{P_U(1 - P_U)}{10 + 21}}$$

$$P_U - .323 = 1.96 \sqrt{\frac{P_U(1 - P_U)}{31}} \tag{3-13}$$

The only difference between Equation 3-12, which was solved for P_L, and Equation 3-13, which is to be solved for P_U, is $+1.96$ or -1.96. Therefore by squaring both sides of Equation 3-13, we obtain the identical quadratic equation obtained for P_L. SInce the solutions to that were .185 and .500, we do not need to solve the equation again. This time we take .500, the higher value, as the value for P_U.

Now we apply our values of P_L and P_U to finding limits within which the true relative risk is likely to be found. First, we substitute Table 3-8 data into Equation 3-4 and get

$$\widehat{RR} = \frac{10/135}{21/470} = 1.66$$

Then, substituting our P_L and P_U values in Equations 3-10 and 3-11, we get

$$RR_L = \frac{P_L}{1 - P_L}\left(\frac{n_2}{n_1}\right) = \frac{.185}{1 - .185}\left(\frac{470}{135}\right) = .79$$

$$RR_U = \frac{P_U}{1 - P_U}\left(\frac{n_2}{n_1}\right) = \frac{.500}{1 - .500}\left(\frac{470}{135}\right) = 3.48$$

The wide confidence limits (.79 and 3.48) of the relative risk (1.66) are a necessary consequence of the small total number (31) of observed cases of myocardial infarction.

The preceding computation of confidence limits for relative risk rests entirely on elementary statistical principles. However it is somewhat annoying to calculate without benefit of a computer program.

Method of Katz et al for Relative Risk

An alternative method that is very much easier to calculate has been suggested by Katz et al [1978]. This method uses a variance formula for ln RR that is derived similarly to that reported by Woolf for ln OR. The formula, which like Woolf's we cannot explain in terms of elementary statistics, is

$$\widehat{\text{var}}(\ln RR) = \frac{b/a}{a+b} + \frac{d/c}{c+d} \tag{3-14}$$

where a, b, c, d are the symbols we have used for the frequencies in a 2×2 table. Applying Equation 3-14 to Table 3-8 data we get

$$\widehat{\text{var}}(\ln RR) = \frac{125/10}{135} + \frac{449/21}{470} = .1381$$

$$1.96\ \text{SE}(\ln RR) = 1.96(.1381)^{1/2} = .7284$$

$$.95 \text{ confidence limits on } \ln RR = \ln 1.6578 \pm .7284$$

$$.95 \text{ confidence limits on } \ln RR = .5055 \pm .7284$$

$$.95 \text{ confidence limits on } \ln RR = -.2229,\ 1.2339$$

$$.95 \text{ confidence limits on } RR = .80,\ 3.43$$

This result is very close to the limits of .79 and 3.48 obtained by solving the quadratic equations in P_L or P_U.

Recalling that the relative risk and the odds ratio are quite similar for rare diseases and noting that Table 3-8 data reflect 16-year incident data of $10/135 = .074$ for those with high cholesterol levels and $21/470 = .045$ for those with low cholesterol levels, we use Table 3-8 data to calculate the estimated odds ratio and 95 percent confidence limits (by Woolf's method) on the true odds ratio, as an additional comparison:

$$\widehat{OR} = \frac{10(449)}{125(21)} = 1.71$$

$$\ln \widehat{OR} = .5368$$

$$\text{SE}(\ln \widehat{OR}) = \left(\frac{1}{10} + \frac{1}{125} + \frac{1}{21} + \frac{1}{449}\right)^{1/2} = .3973$$

$$1.96\ \text{SE}(\ln \widehat{OR}) = .7787$$

$$\ln \widehat{OR} \pm 1.96\ \text{SE}(\ln \widehat{OR}) = -.2419 \text{ and } 1.3155\ (95\% \text{ CL on } \ln OR)$$

$$e^{-.2419} \text{ and } e^{1.3155} = .79 \text{ and } 3.73\ (95\% \text{ CL on } OR)$$

These limits compare quite well with the corresponding values for the relative risk which were .79–3.48 using quadratic equations and .80–3.43 using the method of Katz et al. It should be noted that agreement between relative risk and odds ratio based on longitudinal data can always be increased by shortening the observation period, i.e., splitting it into two more intervals.

Summary

Our presentation of confidence limits for relative risk can be summarized as follows:

a. For risks under .10, the quadratic equation method (as explained on pages 58–62) is appropriate, understandable in terms of elementary statistics, and bothersome to calculate unless programmed for a computer.
b. The variance formula reported by Katz et al [1978] is not explainable at an elementary level but is very easy to compute.
c. For risks less than .10, confidence limits on the odds ratio using Woolf's method can be used as a substitute for limits on the relative risk.
d. By showing the close numerical agreement among these methods we hope to convince you that conceptually simpler techniques are often as "good" as those more difficult to understand. In addition, it is easier to accept procedures you do not fully comprehend when you have observed the similar results obtained with measures you do understand.

As a practical matter, we recommend using method (b) in your future work with respect to relative risks. However this recommendation comes after our strong suggestion that you first work through method (a).

SAMPLE SIZE CALCULATIONS USING ODDS RATIOS

Sample size calculations for retrospective studies use the principles outlined in Chapter 2 for a prospective clinical trial, but some differences are worth noting.

Rarely, if ever, is a retrospective study sample size calculation based on specified alternatives for P, such as P_c and P_e. The investigator is much more likely to calculate the sample size needed to detect a significant difference between cases and controls if the proportion with the suspected risk factor among noncases is P_c and the risk factor is associated with an odds ratio of K or more. As a specific illustration, the investigator may want to know the sample size needed to establish a statistically significant difference between intestinal cancer cases and controls with respect to the proportion who state that they usually eat high-fiber foods fewer than two times per week. This calculation requires an assumption, such as "the proportion of the noncases, which for this disease is almost equivalent to the general public, eating high-fiber foods less frequently than two times per week is about 70 percent." An additional requirement for this calculation is the specification by the investigator of what level of risk the sample should have a high probability of detecting. This can be specified as "low-fiber diets are associated with an odds ratio of 2 or more." It is also necessary to specify the type I error and type II error that apply identically to prospective and retrospective studies.

For prospective studies, all the elements needed for sample size calculation are present: α, β, P_c, and P_e, the latter two being the binominal parameters for the groups being compared. For retrospective studies, we have α, β, P_c, and OR (instead of P_e). However, it is a simple matter to use P_c and OR to derive the P_e implied by them. Using the illustration of the relationship of a low-fiber diet to intestinal cancer, we organize the relevant data into a 2×2 table relating to population data (not sample estimates) as follows:

Diet	Cases	Noncases (controls)
Low-fiber diet (high-fiber food less frequently than 2 times per week)	$100P_e$ A | B	70
Not low-fiber diet (high-fiber food at least 2 times per week)	C | D $100(1 - P_e)$	30
Total	100	100

We have arbitrarily established the table for 100 cases and 100 controls. Any other numbers would serve as well, but 100 is a convenient choice. Since one of the conditions underlying our calculation is that 70 percent of the general public eats a low-fiber diet, and since the general public and noncases of intestinal cancer are almost equivalent, we have designated 70 of the 100 controls as on low-fiber diets. If we now put $100P_e$ (100 times the proportion of cases reporting a low-fiber diet) into cell A and $100(1 - P_e)$ into cell C, we transform the proportions into numbers totalling 100 cases and have completed the 2×2 table. The remaining condition to be used is that the specified odds ratio, i.e., the odds ratio we wish to be able to identify as significantly different from 1.00, if it truly is as specified, is

$$OR = \frac{AD}{BC} = 2$$

Using the data in the table, we can now write

$$\frac{AD}{BC} = \frac{100P_e(30)}{70(100)(1 - P_e)} = 2$$

Solving for P_e, we obtain $P_e = .82$.

Table 3-9. Sample Size Requirements for Prospective and Retrospective Studies[a]

Disease incidence in unexposed group	Frequency of attribute in population (%)	Detectable relative risk	Sample size needed in each group	
			Prospective	Retrospective
1/1000	50	1.2	576 732	2535
		2.0	31 443	177
		4.0	5815	48
1/100	50	1.2	57 100	2535
		2.0	3100	177
		4.0	567	48
1/10	50	1.2	5137	2535
		2.0	266	177
		4.0	42	48

[a] Two-sided $\alpha = .05$; $\beta = .10$.
Source: J. Tonascia, unpublished notes.

If we specify α and β as .05 and .10, respectively, we have all the ingredients for sample size calculation for a retrospective study and can apply the formulas in Chapter 2.

$$P_c = .70 \qquad \alpha = .05$$

$$P_e = .82 \qquad \beta = .10$$

It is probably not at all obvious that if 70 percent of controls and 82 percent of cases eat a low-fiber diet the odds ratio associated with these data is 2. This is precisely why retrospective studies do not formulate their sample size queries using P_c and P_e but use P_c and OR instead. For the reader who is curious, we have calculated sample size for this illustrative retrospective study using Equation 2-6 and found that 288 cases and 288 controls are the numbers required. Good discussions of sample size requirements contrasting prospective and retrospective studies, together with convenient reference tables, can be found in works by Schlesselman [1974 and unpublished] and Walter [1977]. Retrospective studies generally require many fewer subjects than prospective ones to investigate equivalent problems, as illustrated in Table 3-9. This is so because it is not necessary to have as many individuals without disease (for comparison to the cases) as are generated in prospective studies of disease with low or moderate incidence.

APPLICATION TO FRAMINGHAM HEART STUDY DATA

The first step in any analysis should be an examination of the basic data *before* they are adjusted in any way. This will allow you to (1) look for

Table 3-10. Coronary Heart Disease Status by Level of Systolic Blood Pressure

| SBP(mm Hg) | Coronary heart disease | | | |
	On Exam 1 (prevalence cases)	On Exams 2–10 (incidence cases)	Negative	Total
≥165	17	95	201	313
<165	26	173	894	1093
Total	43	268	1095	1406

any errors or inconsistencies that remain after editing, (2) decide the variables for which adjustment is needed, (3) have a clear idea of the crude relationship between the risk factor and the event being studied, and (4) improve your understanding of the results after adjustment. In our use of Appendix data to illustrate the methods discussed in this chapter, we will investigate whether persons with systolic blood pressure of 165 mm Hg or more (SBP ≥ 165) are at increased risk of coronary heart disease. We will follow this same thread in succeeding chapters dealing with other methods of data analysis.

Framingham data relating systolic blood pressure to coronary heart disease are summarized in Table 3-10.

In order to examine the association between elevated blood pressure and the risk of *developing* coronary disease, it is necessary to omit the prevalence cases included in Table 3-10 from the analysis. The prevalence cases had CHD at the study onset and thus were no longer at risk of *developing* it. After excluding the 43 prevalence cases we get Table 3-11 which is a 2×2 table relating systolic blood pressure and coronary disease.

Using data from Table 3-11, the estimated relative risk $(\widehat{RR})$ of disease for those with SBP ≥ 165 is

$$\widehat{RR} = (95/296)/(173/1067) = (.321/.162) = 1.98$$

Table 3-11. Coronary Heart Disease Status after 18 Years by Level of Systolic Blood Pressure among Those Free of CHD on Exam 1

| SBP(mm Hg) | Coronary heart disease | | Total at risk |
	Yes	No	
≥165	95	201	296
<165	173	894	1067
Total	268	1095	1363

The .95 confidence limits, using Katz's method, Equation 3-14, for the variance of ln RR, are computed as follows:

$\ln RR = .6831$

$\text{var}(\ln RR) = (201/95)/296 + (894/173)/1067 = .0120$

$1.96\text{SE}(\ln RR) = 1.96(.0120)^{1/2} = .2147$

.95 confidence limits on $\ln RR = .6831 \pm .2147 = .4684, .8978$

.95 confidence limits on $RR = 1.60$ and 2.45

The quadratic equation method for estimating confidence limits on relative risk requires that the individual risks be small. This is clearly not the case for Table 3-11 data. Recognizing that the quadratic equation method is not suitable for these data, we still use it to see what discrepancy results.

with $95 + 173 = 268$ events, $p = 95/268 = .3545$

$P_L = .3545 - 1.96[P_L(1 - P_L)/268]^{1/2}$

$271.84(P_L)^2 - 193.85P_L + 33.69 = 0$

$$P_L = \frac{193.85 \pm [37,577.82 - (4)(271.84)(33.69)]^{1/2}}{543.68}$$

$$P_L = \frac{193.85 \pm 30.74}{543.68} = .3000, .4131 = .3000$$

$P_U = .4131$

$RR_L = (.3000/.7000)(1067/296) = 1.54$

$RR_U = (.4131/.5869)(1067/296) = 2.54$

These results are different, but not remarkably so, from the 1.60, 2.45 obtained with Katz's method. Because the data do not fit the require-

Table 3-12. Total Cancer Deaths According to Smoking History

Smoking category[a]	Cancer deaths during 18 years		
	Yes	No	Total
Smoker	40	593	633
Nonsmoker	39	733	772
Total	79	1326	1405

[a] Smoking history was unknown for one person.

ments for the quadratic equation approach, we prefer the .95 limits obtained with Katz's method (Equation 3-14).

The estimated odds of disease and .95 confidence limits on the odds ratio, for those with SBP ≥ 165 compared to those with SBP < 165, are

$$\widehat{OR} = \frac{(95)(894)}{(173)(201)} = 2.4424$$

$$\ln \widehat{OR} = .8930$$

$$\text{var}(\ln OR) = [(1/95) + (1/201) + (1/173) + (1/894)] = .0224$$

$$1.96 \, \text{SE}(\ln OR) = 1.96(.0224)^{1/2} = .2933$$

$$\ln OR \pm 1.96 \, \text{SE}(\ln OR) = .8930 \pm .2933 = .5997, \, 1.1863$$

$$.95 \text{ confidence limits on } OR = 1.82 \text{ and } 3.27$$

In the above example, the $\widehat{OR}$ (2.44) was somewhat larger than the $\widehat{RR}$ (1.98). We are not surprised since in this population incidence of CHD over an 18-year period is unfortunately not a rare event (about 20%). OR will be very close to RR only for rare events. During this 18-year period, death from all forms of cancer was a rare event (under 6%); the relevant data are summarized in Table 3-12.

From Table 3-12 we get

$$\widehat{RR} = (40/633)/(39/772) = 1.25$$

$$\widehat{OR} = (40)(733)/(593)(39) = 1.27$$

thus for cancer mortality with a risk of 6.3% for smokers and 5.1% for nonsmokers, the agreement between OR and RR is very good.

One last point. As most statistical analyses are now carried out on computers it is important to check whether the computer is doing what you think it is doing. Compare the total counts from basic tables with totals from more complicated tabulations and, whenever possible, do a few calculations by hand to verify computer operations.

EXERCISES

Ex. 3-1. The Appendix data associating serum cholesterol level of 260 mg/100 ml with 18-year incidence of coronary heart disease are as follows:

Cholesterol level	New case of CHD		Total at risk
	Yes	No	
≥ 260	91	295	386
< 260	177	800	977
Total	268	1095	1363

Use these data to:

a. Calculate the relative risk of acquiring CHD, comparing those with serum cholesterol of 260 or greater to those with levels under 260.
b. Calculate .95 confidence limits on RR by solving the quadratic equations for P_L and P_U and converting the solutions to limits on RR.
c. Calculate .95 confidence limits on RR using the method of Katz et al.
d. Compare the results in (b) and (c) above. Which would you prefer for these data? Why?

Ex. 3-2. If we add the prevalence cases to the data shown in Exercise 3-1, we have:

Serum cholesterol level	Coronary disease first diagnosed			
	Exam 1	Exams 2–10	Not 1–10	Total
⩾260	11	91	295	397
<260	32	177	800	1009
Total	43	268	1095	1406

Repeat the calculations outlined in Exercise 3-1 using the prevalence data on examination 1. How is your estimate of the association between elevated cholesterol and coronary disease changed if based on incidence or prevalence data? Which is more meaningful? Why?

Ex. 3-3. For men aged 45–49 on examination 1, the following table summarizes Framingham Heart Study data relating serum cholesterol (in three classes) to the risk of developing diagnosable coronary heart disease within 18 years.

Serum cholesterol level	Coronary heart disease		
	Yes	No	Total
⩾260	10	26	36
220–259	11	68	79
<220	24	70	94
Total	45	164	209

a. Calculate estimates of OR and RR comparing ⩾260/<220 and 220–259/<220. To do this break up the table into separate 2×2 tables.

b. Calculate .90 confidence limits for the above *OR*'s using Woolf's method.

c. What is your interpretation of these data with respect to the cholesterol/CHD relationship among 45- to 49-year-old men?

Ex. 3-4.

a. Use the Appendix listing to determine the number of (i) CHD incidence cases and (ii) CHD negatives among men aged 60–62 with Framingham Relative Weight (FRW) of 120 or more. Use the Appendix summary tabulations in association with the listing to minimize the labor involved with regard to this or any other exercise that requires counting of Appendix data. Estimate the odds ratio and relative risk related to CHD incidence among 60- to 62-year-old men comparing $FRW \geq 120$ to $FRW < 120$.

b. Estimate the odds ratio and relative risk related to CHD incidence, comparing smokers and nonsmokers among men aged 50–54.

c. Estimate the odds ratio and relative risk related to mortality among men and women aged 60–62 comparing those with diastolic blood pressure of 90 or more to those with diastolic pressure of less than 90.

NOTES

* Some prefer the term *case-control studies*. We are satisfied with either term and use them interchangeably.

† For chronic diseases not characterized by cure, the annual incidence rate in a specified cohort is not identical to $1/k$th the k year rate. A small example may be helpful. If the annual incidence rate was .10 with a starting population at risk of 10 000, the expected number of new cases in each of the first three years would be $.10(10\,000) + .10(9000) + .10(8100) = 2710$. Thus the three-year incidence rate associated with an annual incidence rate of .10 is .271. If the risk is low, the annual incidence rate becomes very close to $1/k$th the k year rate. For the above population with an annual rate of .01, the expected number of cases in the first three years is $.01(10\,000) + .01(9900) + .01(9801) = 297$ for a 3-year rate of .0297. The relationship of incidence and prevalence rates in a closed cohort with stable rates is described by $(1 - P) - (1 - I)^t$ where P is the prevalence rate, I is the incidence rate per time period, and t is the number of time periods equivalent to the average duration of the disease.

4
Attributable Risk

If you "know" that activity A multiplies the risk of lung cancer by 10 and that activity B multiplies the risk of lung cancer by 20 (i.e., $\hat{RR}_A = 10$ and $\hat{RR}_B = 20$), is it correct to infer (assuming very narrow confidence limits on both RR_A and RR_B) that activity B has a greater effect on the public health than activity A? Assuming that a county health department has resources to reduce or eliminate one of these hazards but not both, is an attack on B potentially of greater benefit than one on A? Suppose A were cigarette smoking and B were uranium mining and 40 percent of the adults in the county smoke cigarettes but only .04 percent mine uranium. Although those who mine uranium are at very great relative risk, the effect of this high risk on the community is small because few individuals are exposed to the risk factor. Clearly the effect of a risk factor on community health is related to both relative risk and the percentage of population exposed to the factor.

In a general sense, attributable risk can be defined as the proportionate excess risk of disease that is associated with exposure to a risk factor. It is an epidemiologic concept combining relative risk and risk factor prevalence so as to reflect the fraction of all cases associated with the risk factor. Although there are a number of different formulas that have been used to define attributable risk, they fall into two general classes:

1. attributable risk in the exposed group, and
2. attributable risk in the total population.

As a first step in developing the formulas for attributable risk, the following terms are defined:

I_0 incidence rate among those not exposed to the risk factor

I_r incidence rate among those exposed to the risk factor
I_t incidence rate among the total population
RR relative risk I_r/I_0
P proportion of the population exposed to the risk factor
N size of the population

ATTRIBUTABLE RISK IN EXPOSED GROUP

There are very few instances when an exposure is both necessary and sufficient to cause a disease. As a result, exposure to a risk factor will account for only a fraction of the incidence rate in the exposed group. The incidence rate in the exposed group consists of two components.

Incidence rate not due to exposure (I_0)

                + Incidence rate due to exposure

                      = Incidence rate in exposed group (I_r)

Then if $I_r > I_0$ the excess incidence rate among those exposed to the risk factor, which is a definition of attributable risk (AR), is

$$AR = I_r - I_0 \qquad (4\text{-}1)$$

and the proportion of the incidence rate among those with the risk factor due to association with the risk factor, which is also a definition of attributable risk, is

$$AR = \frac{I_r - I_0}{I_r} \qquad (4\text{-}2)$$

Dividing the right-hand side numerator and denominator of this equation by I_0, we can express that proportion of the incidence rate *among those with the risk factor* "due to" association with the risk factor as

$$AR = \left(\frac{I_r}{I_0} - \frac{I_0}{I_0}\right) \bigg/ \frac{I_r}{I_0} = \frac{RR - 1}{RR} \qquad \text{provided } RR \geqslant 1 \qquad (4\text{-}3)$$

The incidence rate due to the risk factor *among those with the factor is* then

$$I_r \left(\frac{RR - 1}{RR}\right) \qquad \text{provided } RR \geqslant 1 \qquad (4\text{-}4)$$

The number of cases due to association with the risk factor is the term above multiplied by the number in the population having the risk factor

(*NP*):

$$NPI_r\left(\frac{RR-1}{RR}\right) \qquad \text{provided } RR \geqslant 1 \qquad (4\text{-}5)$$

where NPI_r is the total number of cases occurring among those with the risk factor.

ATTRIBUTABLE RISK IN THE TOTAL POPULATION

Using the results from Equation 4-5, attributable risk in the population is the number of cases due to association with the risk factor divided by total cases in the population (or the proportion of total cases due to the risk factor) as described in Equation 4-6

$$AR = \frac{NPI_r[(RR-1)/RR]}{NPI_r + N(1-P)I_0} \qquad \text{provided } RR \geqslant 1 \qquad (4\text{-}6)$$

where $N(1-P)I_0$ is the total number of cases occurring among those without the risk factor.

Dividing each term in Equation 4-6 by NI_0 and simplifying, we get an expression for attributable risk as originally reported by Levin [1953]:

$$AR = \frac{P(RR)[(RR-1)/RR]}{P(RR)+(1-P)} = \frac{P(RR-1)}{1+P(RR-1)} \qquad \text{provided } RR \geqslant 1$$

$$(4\text{-}7)$$

In actual practice we substitute $\hat{RR}$ and p for RR and P, respectively, and obtain Equation 4-8.

$$\hat{AR} = \frac{p(\hat{RR}-1)}{1+p(\hat{RR}-1)} \qquad \text{provided } \hat{RR} \geqslant 1 \qquad (4\text{-}8)$$

A formula for attributable risk in the population which is equivalent to Equation 4-8 was reported by Leviton [1973]. It is

$$\hat{AR} = \frac{\hat{I}_t - \hat{I}_0}{\hat{I}_t} \qquad (4\text{-}9)$$

When the relative risk (or odds ratio) is very high, it strongly suggests that the association so identified is real [Cornfield et al 1959] rather than something spurious derived from various confounding factors (Chapter 5). When the attributable risk is high (the range is from 0 to 1), the risk factor is of importance to the health of the community. Table 4-1 shows

Table 4-1. Association of Relative Risk and Population Attributable Risk for Coronary Heart Disease among Framingham Men Aged 35 to 44 on Initial Examination

Risk factor at initial examination	$\hat{RR}$ at 16-year follow-up[a]	Proportion of population studied with risk factor at initial examination (p)	$\hat{AR}$ using Equation 4-8	Comment
Systolic blood pressure ⩾180	2.8	.02	.03	Uncommon risk factors will rarely lead to a high $\hat{AR}$
Enlarged heart on X-ray	2.1	.10	.10	Compared to cigarette smoking, $\hat{RR}$ somewhat higher but $\hat{AR}$ much lower
Cigarette smoking	1.9	.72	.39	Lowest $\hat{RR}$ in table, but almost 40% of all coronary disease is associated with cigarettes

[a] Relative to those without the risk factor.
Source: Shurtleff 1970.

some examples of the relationship between *RR* and *AR* with respect to risk factors and coronary heart disease among Framingham men [Shurtleff 1970].

Although Equation 4-7 requires *RR* for its calculation, the odds ratio may be used as a substitute if the disease is rare in the population. Other terms that have been used for attributable risk in the total population are attributable fraction [Walter 1976], population attributable risk [Cole and MacMahon 1971], and aetiologic fraction [Miettinen 1974a].

ILLUSTRATIVE CALCULATIONS

Formulas for *AR* are most easily expressed in notation corresponding to the standard notation we have used for the 2×2 table and that we repeat in Table 4-2. Note that the symbols in Table 4-2 are not specific for prospective or retrospective studies. Thus, for a prospective study based on a sample of the general population in which "disease +" represents incident cases (and which is of sufficiently short duration that the dates on which cases occurred can be ignored), the proportion with the risk factor can usually be estimated by $(a + b)/t$. For retrospective studies in which "disease −" refers to controls representing the general population, the proportion with the risk factor can be estimated by $b/(b + d)$. Also, for

Table 4-2. Notation for Cross-Classification of Disease and Risk Factor

Risk factor	Disease		
	+	−	Total
+	a	b	$a + b$
−	c	d	$c + d$
Total	$a + c$	$b + d$	t

prospective data arranged as in Table 4-2, $\hat{RR}$ is derived from $a/(a + b) \div c/(c + d)$. For retrospective data, the relative risk would be estimated, when appropriate, by ad/bc, the odds ratio.

In Exposed Group

To illustrate the calculations, we shall use Equations 4-1, 4-2, 4-3, 4-8, and 4-9 in conjunction with data from a large prospective study of smoking and mortality [Kahn 1966] to estimate AR for lung cancer related to smoking cigarettes. the data are shown in Table 4-3.

The excess incidence rate among those exposed to the risk factor (using Equation 4-1) equals

$$\frac{1116}{701\,768} - \frac{426}{1\,015\,999} = .00159 - .00042 = .00117$$

The proportion of the incidence rate among those with the risk factor (using Equation 4-2) equals

$$\frac{.00117}{.00159} = .736$$

Table 4-3. Current Cigarette Smoking and Mortality among U.S. Veterans

Smoking category	Lung cancer mortality		Total population
	+	−	
Current cigarette smokers	1116 (a)	700 652 (b)	701 768 $(a + b)$
All others	426 (c)	1 015 573 (d)	1 015 999 $(c + d)$
Total	1542 $(a + c)$	1 716 225 $(b + d)$	1 717 767 (t)

Note: person-years of observation in the original report are considered here, and in the text, as if they were separate individuals.
Source: Kahn 1966.

Equation 4-3 is equivalent to Equation 4-2. To use equation 4-3 we first calculate $\hat{R}R$ from Table 4-3 as an estimate of RR. As these are prospective data, $\hat{R}R = (1116/701\,768)/(426/1\,015\,999) = 3.79$. The $\hat{R}R$ of 3.79 is much lower than usually quoted for the relationship between cigarette smoking and lung cancer. Most calculations of this $\hat{R}R$ relate the risk among current cigarette smokers to the risk among those who have never smoked. However, the present calculation relates the risk among current cigarette smokers, including light smokers, to the risk among all others, including ex-smokers, pipe smokers, and cigar smokers. AR (from Equation 4-3) $= (3.79 - 1)/3.79 = .736$, which is equal to the result from Equation 4-2.

In the Total Population

To calculate population attributable risk from Equation 4-8, we need RR and the proportion of the population exposed to the risk factor (p). RR as estimated above is 3.79 and p can be derived from Table 4-3 as

$$p = 701\,768/1\,717\,767 = 0.41$$

When the population is dichotomized, the $\hat{R}R$ refers to the ratio of risk among those with the factor to risk among those without it and the prevalance of the risk factor (p) refers to prevalence in the total population. When two population groups that do not encompass the entire population are contrasted, as, for example, those who are heavy cigarette smokers and those who have never smoked, the $\hat{R}R$ resulting from this more extreme comparison can be used in the formula for $A\hat{R}$, but the risk factor prevalence used with it must be that appropriate to just the two categories being considered. These calculations can be based on the Table 4-2 format if "risk factor $+$" and "risk factor $-$" define the restricted categories. The attributable risk resulting from a nonexhaustive two-category comparison should be understood as the fraction of *the cases in the two limited categories* associated with the high risk factor. For clarity, it is probably best not to aim at attributable risk in the total population when comparing two subcategories that together comprise less than the total. Instead estimate AR in the exposed group based on Equation 4-2 or 4-3 with I_r representing the exposed group (e.g., heavy smokers) and I_0 the reference group (e.g., nonsmokers).

In addition, if the reference category is one such as "never smoked," the cases attributed to smoking would have to be understood as cases in excess of the rate observed for those who had never smoked. Conceptually this excess could be completely eliminated only by converting the population to one that never smoked and not just to a population of ex-smokers.

Inserting the previously calculated values of $\hat{R}R$ and p into Equation

4-8 we get

$$\hat{AR} = \frac{.41(2.79)}{1 + .41(2.79)} = .53$$

Thus we estimate that 53 percent of the lung cancer that occurs in the population under consideration is associated with current cigarette smoking. Since this calculation derived from dichotomizing the complete population data, it is at least imaginable that, if the cigarette smoking–lung cancer association is causal, 53 percent of lung cancer mortality could be eliminated by converting the population from current cigarette smokers to ex-smokers or to pipe or cigar smokers.

Equation 4-9 is an alternative form of Equation 4-8 and produces the same numerical result.

$$\hat{AR} = \left(\frac{1542}{1\,717\,767} - \frac{426}{1\,015\,999} \right) \Big/ 1542/1\,717\,767 = .53$$

Caution: Because of the variety of ways in which attributable risk is expressed, be sure you understand how it has been calculated before using a published report on it. Furthermore, when reporting on attributable risk yourself, define it precisely.

VARIANCE OF POPULATION ATTRIBUTABLE RISK

Using the notation of Table 4-2, RR would be estimated as $[a/(a + b)]/[c/(c + d)]$ for a prospective study and as ad/bc for a case-control study of an uncommon disease. Thus, using the notation in Table 4-2, we require two separate formulas for vâr(AR) [Walter 1978]:

$$\text{vâr}(AR) \text{ for prospective data} = \frac{ct[ad(t - c) + bc^2]}{(a + c)^3(c + d)^3} \qquad (4\text{-}10)$$

$$\text{vâr}(AR) \text{ for retrospective data} = \left[\frac{c(b + d)}{d(a + c)} \right]^2 \left[\frac{a}{c(a + c)} + \frac{b}{d(b + d)} \right]$$

$$(4\text{-}11)$$

To calculate vâr (AR) for a prospective study, we substitute the data of Table 4-3 (which follows the format of Table 4-2) into Equation 4-10.

$$\text{vâr } AR = \frac{426(1\,717\,767)[1116(1\,015\,573)(1\,717\,767 - 426) + 700\,652(426)^2]}{(1116 + 426)^3(426 + 1\,015\,573)^3}$$

$$= .000\,370$$

$$\hat{SE}(AR) = (.000370)^{1/2} = .0192$$

$$1.96\,\hat{SE}(AR) = .038$$

Table 4-4. Retrospective Data Derived from Table 4-3

Smoking category	Lung cancer mortality		Total
	+	−	
Current cigarette smokers	1116 (a)	701 (b)	1817
All others	426 (c)	1016 (d)	1442
Total	1542 ($a + c$)	1717 ($b + d$)	3259

Thus on the basis of this large data set we calculate the 95 percent confidence limits on AR as $.53 \pm .04$, or $.49$ to $.57$.

To illustrate the use of the retrospective formula for vâr(AR), imagine that we have been able to identify all the lung cancer deaths in Table 4-3 as well as a perfectly representative one per 1000 sample of the rest as controls. These data, which are shown in Table 4-4, are essentially identical to the data of Table 4-3 except for the great reduction in the number of those not dying of lung cancer. The point of this illustration is to show how the variance of $\hat{AR}$ changes between prospective and retrospective studies with equivalent relationships. From Table 4-4

$$\hat{RR} \cong \hat{OR} = \frac{1116(1016)}{701(426)} = 3.80$$

$$p = \frac{701}{1717} = .41$$

$$\hat{AR} = \frac{p(\hat{RR} - 1)}{1 + p(\hat{RR} - 1)} = \frac{.41(2.80)}{1 + .41(2.80)} = .53$$

Using Equation 4-11,

$$\text{vâr}(AR) \text{ retrospective} = \left[\frac{426(1717)}{1016(1542)} \right]^2 \left[\frac{1116}{426(1542)} + \frac{701}{1016(1717)} \right]$$

$$= .000458$$

$$1.96 \sqrt{\text{vâr}(AR)} = 1.96(.0214) = .042$$

Although the retrospective variance is about 25 percent larger than the prospective variance, the relative difference in standard errors is only 11 percent. Thus using Tables 4-3 and 4-4 for basic data sources, our comparison is as follows:

	Prospective	Retrospective
$\hat{RR}$	3.79	3.80
p	.41	.41
$\hat{AR}$	.53	.53
95% CL on AR	.49 and .57	.49 and .57

The agreement indicates that the slightly wider confidence limits applicable to the very much smaller (although still quite large) sample size of the retrospective study are not detectable with two significant figures.

ALTERNATIVE FORMULATION OF POPULATION ATTRIBUTABLE RISK

The definition and measurement of attributable risk may be approached in a different way. Suppose 40 percent of all *cases* are in the high-risk category and the proportion of the high-risk incidence rate due to the risk factor, $(I_r - I_0)/I_r$, is 60 percent. Then .40(.60), or 24 percent, of all cases are attributable to the high-risk factor. More generally, using Equation 4-3 and the notation of Table 4-2, this formulation of $\hat{AR}$ can be expressed as

$$\hat{AR} = \left(\frac{a}{a+c}\right)\left(\frac{\hat{RR}-1}{\hat{RR}}\right) \qquad \text{provided } \hat{RR} \geq 1 \qquad (4\text{-}12)$$

Applying Equation 4-12 to Table 4-3 data we get

$$\hat{AR} = \frac{1116\,(2.79)}{1542\,(3.79)} = .53$$

as obtained previously using Equation 4-8.

Equation 4-12 can be recognized as the basis of Equation 4-13, which calculates attributable risk after adjustment for confounding factors by means of the standardized morbidity ratio (*SMR*), which will be explained in Chapter 5 [Miettinen 1974a]. The summation in Equation 4-13 is over each category of the confounding variable(s):

$$\hat{AR} = \sum_i \left(\frac{a_i}{a_i+c_i}\right)\left(\frac{\hat{SMR}_i-1}{\hat{SMR}_i}\right) \qquad \text{provided each } \hat{SMR}_i \geq 1 \quad (4\text{-}13)$$

A NOTE ON CAUSATION

Several times in our discussion we have referred to disease "due to" association with the risk factor. In fact, all the calculations of attributable risk summarize the proportion of disease *associated with* a risk factor. Whether the disease is caused by the risk factor must be determined on other criteria, as outlined in texts on epidemiology [Kelsey et al 1986, Lilienfeld and Lilienfeld 1980, MacMahon and Pugh 1970, Schlesselman 1982]. Direct experimentation to discover whether eliminating the risk factor eliminates the disease associated with it is usually difficult and expensive and is rarely undertaken. More commonly, indirect indicators are relied upon to suggest whether or not a change in risk factor level has resulted in a change in risk.

APPLICATION TO FRAMINGHAM HEART STUDY DATA

Using the data in Table 4-5, we can quantify the excess incidence of coronary heart disease associated with systolic blood pressure of 165 or higher.
In the notation of pages 72–3, this excess 18-year incidence rate is

$$I_r - I_0 = .321 - .162 = .159$$

The *proportion* of the total 18-year incidence rate in the *exposed group* that is associated with exposure is:

$$\frac{I_r - I_0}{I_r} = \frac{.321 - .162}{.321} = .495 = 49.5\%$$

or

$$\frac{RR - 1}{RR} = \frac{1.98 - 1}{1.98} = .495 = 49.5\%$$

We can also measure the 18-year incidence rate *in the total population* that is associated with exposure. This is

$$I_t - I_0 = .197 - .162 = .035$$

Expressed as a proportion of the total population incidence rate, the incidence rate in the total population that is associated with exposure has been called population attributable risk percentage. It is calculated as follows:

$$\frac{I_t - I_0}{I_t} = \frac{.197 - .162}{.197} = .178 = 17.8\%$$

Table 4-5. Development of CHD over 18 Years by Level of SBP

Systolic blood pressure (mm Hg)	Coronary disease		Number at risk	Risk	RR
	+	−			
⩾165	95	201	296	.321	1.98
<165	173	894	1067	.162	1.00
Total	268	1095	1363	.197	—

or

$$\frac{P(RR-1)}{1+P(RR-1)} = \frac{(296/1363)(1.98-1)}{1+(296/1363)(1.98-1)} = \frac{.217(.98)}{1+.217(.98)} = .175 = 17.5\%$$

The slight disagreement is due to rounding. An additional way of expressing the excess risk due to exposure is the *number* of cases attributable to blood pressure of 165 or more.

$$\frac{NPI_r(RR-1)}{RR} = \frac{1363\left(\frac{296}{1363}\right)\left(\frac{95}{296}\right)(1.98-1)}{1.98} \cong 47 \text{ cases}$$

We can summarize these last few computations by stating that in Framingham about 50 cases of coronary heart disease, which is half of the CHD incidence in the high-blood pressure group or about 18 percent of the CHD incidence in the total population, are "due to" systolic blood pressure of 165 or more. We have included alternative formulas using relative risk because retrospective studies do not provide estimates of incidence rates. Do not forget that the usual retrospective study provides estimates of the odds ratio, not the relative risk. Only if the disease is relatively rare in the population can the estimated odds ratio be used as an estimate of the relative risk.

The previous calculations of relative risk and attributable risk of coronary disease associated with elevated blood pressure have all used a single cutpoint, e.g., ≥ 165 compared to <165. Similar calculations are possible when blood pressure is divided into more than two groups. Table 4-6 presents such data with systolic blood pressure in six classes.

It seems reasonable to consider the persons with SBP < 140 as the nonexposed group. Relative risks for the other SBP groups are calculated by comparing their risk to the risk for those with SBP < 140. *Among*

Table 4-6. Eighteen-Year Incidence of Coronary Heart Disease by Systolic Blood Pressure Level

SBP (mm Hg)	Coronary disease				Relative risk
	At risk	+	−	Risk	
≥ 180	158	54	104	.342	2.65
170–179	98	31	67	.316	2.45
160–169	127	29	98	.228	1.77
150–159	181	39	142	.215	1.67
140–149	231	42	189	.182	1.41
<140	568	73	495	.129	1.00
Total	1363	268	1095	.197	—

those with SBP $\geqslant 180$, the proportion of the incidence rate "due to" blood pressure at that level is

$$\frac{I_r - I_0}{I_r} = \frac{.342 - .129}{.342} = .623 = 62.3\%$$

Among those with SBP of 140–149, the proportion of the incidence rate "due to" blood pressure at that level is

$$\frac{I_r - I_0}{I_r} = \frac{.182 - .129}{.182} = .291 = 29.1\%$$

EXERCISES

Ex. 4-1. Use the data in Table 3.1A (page 46) to answer the following questions.

a. What is the excess risk of stroke among cigarette smokers?
b. What percentage of the risk of stroke among cigarette smokers can be attributed to smoking?
c. What percentage of all strokes in the Honolulu Heart Study can be attributed to smoking?

Ex. 4-2. Use Tables 4-3 and 4-7 to answer the following questions about this population of insured war veterans. Use those who are not current cigarette smokers as the reference group.

a. Estimate the relative risk of CHD and lung cancer, respectively, associated with current cigarette smoking.
b. Estimate the excess mortality rate and the population attributable risk associated with cigarette smoking for CHD and for lung cancer.

Table 4-7. Current Cigarette Smoking and Mortality among U.S. Veterans

Smoking category	Coronary disease mortality		Total population[a]
	+	−	
Current cigarette smokers	6 395	695 373	701 768
All others	7 908	1 008 091	1 015 999
Total	14 303	1 703 464	1 717 767

[a] Person-years of observation in the original report are considered here, and in the text, as if they were separate individuals.
Source: Kahn 1966.

c. Estimate the excess number of deaths from CHD and from lung cancer associated with current cigarette smoking

d. Use the above results to comment on CHD and lung cancer as public health problems.

Ex. 4-3. Use Table 4-8 to answer the following:

a. Estimate the relative risk for CHD and for lung cancer comparing all current cigarette smokers to those who have never smoked. Compare these results to the relative risks estimated from Tables 4-3 and 4-7 and comment on any differences.

b. Comparing those who smoke more than 39 cigarettes/day to those who have never smoked, compute the excess mortality rate, for lung cancer and CHD, as a proportion of the exposed rate.

c. Using never smoked as the reference category, estimate the annual excess number of deaths at age 65–74 for each of the smoking categories in this population. Which smoking category is the greatest public health problem and why?

Ex. 4-4.

a. Compute the excess 18-year risk of coronary disease for each of the following systolic blood pressure categories, using the data in Table 4-6, with SBP < 140 defined as the nonexposed group: (i) $\geqslant 180$, (ii) 170–179, (iii) 160–169, (iv) 150–159, and (v) 140–149.

b. Express the excess 18-year risk in each of the exposed groups as a proportion of the total risk in that group.

c. How does excess risk vary with systolic blood pressure level?

Table 4-8. Current Cigarette Smoking and Mortality among U.S. Veterans Aged 65–74

	Annual risk of death per 100,000		Total population[a]
Smoking category	Lung cancer	CHD	
Current cigarette smokers			
Total	281	1559	207 895
>39/day	606	1955	8 937
21–39/day	447	1701	50 045
10–20/day	256	1577	101 731
<10/day	132	1374	37 130
Never smoked or			
occasional only	30	1015	171 211

[a] Person-years of observation in the original report are considered here, and in the text, as if they were separate individuals.
Source: Kahn 1966.

5
Adjustment of Data Without Use of Multivariate Models

Often, in analyzing epidemiologic data, the investigator wishes to adjust for the effect of some variable so that the effect of other variables can be seen more clearly. Consider the simple example of an investigation to determine whether or not gray hair is related to mortality risk. The following two facts stand out:

1. Those with gray hair have a higher death rate than others.
2. Those with gray hair are older than others.

Because of fact 2, the interpretation of fact 1 is unclear. The possible association of gray hair with mortality risk is entangled with the effect of age on mortality risk. Methods for adjusting data to overcome this entanglement are among the common tools used by epidemiologists. The purpose of data adjustment is to disentangle the relationship so that we can evaluate a variable's effect free from confusion and distortion. For the gray hair investigation, adjustment would permit us to determine whether *persons of the same age* who have or do not have gray hair have different mortality risks.

CONFOUNDING

Variables whose effect is entangled with the effect of other variables are known as *confounders,* and it is for such variables that data adjustment is needed. In order for a variable to be a confounder, it must be related to the disease or condition of interest *and* to the risk factor being investigated [Miettinen 1970]. Stated more exactly, it must be related to the disease or condition of interest *and* to the risk factor being

investigated after adjustment for all other risk factors under consideration [Fisher and Patil 1974]. However, if the potential confounding
variable is truly related *only to the disease of interest,* it may still be
desirable to adjust for it [Mantel and Haenszel 1959, Mantel 1986]. There
are two reasons why this is so.

1. The adjustment may reduce the sampling variance of the comparison
   being investigated.
2. Under admittedly unlikely conditions, the crude estimate of the odds
   ratios (OR) can be severely biased even though the potential
   confounder is unrelated to the risk factor (RF) being studied.
   Consider the following data [Mantel 1988].

	Cases	Noncases	Total	OR	Risk difference
Stratum 1					
RF$^+$	10	90	100		
RF$^-$	5	95	100	2.11	.05
Stratum 2					
RF$^+$	95	5	100		
RF$^-$	90	10	100	2.11	.05
Total					
RF$^+$	105	95	200		
RF$^-$	95	105	200	1.22	.05

The stratifying variable (i.e., potential confounder) is unrelated to the
risk factor. This is evident from the identical distribution of risk factor
positives and risk factor negatives within each stratum. Also evident is
the unsatisfactory estimate of the odds ratio derived from the total data
without adjustment. This compares poorly to adjusted estimates that are
obtainable from weighting the stratum-specific data. Finally, note that the
unadjusted *risk difference* is unbiased. For this latter statistic to be
biased, potential confounders must be related to *both* the disease and risk
factor being studied.

The foregoing illustration of a confounding variable related only to the
disease and not to the risk factor uses unreal data. For all practical
purposes, we stand by the usual definition of confounder as a variable
related to both disease and risk factor. However, the artificial example
presented here provides one more demonstration that "all generalizations
(including this one) are false." Nevertheless, there may be a benefit in
adjusting for variables that are substantially related to disease only and
you should not think it wrong to do so.

A very common application of adjustment to remove confounding, and
the one we will use to begin our illustration of this topic, is the age
adjustment of mortality rates. This permits comparison of mortality risk

for various groups free from the distortion introduced by one group having a different age distribution than another. Our first example of confounding uses vital statistics rates, wherein the condition of interest is the death rate and the risk factor to be evaluated is geographic area. When age is associated with area, i.e., the population of one area is much younger (or older) than another, the association of area with mortality risk is confounded by the association of age with mortality risk. If areas differ, as they probably do, in the proportion of the population reading two or more books a year, adjustment of mortality rates to eliminate confounding with this literary variable is unnecessary since reading is (presumably) not related to mortality risk.

We shall discuss two types of age adjustment in relation to mortality rates: direct adjustment and indirect adjustment. The following notation is for sample data and is applicable to both methods:

a	area a
b	area b
s	area chosen as a reference standard
n_{ia}	number of individuals in ith age class of area a
n_{ib}	number of individuals in ith age class of area b
n_{is}	number of individuals in ith age class of standard area
x_{ia}	number of deaths in ith age class of area a (similarly for b and s)
$p_{ia} = \dfrac{x_{ia}}{n_{ia}}$	death rate in ith age class of area a (similarly for b and s)

DIRECT ADJUSTMENT
Definition

The basic idea of direct adjustment, or direct standardization, is to suppose that both area a and area b have the age distribution of the standard area instead of the age distributions they actually have. Standardized rates are then calculated for each area, making use of the standard age distribution. These adjusted rates are then compared, and any difference between them can no longer be due to difference in age distribution because age has been taken into account.

The estimated mortality rates for areas a and b calculated by the direct method are

$$D\hat{S}R_a = \text{directly standardized mortality rate for area a}$$

$$= \frac{\sum\limits_i p_{ia} n_{is}}{\sum\limits_i n_{is}} \tag{5-1}$$

$$D\hat{S}R_b = \text{directly standarized mortality rate for area b}$$

$$= \frac{\sum_i p_{ib}n_{is}}{\sum_i n_{is}} \tag{5-2}$$

Since $\sum_i n_{is}$ is a constant, these equations can also be written in the form

$$D\hat{S}R_a = \sum_i p_{ia}\left(\frac{n_{is}}{\sum_i n_{is}}\right)$$

$$D\hat{S}R_b = \sum_i p_{ib}\left(\frac{n_{is}}{\sum_i n_{is}}\right) \tag{5-3}$$

Thus in each area the age-specific mortality rate for the ith age group has been multiplied by $\left(n_{is}/\sum_i n_{is}\right)$ and the product then summed over all ages. This is equivalent to obtaining a weighted combination of the age-specific mortality rates using *exactly the same weighting factors* in each area.

Choice of Standard Population

If a different standard population had been chosen, a different weighting of age-specific rates would have resulted. Much has been written about the choice of standard populations, emphasizing that in extreme cases the choice of different standard populations can lead to different results. It is even possible that with one standard population the standardized mortality rate for area a will be larger than for area b and with another standard population the standardized mortality rate for b will be larger than for a. The following factors should be considered in choosing a standard population:

1. Select a population that is relevant to the data.
2. Within wide ranges of choice, the population chosen as a standard usually does not make much difference.
3. Understand fully what you are doing in calculating directly standardized rates. If the age-specific rates for area a are greater than for area b at young ages and the opposite is true at older ages, a population giving more weight to younger than to older ages will result in the directly standardized rate for area a exceeding that for area b. A

population giving more weight to older than to younger ages will have the opposite result. Obviously the combining of age-specific data into a standardized overall rate is a convenience. However, do not forget that the age-specific data are the "facts" and that their combination into a weighted average, although often useful, is simply an attempt to summarize these facts into one index.

Since the choice of a particular standard population is somewhat arbitrary, we suggest considering, when two areas are to be standardized, a standard population that relates to the variance of the difference between standardized rates for areas a and b. For each age-specific comparison $p_{ia} - p_{ib}$, the variance of the difference under the null hypothesis is proportional to

$$\frac{1}{n_{ia}} + \frac{1}{n_{ib}}$$

By using the *inverse* of this quantity,

$$\frac{1}{(1/n_{ia}) + (1/n_{ib})} = \frac{n_{ia}n_{ib}}{n_{ia} + n_{ib}}$$

as a population size or weighting factor for the ith age class, we tend to give more weight to age-specific comparisons with small sampling variance and less weight to age-specific comparisons with large sampling variance.

Some common alternative choices for a standard population include total population of the groups to be compared, the population of one of the groups in the comparison, a large population (such as that of the United States), and weighting factors inversely proportional to the variance of the difference between areas. The last is useful when only two groups are being compared. If several groups are being standardized, the variance of the difference between p_{ia} and p_{ib} relates to n_{ia} and n_{ib} and the variance of the difference between p_{ia} and p_{ic} necessarily involves n_{ia} and n_{ic}. Thus weighting factors inversely proportional to the variance of the difference will vary depending on the specific groups being compared, and such factors become impractical for direct standardization of more than two areas.

Illustrative Computation

To illustrate direct standardization methods with a specific example, we use the data in Tables 5-1 and 5-2 on 1970 mortality rates in California and Maine [U.S. Bureau of the Census 1970, National Center for Health Statistics 1970] to compare mortality risk in these two states. In what

Table 5-1. 1970 Mortality Data to Illustrate Direct and Indirect Adjustment

Age (i)	United States (standard population s)		California (a)		Maine (b)	
	Pop. in thousands $(n_{is}/1000)$	Number of deaths (x_{is})	Pop. in thousands $(n_{ia}/1000)$	Number of deaths (x_{ia})	Pop. in thousands $(n_{ib}/1000)$	Number of deaths (x_{ib})
<15	57 900	103 062	5 524	8 751	286	535
15–24	35 441	45 261	3 558	4 747	168	192
25–34	24 907	39 193	2 677	4 036	110	152
35–44	23 088	72 617	2 359	6 701	109	313
45–54	23 220	169 517	2 330	15 675	110	759
55–64	18 590	308 373	1 704	26 276	94	1 622
65–74	12 436	445 531	1 105	36 259	69	2 690
75+	7 630	736 758	696	63 840	46	4 788
Total (excluding unknown ages)	203 212	1920 312	19 953	166 285	992	11 051

Sources: U.S. Bureau of the Census 1970 and National Center for Health Statistics 1970.

follows, we shall use the symbol w_i to represent $n_{is}\Big/\sum_i n_{is}$ or any alternative form of the standard population in the ith age class.

In Table 5-2 the standard weighting factors based on the United States population are calculated as the proportion that each age class in the standard is to the total, e.g., for under age 15, $w_{<15} = 57\,900/203\,212 = .285$. The standard weighting factors that are inversely proportional to the variance of the difference between p_{ia} and p_{ib} are the product of n_{ia} and n_{ib} divided by their sum. For example, for age <15,

$$w_{<15} = \frac{5\,524\,000(286\,000)}{5\,524\,000 + 286\,000} \cong 272\,000$$

Note that in this instance we use the full sample size in each state rather than $n_i/1000$. For directly standardized weighting factors, it was immaterial. Dividing numerator and denominator by 1000 does not affect w_i. For "inverse variance" weighting factors, however, using the actual sample size rather than the sample size in thousands does affect w_i. It increases it 1000-fold. Multiplying each w_i by 1000 does not affect $D\hat{S}R$, but it does affect vâr(DSR). Perhaps the first thing to note in Table 5-2 is that, without adjustment for age, the mortality rate for Maine is higher than for California:

Crude rate per 1000 for California (a)	8.3
Crude rate per 1000 for Maine (b)	11.1
Relative risk (Maine/California)	11.1/8.3 = 1.34

Table 5-2. Summary Statistics Derived from Table 5-1

Age (i)	Weights for direct standardization		Age-specific rate[a]			Under the null hypothesis	
	Based on standard population $\left(w_i = \dfrac{n_{is}}{\sum_i n_{is}}\right)$	Inversely proportional to variance of $p_{ia} - p_{ib}$ $\left[w_i = \dfrac{1}{(1/n_{ia} + 1/n_{ib})} = \dfrac{n_{ia}n_{ib}}{n_{ia} + n_{ib}}\right]$	U.S. (p_{is})	California (p_{ia})	Maine (p_{ib})	Pooled rate for Maine and California[a] $\left(p_i = \dfrac{n_{ia}p_{ia} + n_{ib}p_{ib}}{n_{ia} + n_{ib}}\right)$	Estimated variance within age classes[a] (p_iq_i)
<15	.285	272 000	1.8	1.6	1.9	1.6	.0016
15–24	.174	160 000	1.3	1.3	1.1	1.3	.0013
25–34	.123	106 000	1.6	1.5	1.4	1.5	.0015
35–44	.114	104 000	3.1	2.8	2.9	2.8	.0028
45–54	.114	105 000	7.3	6.7	6.9	6.7	.0067
55–64	.091	89 000	16.6	15.4	17.3	15.5	.0153
65–74	.061	65 000	35.8	32.8	39.0	33.2	.0321
75+	.038	43 000	96.6	91.7	104.1	92.5	.0839
Total	1.000	944 000	—	—	—	—	—
Crude rates	—	—	9.4	8.3	11.1	—	—

[a] All rates are per 1000 population.

Direct adjustment (as in Equation 5-3) using the United States population for standard weighting factors results in

$$D\hat{S}R_a = 8.8 \text{ per } 1000 \text{ (using standard population weighting factors)}$$

$$D\hat{S}R_b = 9.9 \text{ per } 1000 \text{ (using standard population weighting factors)}$$

Note that removing the confounding effect of age reduces the relative risk (Maine/California) from 1.34 to $9.9/88 = 1.12$.

If instead of using standard population weighting factors in Equation 5-3 we use factors inversely proportional to the variance of $p_{ia} - p_{ib}$, we would have

$$D\hat{S}R_a = 9.8 \text{ per } 1000 \text{ (using weighting factors inversely proportional}$$
$$\text{to variance)}$$

$$D\hat{S}R_b = 11.0 \text{ per } 1000 \text{ (using weighting factors inversely proportional}$$
$$\text{to variance)}$$

With these weighting factors, the relative risk (Maine/California) is $11.0/9.8 = 1.12$, unchanged from that obtained using the standard population as a source of constant weighting factors. It is interesting to observe that, when the different standards are used, the adjusted rates do differ but their ratio remains the same. Of course, a mortality rate that has been standardized by the direct method is not meaningful by itself; it has meaning only when compared with another mortality rate that has been similarly standardized.

Variance of the Difference Between Rates

We begin by recalling three rules related to the calculation of variances (Equations 1-9, 1-10, and 1-17):

1. The variance of the difference between independent variables is the sum of their variances: $\text{var}(x - y) = \text{var}(x) + \text{var}(y)$.
2. The variance of a variable multiplied by a constant is the variance of the variable multiplied by the constant squared: $\text{var}(Kx) = K^2 \text{var}(x)$.
3. The estimated variances of p_{ia} and p_{ib} are $p_i q_i / n_{ia}$ and $p_i q_i / n_{ib}$, respectively, where p_i is the estimate of the parameter under the null hypothesis and is computed as the weighted average of p_{ia} and p_{ib}:

$$p_i = \frac{n_{ia} p_{ia} + n_{ib} p_{ib}}{n_{ia} + n_{ib}}$$

We shall use these rules to calculate the variance of the difference between two directly standardized rates.

We want $\hat{var}(DSR_a - DSR_b)$, which, using Equation 5-2, can be written

$$\hat{var}\left(\frac{\sum\limits_i p_{ia}w_i}{\sum\limits_i w_i} - \frac{\sum\limits_i p_{ib}w_i}{\sum\limits_i w_i}\right)$$

with each term divided by $\sum w_i$ to cover instances wherein $\sum w_i \neq 1$. Applying Equations 1-9, 1-10, and 1-17,

$$\hat{var}(DSR_a - DSR_b) = \frac{\sum\limits_i p_i q_i w_i^2}{\left(\sum\limits_i w_i\right)^2 n_{ia}} + \frac{\sum\limits_i p_i q_i w_i^2}{\left(\sum\limits_i w_i\right)^2 n_{ib}}$$

which can be written

$$\hat{var}(DSR_a - DSR_b) = \frac{\sum\limits_i p_i q_i w_i^2}{\left(\sum\limits_i w_i\right)^2}\left(\frac{1}{n_{ia}} + \frac{1}{n_{ib}}\right) \qquad (5\text{-}4)$$

If we are using weighting factors inversely proportional to the variance of $p_{ia} - p_{ib}$, however, then

$$\frac{1}{n_{ia}} + \frac{1}{n_{ib}} = \frac{1}{w_i}$$

and

$$\hat{var}(DSR_a - DSR_b) = \frac{\sum\limits_i p_i q_i w_i^2}{\left(\sum\limits_i w_i\right)^2}\left(\frac{1}{w_i}\right)$$

so that

$$\hat{var}(DSR_a - DSR_b) = \frac{\sum\limits_i p_i q_i w_i}{\left(\sum\limits_i w_i\right)^2} \qquad (5\text{-}5)$$

If inverse variance weighting factors are not used, then the simplification embodied in Equation 5-5 does not apply. Whatever the choice of weighting factors the variance of the difference between directly standardized rates can be estimated by Equation 5-4.

Using Equation 5-4 for the variance of the difference between the adjusted rates for California and Maine based on *standard* population weighting factors we have

$$\text{vâr}(DSR_a - DSR_b) = \frac{\sum_i p_i q_i w_i^2}{\left(\sum_i w_i\right)^2}\left(\frac{1}{n_{ia}} + \frac{1}{n_{ib}}\right)$$

If $\sum_i w_i = 1$, this becomes

$$\sum_i p_i q_i w_i^2 \left(\frac{1}{n_{ia}} + \frac{1}{n_{ib}}\right)$$

Substituting Table 5-2 data beginning with age class under 15 and age class 15 to 24 leads to

$$.0016(.285)^2\left(\frac{1}{272\,000}\right) + .0013(.174)^2\left(\frac{1}{160\,000}\right) + \cdots$$

Note: in Table 5-2, the column "Weights inversely proportional to variance . . . " shows

$$\frac{1}{(1/n_{ia}) + (1/n_{ib})}$$

The reciprocal of that quantity provides $(1/n_{ia}) + (1/n_{ib})$, as wanted for Equation 5-4.

Completing this summation over all age classes leads to

$$\text{vâr}(DSR_a - DSR_b) = .000000008196$$
$$\text{SÊ}(DSR_a - DSR_b) = .000091$$

(for standard population weighting factors). Remember that $D\hat{S}R$ values have been written as "per thousand," thus a $D\hat{S}R_a$ value of 8.8/1000 actually equals .0088 and a $D\hat{S}R_b$ value of 9.9/1000 = .0099. Their difference, $.0088 - .0099 = -.0011$, when divided by the standard error of the difference, which is .000091, permits a test of the null hypothesis that this difference is simply a chance departure from zero. For this test we use

$$z = \frac{\text{difference} - \text{expected value of difference under } H_0}{\text{SÊ of difference}} = \frac{-.0011 - 0}{.000091}$$

$$= -12$$

This z value is far beyond the limits of chance fluctuation and suggests a differential mortality risk between Maine and California, apart from any differences in age structure of the two populations.

Using Equation 5-5 to calculate the variance of the difference between California and Maine adjusted rates based on weighting factors inversely proportional to the variance of $p_{ia} - p_{ib}$, we have

$$\text{vâr}(DSR_a - DSR_b) = \sum_i p_i q_i w_i \bigg/ \left(\sum_i w_i\right)^2 = [.0016(272\,000)$$

$$+ .0013(160\,000) + \ldots]/(944\,000)^2$$

$$\text{vâr}(DSR_a - DSR_b) = 000000009934$$

$$\hat{\text{SE}}(DSR_a - DSR_b) = .000100$$

Again shifting from rate per 1000 to straight proportions, $DSR_a - DSR_b$ for inverse variance weighting factors is $.0098 - .0110 = -.0012$ and the test of the null hypothesis that both areas have the same risk with observed differences simply due to chance fluctuation is

$$z = \frac{-.0012 - 0}{.000100} = -12$$

as before. Thus, both sets of weighting factors lead to the same conclusion: Maine has a higher mortality risk than California, after adjusting for age.

It should be noted that large data sets such as these almost always show significant differences. Keep in mind that *significance* (which is equivalent to *unusualness*) depends on the difference in relation to its standard error and that the latter depends on *sample size*. For very large samples, even the most trivial differences will be statistically significant.

INDIRECT ADJUSTMENT
Definition

Sometimes direct adjustment, or standardization, cannot be carried out because the age-specific rates in the groups to be standardized are not available or, in at least some age classes, are based on such small numbers as to be completely unreliable. Indirect standardization does not require area age-specific rates but does require

1. Age distribution of each group to be standardized
2. Total deaths in each group to be standardized
3. Age-specific rates for a standard population

The indirect method uses items 1 and 3 to calculate how many deaths would be expected in each group if the age-specific rates of the standard population were applicable. This expectation is then compared with the actual number of deaths in the group. This observed/expected ratio is a relative, indirect, age-adjusted rate and is (often multiplied by 100) frequently referred to as a standardized mortality ratio (SMR). By using the notation defined at the beginning of this chapter, we shall see how SMR is related to the indirectly standardized rate (ISR):

$$\frac{\sum_i p_{is} n_{ia}}{\sum_i n_{ia}} = \begin{array}{l}\text{crude rate in area a if age-specific rates of the} \\ \text{standard population are applied}\end{array}$$

$$\frac{\sum_i p_{is} n_{is}}{\sum_i n_{is}} = \text{crude rate in standard population}$$

The ratio of the crude rate in the standard population to the crude rate in area a if age-specific rates of the standard population are applied is

$$\frac{\sum_i p_{is} n_{is}}{\sum_i n_{is}} \left(\frac{\sum_i n_{ia}}{\sum_i p_{is} n_{ia}} \right) = \text{standardizing factor}$$

Note how this standardizing factor, which varies from group to group only because of differences in age distribution, adjusts for differences in age distribution. If the population of area a is very much older than the standard population, so that using *the same age-specific rates* as the standard the crude rate for area a is double the crude rate for the standard, than the standardizing factor will be $\frac{1}{2}$. Similarly, if the population of area a is much younger than the standard, so that using *same age-specific rates* as the standard the crude rate for area a is one-half that for the standard, then the standardizing factor will be 2. Thus the age distribution is evaluated in relation to the standard, and the standardizing factor increases the crude rate for an area with a population younger than the standard and decreases it for an area with a population older than the standard. The indirect age-adjusted rate is finally the crude rate to be standardized multiplied by the standarizing factor.

$$\text{crude rate} \times \text{standardizing factor}$$

$$\begin{array}{l}\text{Indirect} \\ \text{standardized} = \\ \text{rate} (I\hat{S}R_a)\end{array} \left(\frac{\sum_i p_{ia} n_{ia}}{\sum_i n_{ia}} \right) \left(\frac{\sum_i p_{is} n_{is}}{\sum_i n_{is}} \times \frac{\sum_i n_{ia}}{\sum_i p_{is} n_{ia}} \right) \qquad (5\text{-}6)$$

Note that the crude rate for area a has been written in Equation 5-6 as if we had individual age-specific rates, p_{ia}. In fact, we often do not. It is the sum of all $p_{ia}n_{ia}$, i.e., the total number of deaths, that we must know.

By cancelling and rearranging terms, Equation 5-6 can be written in the form

$$I\hat{S}R_a = \left(\frac{\sum_i p_{ia}n_{ia}}{\sum_i p_{is}n_{ia}} \right)\left(\frac{\sum_i p_{is}n_{is}}{\sum_i n_{is}} \right)$$

$$= \frac{\text{observed cases in area a}}{\substack{\text{expected cases if standard} \\ \text{rates applied to population a}}} \cdot \substack{\text{crude rate in} \\ \text{standard area}} \qquad (5\text{-}7)$$

The ISR for area b is identical to that given in Equation 5-7 for area a except that p_{ib} and n_{ib} substitute for p_{ia} and n_{ia}, respectively:

$$I\hat{S}R_b = \left(\frac{\sum_i p_{ib}n_{ib}}{\sum_i p_{is}n_{ib}} \right)\left(\frac{\sum_i p_{is}n_{is}}{\sum_i n_{is}} \right), \qquad (5\text{-}8)$$

Comparing $I\hat{S}R_b$ and $I\hat{S}R_a$ in Equations 5-8 and 5-7, we can see that differences relate to the left factor only. In this factor, the numerator is the number of observed deaths in the area being considered and the denominator is the number of deaths expected in that area if standard rates applied. This term, by itself, is a frequently used statistic. It is called standard mortality (or morbidity) ratio, often abbreviated as SMR.

the standard rates are being combined according to the age,
a b in $I\hat{S}R_b$ and according to the age structure of area a in
direct age-adjusted rates for different areas do not all
weighting factors (as would be true for directly
ically incorrect to compare $I\hat{S}R_a$ with $I\hat{S}R_b$.
compared with $\sum_i p_{is}n_{ia}$ and $\sum_i p_{ib}n_{ib}$ can

because exactly the same set of

the comparison. Thus, each
the standard. Although,
pare indirectly adjusted
actical examples in which
error.
ed earlier, is the standardized
direct, age-standardized rate. To
ate, simply multiply by the crude

rate of the standard population. Recalling that $p_{ia}n_{ia} = x_{ia}$, we can rewrite Equation 5-7 in the form

$$I\hat{S}R_a = \left(\frac{\sum\limits_i x_{ia}}{\sum\limits_i p_{is}n_{ia}}\right)\left(\frac{\sum\limits_i p_{is}n_{is}}{\sum\limits_i n_{is}}\right) \tag{5-9}$$

Variance of Indirectly Adjusted Rates

To estimate the variance of $I\hat{S}R_a$ as shown in Equation 5-9, we shall consider x_{ia} as the only sampling variable since n_{ia} and n_{is} are fixed from sample to sample and p_{is}, which is used for standardization of several areas, can be presumed to be known exactly. Standard rates are frequently based on very large numbers so that even if it is incorrect to regard them as constant from sample to sample, the sampling error is generally very small relative to that for $p_{ia} = x_{ia}/n_{ia}$. Under these conditions, the variance of Equation 5-9 is

$$\text{var}(I\hat{S}R_a) = \frac{\sum\limits_i n_{ia}P_{ia}Q_{ia}}{\left(\sum\limits_i p_{is}n_{ia}\right)^2}\left(\frac{\sum\limits_i p_{is}n_{is}}{\sum\limits_i n_{is}}\right)^2 \tag{5-10}$$

When, as is usual, $p_{ia}q_{ia}$ is substituted for the unknown parameter $P_{ia}Q_{ia}$, we no longer have var$(I\hat{S}R_a)$, but an estimate of it:

$$\hat{\text{var}}(ISR_a) = \frac{\sum\limits_i n_{ia}p_{ia}q_{ia}}{\left(\sum\limits_i p_{is}n_{ia}\right)^2}\left(\frac{\sum\limits_i p_{is}n_{is}}{\sum\limits_i n_{is}}\right)^2 \tag{5-11}$$

Variance of Standardized Mortality Ratio (SMR)

The first term on the right-hand side of Equation 5-9 is $S\hat{M}R$, have referred to previously. Although it is a component of an standardized rate, it is also frequently used alone as a met adjustment. As can be seen from Equation 5-9, the $S\hat{M}R$ for ratio of the observed cases in the area divided by the exp the area if the specific rates from the standard populati Since ISR_a is identical to SMR_a except for a consta variances of ISR_a and SMR_a are also identical exc multiplier. Thus, the variance of SMR_a is exactly a omitting the constant multipler:

$$\left(\frac{\sum\limits_i p_{is} n_{is}}{\sum\limits_i n_{is}} \right)^2$$

which is the square of the crude rate in the standard population, and

$$\text{vâr}(SMR_a) = \frac{\sum\limits_i n_{ia} p_{ia} q_{ia}}{\left(\sum\limits_i p_{is} n_{ia} \right)^2} \qquad (5\text{-}12)$$

If the p_{ia} are small, as they often are, the q_{ia} will be close to unity and

$$\sum_i n_{ia} p_{ia} q_{ia} \cong \sum_i n_{ia} p_{ia}$$

In this event,

$$\text{vâr}(ISR_a) \simeq \frac{\sum\limits_i n_{ia} p_{ia}}{\left(\sum\limits_i p_{is} n_{ia} \right)^2} \left(\frac{\sum\limits_i p_{is} n_{is}}{\sum\limits_i n_{is}} \right)^2 \qquad (5\text{-}13)$$

and the estimated variance of SMR_a is approximately

$$\text{vâr}(SMR_a) \cong \frac{\sum\limits_i n_{ia} p_{ia}}{\left(\sum\limits_i p_{is} n_{ia} \right)^2}$$

This is exactly (observed deaths)/(expected deaths)^2, and since (observed deaths)/(expected deaths) = $S\hat{M}R$, the estimated variance of SMR when p_i are small is then

$$\text{vâr}(SMR) \cong \frac{S\hat{M}R}{E} \qquad (5\text{-}14)$$

$$\hat{SE}(SMR) \cong \sqrt{\frac{S\hat{M}R}{E}} \qquad (5\text{-}15)$$

where E is the number of expected deaths. You may also encounter $\hat{SE}(SMR)$ expressed in a different way:

$$\hat{SE}(SMR) \cong \frac{S\hat{M}R}{\sqrt{O}} \qquad (5\text{-}16)$$

where O is the number of observed deaths. At first glance Equation 5-16 seems to be in disagreement with Equation 5-15, but the exact equivalence of these two equations can be shown as follows. Recall that $SMR = O/E$; then

$$\frac{\sqrt{S\hat{M}R}}{\sqrt{E}} = \frac{\sqrt{O}/\sqrt{E}}{\sqrt{E}} \qquad (5\text{-}15')$$

$$= \frac{\sqrt{O}/\sqrt{E}}{\sqrt{E}} \left(\frac{\sqrt{O}/\sqrt{E}}{\sqrt{O}/\sqrt{E}}\right)$$

$$= \frac{O/E}{\sqrt{O}} = \frac{S\hat{M}R}{\sqrt{O}} \qquad (5\text{-}16')$$

Confidence Limits for Standardized Mortality Ratio (*SMR*)

The standard mortality or morbidity ratio (*SMR*) does not have a symmetrical distribution, ranging from 1 to 0 when indicating reduced risk and from 1 upward without limit when indicating increased risk. Thus, it may not be a normally distributed variable unless based on a large number of cases. When the expected number of cases is "large," perhaps 25 or more, using the standard error of *SMR* as if it applied to a normal distribution should not be seriously misleading. However, if the number of cases expected were 5 or less, the assumption that the normal approximation is valid may be completely unwarranted. When the number of expected cases is 6–24, be cautious and seek statistical advice.

Three methods for calculating confidence limits on *SMR* are illustrated for an *SMR* equal to 1.67 based on 19 observed and 11.36 expected events. All three presume that the observed number of events is from a Poisson distribution and that the expected number of events is not subject to sampling error. They are presented in decreasing order of accuracy.

1. Using a table of confidence limits for the Poisson parameter [Documenta Geigy 1970, Schoenberg 1983] we find that 19 observed cases is compatible (at .95 confidence) with a parameter as small as 11.44 and as large as 29.67. Dividing each of these by our expected number of 11.36, we get .95 limits on *SMR* of 1.01 and 2.61.
2. If such a table is not available, we will assume that the shape of the Poisson distribution is approximately normal but at the same time

make use of the following: (a) equality of the Poisson mean and variance and (b) the true sampling variance (rather than an estimate based on sample observations). These factors are represented in the equations below that relate the upper (λ_U) and lower (λ_L) .95 confidence limits for the Poisson parameter to the observed number of events.

$$19 + 1.96(\lambda_U)^{1/2} = \lambda_U$$
$$19 - 1.96(\lambda_L)^{1/2} = \lambda_L$$

where $19 =$ observed number of events and $\lambda_U = .95$ upper limit and $\lambda_L = .95$ lower limit on λ.

These equations state that with .95 confidence, the parameter λ will not be larger than the observed number plus 1.96 standard errors of the sampling distribution of observed events nor will λ be smaller than the observed number less 1.96 standard errors of the sampling distribution of observed events. Recognizing that the above are quadratic equations in $\lambda^{1/2}$ and putting them in the standard form $ax^2 + bx + c = 0$, we have

$$\lambda_U - 1.96(\lambda_U)^{1/2} - 19 = 0$$

where $a = 1$, $b = -1.96$, and $c = -19$, then

$$(\lambda_U)^{1/2} = [-b \pm (b^2 - 4ac)^{1/2}]/2a = \{1.96 \pm [3.84 - (4)(1)(-19)]^{1/2}\}/2$$
$$= [1.96 \pm 8.94]/2 = -3.49, 5.45$$
$$\lambda_U = 12.18, 29.70$$

Solving the equation in λ_L results in an identical solution to that for λ_U so that $\lambda_L = 12.18$ and $\lambda_U = 29.70$. Dividing each of these by the fixed expected number of events we get .95 limits on *SMR* of 1.07 and 2.61 close to those obtained with Poisson tables.

3. Instead of using the known equivalence of the Poisson mean and variance, and the true sampling variance we could let the mean and variance of the sampling distribution be independent. In addition we could estimate the sampling variance based on sample data as in Equation 5-15. Taken together with the assumption that sample values of *SMR* are normally distributed, this leads to the following equations and estimated confidence limits of .92 and 2.42.

$$SMR + 1.96(SMR/E)^{1/2} = SMR_U = 1.67 + 1.96(.383) = 2.42$$
$$SMR - 1.96(SMR/E)^{1/2} = SMR_L = 1.67 - 1.96(.383) = 0.92$$

Method 3, which relies on assumed normality and estimated variances, would perform better with larger numbers. If the *SMR* had been calculated from 190/113.6, exactly 10 times the numbers used up to this point, confidence limits using method 3 would be

$$1.67 + 1.96(1.67/113.6)^{1/2} = 1.91$$
$$1.67 - 1.96(1.67/113.6)^{1/2} = 1.43$$

For these same numbers (190 and 113.6) the .95 limits on *SMR* obtained from the Poisson tables are 1.93 and 1.44. Almost always estimates based on the normality assumption are more correct when based on larger numbers.

Illustrative Computation

We shall use Tables 5-1 and 5-2 data to illustrate how to calculate Maine and California rates adjusted for age by the indirect method. Remember that for indirect adjustment it is not strictly correct to compare the Maine rate with the California rate. However, each can be properly compared to the standard population. Using Equation 5-9 and United States rates for a standard,

$$I\hat{S}R_a = \left(\frac{\sum_i x_{ia}}{\sum_i p_{is}n_{ia}}\right)\left(\frac{\sum_i p_{is}n_{is}}{\sum_i n_{is}}\right)$$

$$= \frac{166\ 285}{.0018(5\ 524\ 000) + \ldots + .0966(696\ 000)}(.0094)$$

$$= \frac{166\ 285}{178\ 253}(.0094) = .0088$$

Similarly

$$I\hat{S}R_b = \frac{11\ 051}{10\ 524}(.0094) = .0099$$

After indirect adjustment, the California and Maine rates are identical to the rates obtained by direct adjustment using the United States population as a standard. Of course, this will not always be true, but differences will usually be slight. Using Equation 5-11,

$$\text{vâr}(ISR_a) = \frac{5\ 524\ 000(.0016)(.9984) + \cdots + 696\ 000(.0917)(.9083)}{(178\ 253)^2}(.0094)^2$$

$$= \frac{158\ 410}{(178\ 253)^2}(.0094)^2 = .000000000441$$

$$\hat{SE}(ISR_a) = .000021$$

$$\hat{var}(ISR_b) = \frac{286\,000(.0019)(.9981) + \cdots + 46\,000(.1041)(.8959)}{(10\,524)^2}(.0094)^2$$

$$= \frac{10\,424}{(10\,524)^2}(.0094)^2 = .000000008316$$

$$\hat{SE}(ISR_b) = .000091$$

Using the approximation in Equation 5-13 dependent on small p_{ia} and p_{ib},

$$\hat{var}(ISR_a) \cong \frac{\sum_i x_{ia}}{\left(\sum_i p_{is} n_{ia}\right)^2}\left(\frac{\sum_i p_{is} n_{is}}{\sum_i n_{is}}\right)$$

$$= \frac{166\,285}{(178\,253)^2}(.0094)^2 = .000000000462$$

$$\hat{SE}(ISR_a) = .000022$$

$$\hat{var}(ISR_b) \cong \frac{11\,051}{(10\,524)^2}(.0094)^2 = .000000008816$$

$$\hat{SE}(ISR_b) \cong .000094$$

We compare below the standard errors of the indirectly adjusted mortality rates computed by Equations 5-11 and 5-13:

	$\hat{SE}(ISR_a)$	$\hat{SE}(ISR_b)$
Equation 5-11	.000021	.000091
Equation 5-13	.000022	.000094

Note how close the computed standard errors derived from the low p value approximation (Equation 5-13) are to the more accurate estimates (Equation 5-11). This excellent agreement is due to the small p values in our example.

This completes our calculation of indirectly adjusted rates and their standard error based on data in Tables 5-1 and 5-2. The SMR is an element of the indirectly standardized rate, and we now compute these ratios and their standard error. Using the first term in Equations 5-7 and

5-8, we get

$$S\hat{M}R_a = \frac{\sum_i p_{ia}n_{ia}}{\sum_i p_{is}n_{ia}} = \frac{166\,285}{178\,253} = .933$$

$$S\hat{M}R_b = \frac{\sum_i p_{ib}n_{ib}}{\sum_i p_{is}n_{ib}} = \frac{11\,051}{10\,524} = 1.050$$

The estimated variance of SMR is obtained from Equation 5-12 or, under the small p_i approximation, from Equation 5-14:

$$\text{vâr}(SMR_a) \text{ using Equation 5-12} = \frac{\sum_i n_{ia}p_{ia}q_{ia}}{\left(\sum_i p_{is}n_{ia}\right)^2} = \frac{158\,410}{(178\,253)^2} = .000004986$$

$$\text{vâr}(SMR_a) \text{ using Equation 5-14} = \frac{S\hat{M}R_a}{E} = \frac{S\hat{M}R_a}{\sum_i p_{is}n_{ia}} = \frac{.93}{178\,253}$$

$$= .000005217$$

$$\text{vâr}(SMR_b) \text{ using Equation 5-12} = \frac{10\,424}{(10\,524)^2} = .000094118$$

$$\text{vâr}(SMR_b) \text{ using Equation 5-14} = \frac{1.05}{10\,524} = .000099772$$

Taking the square roots of these variances, we compare the standard errors of SMR obtained by the two formulas and see that they are very similar:

	$\hat{SE}(SMR_a)$	$\hat{SE}(SMR_b)$
Equation 5-12	.0022	.0097
Equation 5-14	.0023	.0100

We previously stated that it is technically incorrect to compare the indirectly adjusted rates for the two areas. The same limitation applies to a comparison of SMR values. With full awareness of this limitation, it is interesting to note that using Table 5-1 data and the United States as the standard, $S\hat{M}R_b/S\hat{M}R_a = 1.125$, $I\hat{S}R_b/I\hat{S}R_a = 1.125$ (the ratio of two SMR values will always be identical to the ratio of the corresponding ISR values), and $D\hat{S}R_b/D\hat{S}R_a = 1.125$. These are all in contrast to the corresponding ratio of crude rates, which is 1.337.

GENERAL APPLICATION OF DIRECT AND INDIRECT ADJUSTMENT

Although our illustration of direct and indirect adjustment has related to mortality rates and age, students should realize that the procedures are equally applicable to morbidity rates and to adjustment for variables other than age, e.g. race, sex, or smoking status.

CONFOUNDING VARIABLES IN 2 × 2 TABLES

Tables 5-3 and 5-4 show data relating age, systolic blood pressure, and prevalence of myocardial infarction from a sample of the Israeli Ischemic Heart Disease Study population. We see that the odds ratios for disease comparing those with the factor and those without are 3.44 for age (Table 5-3) and 1.88 for blood pressure (Table 5-3). The odds ratio for higher blood pressure comparing older persons to younger is 3.04 (Table 5-4). If our major interest is in estimating the odds ratio relating systolic blood pressure to myocardial infarction, age is a confounding variable because it is related both to the disease of interest, myocardial infarction, and to the risk factor we wish to evaluate, systolic blood pressure. Thus the odds ratio of 1.88 relating elevated blood pressure to myocardial infarction risk reflects not only the association of blood pressure and myocardial infarction but also the association of age and myocardial infarction.

Table 5-3. Relationship of Age and Systolic Blood Pressure to Prevalence of Myocardial Infarction in a Sample of Individuals in the Israeli Ischemic Heart Disease Study

	Myocardial infarction	
	Present	Absent
Age $\geqslant 60$	15	188
Age < 60	41	$1767(\hat{OR} = 3.44)$
SBP $\geqslant 140$	29	711
SBP < 140	27	$1244(OR = 1.88)$
Total	56	1955

Source: unpublished data from the Israeli Ischemic Heart Disease Study.

Table 5-4. Relationship of Systolic Blood Pressure to Age in a Sample of Individuals in the Israeli Ischemic Heart Disease Study

	Age $\geqslant 60$	Age < 60	Total
SBP $\geqslant 140$	124	616	740
SBP < 140	79	1192	1271
Total	203	1808	2011
			$\hat{OR} = 3.04$

Source: unpublished data from the Israeli Ischemic Heart Disease Study.

Stratification to Control Confounding

One obvious way to reduce the confounding effect of age is to look at the date in separate strata by age. Table 5-5 presents the data relating systolic blood pressure and myocardial infarction after they have been subdivided into age classes.

Definition of Interaction. The odds ratios in Table 5-5 relating elevated blood pressure to risk—.95 for those age 60 and over and 1.87 for those under age 60—suggest a relationship between variables that we have not previously discussed. What meaning can be attached to an odds ratio relating high blood pressure to risk of disease if this odds ratio is different at different ages? Naturally the overall odds ratio can be viewed as an average derived from a combination of odds ratios for specific age classes. However, such an average would be interpreted one way if the

Table 5-5. Prevalence of Myocardial Infarction by Systolic Blood Pressure and Age

	MI cases	MI negative	Total
Age $\geqslant 60$			
SBP $\geqslant 140$	$9(a_1)^a$	$115(b_1)$	$124(m_{11})$
SBP < 140	$6(c_1)$	$73(d_1)$	$79(m_{21})$
Total	$15(n_{11})$	188	$203(t_1)$
			$\hat{OR} = 0.95$
Age < 60			
SBP $\geqslant 140$	$20(a_2)$	$596(b_2)$	$616(m_{12})$
SBP < 140	$21(c_2)$	$1171(d_2)$	$1192(m_{22})$
Total	$41(n_{12})$	1767	$1808(t_2)$
			$\hat{OR} = 1.87$

[a] Letters in parentheses are used in the text discussion of these data.
Source: unpublished data from the Israeli Ischemic Heart Disease Study.

items included were all sample estimates of the same odds ratio subject only to random variation and another way if the odds ratios being averaged were truly different. If the association of blood pressure and risk is different at different ages (beyond the range of variation we can assign to chance), we say that there is *interaction* between age and blood pressure in relation to risk of disease. Miettinen suggests *effect modification* as a better description than interaction [Miettinen 1974b]. However, since *effect modification* implies a real effect requiring data beyond those of the associations we are discussing and since *interaction* is a quite common term in the statistical and epidemiologic literature, we shall continue using it.

Interaction can be defined more precisely. For simplicity, we shall do this with respect to mortality rates as related to attribute variables A and B. We define four mortality rates as follows:

AB mortality rate associated with variables A and B when both are present

aB mortality rate associated with variable B present but A is absent

Ab mortality rate associated with variable A present but B is absent

ab mortality rate associated with variables A and B when both are absent

Using the above notations, interaction between A and B can be defined as the existence of nonzero values of

$$(AB - aB) - (Ab - ab)$$

This difference of differences compares the arithmetic effect of A on mortality rate when B is present $(AB - aB)$ with the arithmetic effect of A on mortality rate when B is absent $(Ab - ab)$. If $AB - aB = Ab - ab$, we say there is *no interaction* between A and B. More exactly, if we do not detect a significant difference between sample estimates of $AB - aB$ and $Ab - ab$, we can say we have no evidence of interaction.

Interaction can be defined with respect to alternative scalings of data [Kupper and Hogan 1978], for example, a logarithmic effect: $(\log AB - \log aB) - (\log Ab - \log ab)$. This is zero if $AB/aB = Ab/ab$. Absence of interaction on a logarithmic scale suggests that the ratio effect of A is unchanged whether B is present or not. Thus if A increases mortality rate by .10 whether or not B is present, then interaction between A and B is not present *when interaction is defined arithmetically*. However, if the increase of .10 is from .05 to .15 with B absent and from .20 to .30 with B present, AB interaction exists if it is defined on a logarithmic scale because the ratios .15/.05 and .30/.20 are unequal. Rothman has suggested a probability scale as biologically appropriate [Rothman 1974]. Additional discussion may be found in Schlesselman [1982].

A final comment about interaction. If the effect of high blood pressure on mortality is considerable at younger ages and less so at older ages, that is a fact of nature we should try to uncover. It is not something we want to eliminate by clever transformation of the measurement scale [Rothman 1976]. Interaction between age and blood pressure is separate and distinct from confounding between age and blood pressure. If we do not properly control the latter, we overstate the effect of elevated blood pressure on mortality risk (because those with elevated pressure are older than those without it). To recapitulate the discussion of the relationship of age, blood pressure and risk:

1. Elimination of confounding between age and blood pressure with respect to risk results in better estimates of the overall association of blood pressure and risk.
2. If interaction between age and blood pressure is present, this estimate of the overall association between blood pressure and risk is not applicable to all age groups

Mantel–Haenszel Procedure to Control Confounding

We now return to the data of Table 5-5 with estimated odds ratios for each of two age classes. The Mantel–Haenszel (M–H) procedure [Mantel and Haenszel 1959] can combine the odds ratios for separate strata into an overall summary estimate of the odds ratio relating blood pressure and risk of myocardial infarction. The advantage of this M–H overall odds ratio over the odds ratio for the same disease and risk factor given in Table 5-3 is that the confounding effect of age (with respect to two age classes) is eliminated. If there is a common odds ratio, the M–H procedure estimates it. If there is no common odds ratio (i.e., interaction is present), the M–H procedure provides a weighted average of the separate odds ratio. The overall odds ratio using the M–H procedure is estimated as follows:

$$\hat{OR}(\text{overall}) = \frac{\sum_i a_i d_i / t_i}{\sum_i b_i c_i / t_i} \tag{5-17}$$

where t_i is the total number of individuals and $a_i d_i$ and $b_i c_i$ are the cross-product terms for the ith 2×2 table arranged as in Table 3-3. For the data in Table 5-5 this is

$$\frac{(9 \times 73)/203 + (20 \times 1171)/1808}{(115 \times 6)/203 + (596 \times 21)/1808} = 1.57$$

Thus, instead of estimating 1.88 as the odds ratio relating elevated systolic blood pressure to myocardial infarction prevalence, we now estimate it as 1.57 after removing part of the confounding effect of age. Presumably, the effect of age has not been eliminated entirely because *within* the age classes ≥60 and <60 the persons with elevated blood pressure are likely to be older than the others. If this residual confounding is considered important, it can be dealt with by constructing additional age strata using narrower intervals or by multivariate methods (described in Chapter 6).

See Chapter 8 for a procedure, similar to M–H, to estimate the common relative risk from person-year data.

Matching Data in 2 × 2 Tables

Another method for removing the confounding effects of age on the association of systolic blood pressure with myocardial infarction is to match each infarction case with one or more randomly chosen controls *of the same age as the case.** Using unpublished data, we selected one control per case by picking an individual of the same age as the myocardial infarction case but without any history of myocardial infarction from a list of Israel Ischemic Heart Study participants arranged by age and serial number. The serial numbers were assigned in a way completely unrelated to age or blood pressure, and thus the qualifying individual with the next higher serial number than the case was a satisfactory choice. Data for the 56 *pairs* of matched cases and controls are summarized in Table 5-6. Note that Table 5-6 relates to pairs of individuals and not to single persons, i.e., 15 cases *and* 15 age-matched controls are represented by the 15 in the upper left corner of the table. Because Table 5-6 counts pairs and not individuals, the cells have different meaning than the cells in the 2 × 2 tables we have seen up to this point. For this reason the estimation of an odds ratio based on matched

Table 5-6. Relationship of Systolic Blood Pressure to Myocardial Infarction: Paired Case-Control Data Matched by Age

	Controls		
Cases	SBP ≥ 140	SBP < 140	Total
SBP ≥ 140	15	13	28
SBP < 140	11	17	28
Total	26	30	56

$$OR = \frac{13}{11} = 1.18$$

Source: unpublished data from the Israeli Ischemic Heart Disease Study.

data is different from the usual calculation using the cross-products ratio. Before discussing the formula, it will be helpful to consider what information is provided about the relationship between systolic blood pressure and myocardial infarction by the 32 pairs in Table 5-6 (15 + 17), wherein the case and the control are in the *same* blood pressure category.

If you wish to study whether systolic blood pressure ≥140 is positively associated with myocardial infarction, you cannot do so in a population in which everyone has systolic blood pressure ≥140. The 32 pairs with case and control in the same blood pressure category similarly provide no basis for learning about how blood pressure might be related to myocardial infarction. If all individuals in a sample have high blood pressure or all have low blood pressure, it is impossible to learn from such a sample what might be the association between systolic blood pressure and myocardial infarction if blood pressure differences existed.

Another illustration may be useful. If you wish to discriminate between two swimmers as to which has a greater ability to swim long distances and you are given the following data on paired trials:

Trial 1   Both finished the prescribed course.
Trial 2   Both finished the prescribed course.
Trial 3   Neither finished the prescribed course.
Trial 4   A finished but B did not.

it should be clear that no judgment can be made as to greater endurance of one swimmer over the other from trials 1 through 3. Only trial 4, where there is a difference between the members of the pair, provides evidence as to possible difference between them. Similarly with the matched data. Pairs with both case and control having the risk factor or pairs with neither having the risk factor provide no information regarding the odds ratio. Data from a matched case-control study can be arranged as in Table 5-7, in which f is the number of *pairs* with both case and control factor positive, g is the number of *pairs* with the case factor positive and the control factor negative, etc. To emphasize that these are paired data, we use the symbols f, g, h, j for cells of this 2×2 table to distinguish them from the a, b, c, d symbols we have used to represent unpaired data.

Table 5-7. Case-Control Data for Matched Pairs

	Controls	
Cases	Risk factor +	Risk factor −
Risk factor +	f	g
Risk factor −	h	j

Table 5-8. Conversion of Paired Data to Unpaired Equivalent When Both Case and Control Are Positive for Risk Factor

	Paired data			Unpaired equivalent		
	Controls					
Cases	Risk factor +	Risk factor −	Risk factor	Cases	Controls	
Risk factor +	1	0	+	1 (a)	1 (b)	
Risk factor −	0	0	−	0 (c)	0 (d)	
				$ad = 0, bc = 0,$		
				$t = 2$		

With data as in Table 5-7, the estimated odds ratio relating positive factor to presence of disease based on matched pairs (MP) is

$$\hat{OR}(\text{MP}) = \frac{g}{h} \qquad (5\text{-}18)$$

For the data in Table 5-6,

$$\frac{g}{h} = \frac{13}{11} = 1.18$$

As previously discussed, f and j contribute nothing to odds ratio estimation.

Recalling the M–H formula (Equation 5-17) for the overall odds ratio and applying it to matched pair data in which each pair is treated as a separate stratum also results in the ratio g/h as the estimated odds ratio for paired data. To see this, the paired data first have to be changed to their unpaired equivalent, as shown in Tables 5-8 through 5-11. The

Table 5-9. Conversion of Paired Data to Unpaired Equivalent When Case Is Risk-Factor-Positive and Control Is Risk-Factor-Negative

	Paired data			Unpaired equivalent		
	Controls					
Cases	Risk factor +	Risk factor −	Risk factor	Cases	Controls	
Risk factor +	0	1	+	1 (a)	0 (b)	
Risk factor −	0	0	−	0 (c)	1 (d)	
				$ad = 1, bc = 0,$		
				$t = 2$		

Table 5-10. Conversion of Paired Data to Unpaired Equivalent When Case Is Risk-Factor-Negative and Control Is Risk-Factor-Positive

	Paired data			Unpaired equivalent	
	Controls				
Cases	Risk factor +	Risk factor −	Risk factor	Cases	Controls
Risk factor +	0	0	+	0 (a)	1 (b)
Risk factor −	1	0	−	1 (c)	0 (d)
				$ad = 0, bc = 1,$	
				$t = 2$	

M–H formula for $\hat{OR}$,

$$\frac{\sum_i a_i d_i / t_i}{\sum_i b_i c_i / t_i}$$

applied to the data in Tables 5-8 to 5-11 will

1. Have zero added to the numerator and to the denominator for each pair with case and control alike ($a_i d_i = 0$, $b_i c_i = 0$, $t_i = 2$), as in Tables 5-8 and 5-11.
2. Have $\frac{1}{2}$ added to the numerator for each pair with the case positive and the control negative for the risk factor ($a_i d_i = 1$, $b_i c_i = 0$, $t_i = 2$), as in Table 5-9. There are g pairs of this type.
3. Have $\frac{1}{2}$ added to the denominator for each pair with the case negative and the control positive for the risk factor ($a_i d_i = 0$, $b_i c_i = 1$, $t_i = 2$), as in Table 5-10. There are h pairs of this type.
4. Consequently equal $(g/2)/(h/2) = g/h$, as in Equation 5-18.

Table 5-11. Conversion of Paired Data to Unpaired Equivalent When Both Case and Control Are Negative for Risk Factor

	Paired data			Unpaired equivalent	
	Controls				
Cases	Risk factor +	Risk factor −	Risk factor	Cases	Controls
Risk factor +	0	0	+	0 (a)	0 (b)
Risk factor −	0	1	−	1 (c)	1 (d)
				$ad = 0, bc = 0,$	
				$t = 2$	

Summary

To recapitulate, we estimated the odds ratio for the association of myocardial infarction to elevated systolic blood pressure as 1.88 with no adjustment for confounding by age and as 1.57 after partially adjusting for age by stratifying the data into age $\geqslant 60$ and age < 60. When we adjusted by means of individual matching on age, necessarily using only a subset of the full sample, the odds ratio was 1.18. Of course, sampling error is implicit in all these calculations, and it is possible that a method of adjustment that on average lowers an estimated odds ratio by reducing the effect of a confounding variable may in a specific instance actually raise it.

Before additional discussion of these estimated odds ratios for the relationship of myocardial infarction prevalence to elevated systolic blood pressure, it is first necessary to consider their relationship to odds ratios for myocardial infarction *incidence* in relation to elevated systolic blood pressure. Chapter 3 stressed that retrospective case-control studies are necessarily restricted to the use of prevalent cases. Because myocardial infarction is a disease with a high fatality rate, with sudden death as a not uncommon first manifestation, it should be obvious that the odds for *being* a case or *not being* a case based on existing cases may be quite different from the odds for *becoming* a case or *not becoming* a case based on prospective incidence data. In fact, incidence data from the same Israel Ischemic Heart Disease Study sample we have used here for prevalence associations do indicate larger odds ratios relating systolic blood pressure and incidence of myocardial infarction (adjusted for age) than those for prevalence. This may or may not be an important distinction for other diseases, and we include this comment to remind the reader to always consider the potential differences between data obtained prospectively and those obtained retrospectively.

CONFIDENCE LIMITS FOR ADJUSTED ODDS RATIOS
Woolf's Method

To discuss confidence limits for adjusted odds ratios, it is necessary to return to unmatched data in the (by now familiar) format of Table 3-3, except that we use a_i, b_i, c_i, and d_i to indicate sample data for the ith stratum. We shall use Woolf's method [Woolf 1955] to derive confidence limits on an overall estimate of the odds ratio and also to test whether or not interaction is present. For data sets as large as are usually available in high-quality epidemiologic studies, Woolf's method can be expected to give good results. However, other methods are available, including many programmed for a desk calculator [Abramson and Peretz 1983, Rothman and Boice 1979]. For small data sets a statistician's advice will be helpful. In a later section we shall compare various alternative methods for calculating confidence limits on odds ratios, with particular attention to the size of the data set required for satisfactory results. If the reader will accept the estimated variance of $\ln \hat{OR}$ given by Woolf as

$$\frac{1}{a} + \frac{1}{b} + \frac{1}{c} + \frac{1}{d}$$

the remainder of his method for computing confidence intervals can be easily derived.

Logarithms are used to calculate confidence limits on odds ratios because they introduce approximate normality into the otherwise extremely skewed distribution of all possible sample odds ratios. Thus, while an $\hat{OR}$ of 3 is farther from its expected value of unity (under the null hypothesis) than is an $\hat{OR}$ of $1/3$, $\ln 3$ ($=1.0986$) is exactly as far from its expected value of zero (under the null hypothesis) as is $\ln(1/3)$ ($= -1.0986$). In combining $\ln \hat{OR}_i$ values for individual strata into a single overall estimate, it is sensible to give more weight to those $\ln \hat{OR}_i$ that are estimated with greater precision. An easy way to accomplish this is to weight each $\ln \hat{OR}_i$ by

$$\left(\frac{1}{a_i} + \frac{1}{b_i} + \frac{1}{c_i} + \frac{1}{d_i}\right)^{-1}$$

the reciprocal of its estimated variance. If we designate this reciprocal as w_i, we have

$$\ln \hat{OR} = \frac{\sum\limits_i w_i \ln \hat{OR}_i}{\sum\limits_i w_i} \tag{5-19}$$

Making use of Equations 1-8 and 1-10, the variance of $\ln OR$ is

$$\hat{var}(\ln OR) = \frac{\sum\limits_i w_i^2 [\hat{var}(\ln OR_i)]}{\left(\sum\limits_i w_i\right)^2}$$

But since

$$w_i = \frac{1}{\hat{var}(\ln OR_i)} \qquad \hat{var}(\ln OR_i) = \frac{1}{w_i}$$

and

$$\text{vâr}(\ln OR) = \frac{\sum_i w_i^2(1/w_i)}{\left(\sum_i w_i\right)^2} = \frac{\sum_i w_i}{\left(\sum_i w_i\right)^2} = \frac{1}{\sum_i w_i} \qquad (5\text{-}20)$$

the estimated standard error of $\ln \hat{OR}$ is then $1/\sqrt{\sum w_i}$, and 95 percent confidence limits on $\ln OR$ are

$$\ln \hat{OR} \pm 1.96\left(\frac{1}{\sqrt{\sum_i w_i}}\right) \qquad (5\text{-}21)$$

After finding the 95 percent confidence limits on $\ln OR$, the corresponding antilogs

$$e^{\ln \hat{OR} - (1.96/\sqrt{\sum w_i})} \qquad e^{\ln \hat{OR} + (1.96/\sqrt{\sum w_i})} \qquad (5\text{-}22)$$

are the 95 percent confidence limits on OR.

Test for Interaction

If we are thinking about combining odds ratios from separate strata, it is useful to test for interaction. Consider the data in Table 5-5. The odds ratios for the two strata are .95 and 1.87. Perhaps the odds ratio of .95 reflects a true odds ratio of 1.00 for age <60 and the odds ratio of 1.87 reflects a true odds ratio of 2.00 for age ≥60. If the underlying odds ratios for individual strata are really different, do we want to calculate an overall average value? In any event, we should determine whether or not the strata odds ratios reflect basic differences. A test for interaction on Table 5-5 data (i.e., is the effect of blood pressure on risk different at different ages?) will answer the question as to whether it is desirable to combine individual odds ratios.

A systematic summary of Table 5-5 data, which we shall use to test for interaction and also to compute confidence limits, can be prepared as shown in Table 5-12. Using these summary data from Table 5-12, we

Table 5-12. Systematic Summary of Functions of Data Taken from Table 5-5

Stratum	$\hat{OR}_i$	$\ln \hat{OR}_i$	$\text{vâr}(\ln OR_i)$	$1/\text{vâr}(\ln OR_i) = w_i$
1	.95	−.0513	$\frac{1}{9} + \frac{1}{6} + \frac{1}{115} + \frac{1}{73} = .300$	3.33
2	1.87	.6259	$\frac{1}{20} + \frac{1}{21} + \frac{1}{596} + \frac{1}{1171} = .100$	10.00

have

$$\ln \hat{OR} = \frac{3.33(-.0513) + 10.00(.6259)}{3.33 + 10.00} = .4567$$

$$\hat{OR} = e^{.4567} = 1.58$$

To test for interaction, we use Equation 1-22 for χ^2_{k-1}. This helps us to determine if the individual $\ln \hat{OR}_i$ for each stratum differs from $\ln \hat{OR}$ by more than can be explained by random variation. For this specific problem, χ^2 is computed as follows:

$$\chi^2_{2-1} = \sum_{i=1}^{2} \frac{(\ln \hat{OR}_i - \ln \hat{OR})^2}{var(\ln \hat{OR}_i)}$$

Our test for interaction on the two odds ratios shown in Table 5-5 data is then

$$\chi^2_1 = \frac{(-.0513 - .4567)^2}{.300} + \frac{(.6259 - .4567)^2}{.100} = 1.15$$

Since the probability of a χ^2_1 value of 1.15 or greater is more than 20 percent, we lack evidence that the odds ratios in Table 5-5, different as they are (.95 and 1.87), are not sample values from the same population. Thus, the overall odds ratio of 1.58 may be interpreted as indicating the general relationship between systolic blood pressure elevation and risk of myocardial infarction.

Of course, it should be recognized that with only 15 cases of myocardial infarction in the age ≥ 60 group, the ability of our interaction test to detect, in the odds ratios in different strata, a difference greater than can be accounted for by chance is quite modest. The technical term for the ability of sample data to detect differences if they exist is *power*. Obviously, other factors being equal, the smaller the sample, the less power $(1 - \beta)$ to detect differences if they are present.

Since we lack evidence of interaction, it is certainly reasonable to make use of the overall estimates of OR previously calculated. We illustrate the calculation of confidence limits for $\ln \hat{OR}$ using Equation 5-21 and Table 5-5 data as summarized in Table 5-12:

$$\ln \hat{OR} = .4567$$

$$\hat{SE}(\ln OR) = \frac{1}{(\sum w_i)^{1/2}} = \frac{1}{(3.33 + 10.00)^{1/2}} = .2739$$

$$95\% \text{ CL on } \ln OR = .4567 \pm 1.96(.2739) = -.0801 \text{ and } .9935$$

$$95\% \text{ CL on } OR = e^{-.0801} \text{ and } e^{.9935} = .92 \text{ and } 2.70$$

Significance Test-Based Limits

We now discuss an alternative to Woolf's method for calculating confidence limits on an overall odds ratio derived from a combination of odds ratios for separate strata. This procedure, which is based on a significance test, was suggesed by Miettinen [1976a], and we shall use it in combination with the M–H procedure [Mantel and Haenszel 1959] for estimating an overall odds ratio and testing it for significance.

Mantel–Haenszel Summary χ^2. First consider the M–H χ^2 test (one degree of freedom) on the data in a set of 2×2 tables. The χ_1^2 indicates whether or not the data are unusual in terms of deviation from expectation under the null hypothesis, which is that disease and risk factor are related only by chance. Any other χ_1^2 test of the *same data* with respect to the *same null hypothesis* should indicate the same degree of unusualness, i.e., the same χ_1^2 value. If the sample size is adequate, any test of departure from the null hypothesis should lead to the same χ_1^2 value because with only one degree of freedom it is not possible to measure departure from expectation in more than one basic way. Thus, whether, as in the M–H χ_1^2 test, relating $\sum a_i$ to $E(\sum a_i)$ and dividing by $\mathrm{var}(\sum a_i)$ or, as we now propose, relating $\ln \hat{OR}$ to $E(\ln \hat{OR})$ and dividing by $\mathrm{var}(\ln \hat{OR})$, χ_1^2 based on the same data should be equivalent. We are now ready to describe in detail and calculate the M–H χ_1^2 for Table 5-5 data.

The overall significance test for a set of 2×2 tables suggested by Mantel and Haenszel [1959] is

$$\chi_1^2 = \frac{[|\sum a_i - E(\sum a_i)| - \frac{1}{2}]^2}{\mathrm{var}(\sum a_i)} \qquad (5\text{-}23)$$

This formula is basically the same as Equation 1-21 with

$$x = \sum a_i$$

$$E(x) = E\left(\sum a_i\right) = \sum (Ea_i)$$

$$\mathrm{var}(x) = \mathrm{var}\left(\sum a_i\right) = \sum [\mathrm{var}(a_i)]$$

Note that because the a_i in separate strata are independent, the variance of the sum of the a_i values equals the sum of the variances of the a_i values. In addition, the expected value of a sum is always the sum of the expected values, whether or not the variables are independent. If we use the notation of Table 3-3 we have

$$x = \sum a_i$$

$$E(x) = E\left(\sum a_i\right) = \sum (Ea_i) = \sum \left(n_{1i}\frac{m_{1i}}{t_i}\right)$$

i.e., under the null hypothesis, the expected number of cases in stratum i with risk factor present equals the total number of cases (n_{1i}) multiplied by the proportion with the risk factor among cases and noncases combined (m_{1i}/t_i). Under the assumption that row and column totals in each stratum are fixed and not subject to sampling error, the variance of a_i is

$$n_{1i}\left(\frac{m_{1i}}{t_i}\right)\left(\frac{m_{2i}}{t_i}\right)\left(\frac{t_i - n_{1i}}{t_{i-1}}\right)$$

The above is analogous to the variance of a binomial sum, given in Equation 1-18, but with the finite correction factor added; thus

$$np(1-p)\left(\frac{N-n}{N-1}\right)$$

For the data at hand

$$n = n_{1i}$$

$$p = m_{1i}/t_i$$

$$(1-p) = m_{2i}/t_i$$

$$N = t_i$$

then

$$\sum \text{var}(a_i) = \sum n_{1i}\left(\frac{m_{1i}}{t_i}\right)\left(\frac{m_{2i}}{t_i}\right)\left(\frac{t_i - n_{1i}}{t_i - 1}\right)$$

The final element in Equation 5-23 is the reduction of the absolute value of the difference between $\sum a_i$ observed and $\sum a_i$ expected by one-half before squaring. This represents the continuity correction for χ^2 intended to make the integral values in a 2×2 table fit more closely to the continuous variable represented by the χ^2 distribution. This continuity correction is due to Yates [1934].

To compute the M–H summary odds ratio and χ_1^2 test pertaining to it, we use the data of Table 5-5 according to the labeling shown therein. Then, as previously calculated,

$$\hat{OR}_{M-H} = \frac{\Sigma\, a_i d_i / t_i}{\Sigma\, b_i c_i / t_i} = \frac{9(73)/203 + 20(1171)/1808}{115(6)/203 + 596(21)/1808} = 1.57$$

and for the M–H χ_1^2

$$x = \Sigma\, a_i = 9 + 20 = 29$$

$$E(x) = \Sigma\,(Ea_i) = \frac{15(124)}{203} + \frac{41(616)}{1808} = 23.13$$

$$\mathrm{var}(x) = \mathrm{var}\left(\Sigma\, a_i\right) = \Sigma\,(\mathrm{var}\,a_i) = 15\left(\frac{124}{203}\right)\left(\frac{79}{203}\right)\left(\frac{203-15}{203-1}\right)$$

$$+\, 41\left(\frac{616}{1808}\right)\left(\frac{1192}{1808}\right)\left(\frac{1808-41}{1808-1}\right) = 12.32$$

$$\chi_1^2 = \frac{[|29 - 23.13| - \frac{1}{2}]^2}{12.32} = 2.34$$

Miettinen's Test-Based Limits. We now use the value of $\chi_1^2 = 2.34$ as equal to another χ_1^2, one that, at least conceptually, could have been calculated from these data, namely

$$\chi_1^2 = \frac{[\ln \hat{OR}_{M-H} - E(\ln \hat{OR}_{M-H})]^2}{\mathrm{var}(\ln \hat{OR}_{M\ H})} = 2.34$$

Because we do not know the formula for $\mathrm{var}(\ln \hat{OR}_{M-H})$, we cannot calculate the above directly. However, the use of χ_1^2 from another significance test on these data allows us to proceed as follows. Since the $\hat{OR}_{M-H}$ was 1.57, $\ln \hat{OR}$ can be calculated as $\ln 1.57 = .4511$. Under the null hypothesis, the expected value of $\hat{OR}_{M-H} = 1$ and thus the expected value of $\ln \hat{OR}_{M-H}$ is zero and we have

$$\chi_1^2 = \frac{(.4511 - 0)^2}{\mathrm{var}(\ln \hat{OR}_{M-H})} = 2.34$$

This equation can then be solved for $\mathrm{var}(\ln \hat{OR}_{M-H})$, which is found to equal .0870. Note that this value for $\mathrm{var}(\ln \hat{OR}_{M-H})$ has been derived not directly from any considerations as to the sampling distribution of $\ln \hat{OR}_{M-H}$ but from the equivalence of two possible expressions for χ_1^2

based on departure of Table 5-5 data from the null hypothesis. Because of the manner in which we obtained it, this variance of $\ln \hat{OR}_{M-H}$ is strictly applicable only under null hypothesis conditions, i.e., $OR_{M-H} = 1$ and $\ln OR_{M-H} = 0$ [Halperin 1977]. As a practical matter, it has been found useful over a fairly wide range of departures from the null hypothesis, and you need not hesitate to use it.

Greenland [1984] considers that test based limits are unsatisfactory for odds ratios greater than 10.0 or less than .1. This is a reasonable limitation and also one without much practical consequence due to the rarity of odds ratios greater than 10.0. He also states that test based confidence limits are better suited to odds ratios than to statistics on risk differences.

With $\text{var}(\ln \hat{OR}_{M-H})$ as .0870, the standard error of $\ln \hat{OR}_{M-H}$ is $(.0870)^{1/2} = .2950$ and 95 percent confidence limits on $\ln \hat{OR}_{M-H}$ can be estimated as

$$\ln \hat{OR}_{M-H} \pm 1.96(.2950) = .4511 \pm .5782$$

$$95\% \text{ CL on } \ln OR_{M-H} = -.1271 \text{ and } 1.0293$$

$$95\% \text{ CL on } OR_{M-H} = e^{-.1271} \text{ and } e^{1.0293} = .88 \text{ and } 2.80$$

Comparison of Alternatives. Note the close agreement between Miettinen's method (using M–H χ^2) and Woolf's method for estimating a common odds ratio and its confidence limits. For the common odds ratio Woolf's method estimated 1.58 and the M–H procedure estimated 1.57. The 95 percent confidence limits derived from Woolf's method were .92 and 2.70, versus .88 and 2.80 from Miettinen's test-based procedure using the M–H summary odds ratio and χ_1^2 test for significance. A point to emphasize is that the essential equivalence of the two approaches in this particular instance relates to 2×2 tables with cells as small as 6 and 9. If the basic data were more substantial, we would expect even closer agreement. As an indication of this, if all cell frequencies in Table 5-5 were doubled, the confidence limits on OR using Woolf's method would be 1.08 and 2.31, barely distinguishable from the 1.06 and 2.32 obtained from the test-based procedure of Miettinen.

The close agreement between the M–H procedure and Woolf's method is typical for data sets of moderate size or larger. Although not derived that way, the M–H procedure can be thought of as weighting each OR_i by $b_i c_i / t_i$ whereas Woolf's method weights each $\ln OR_i$ by the inverse of its estimated variance. The general equality of results indicates that the M–H procedure is somehow similar to inverse variance weighting. An advantage of the M–H procedure is that it can be followed even if some cells are zero. With zero cells present, Woolf's method is indeterminate unless the cell values are changed.

Although one analysis [Gart 1982] concludes that the Cornfield method referred to in Chapter 3 is superior to both Woolf's method and Miettinen's test-based method for estimating confidence limits on odds ratios derived from single 2×2 tables, the data shown in that report agree completely with our own experience that differences are not important. The only large difference reported among the three methods is for the inverval .18 and 5.49 versus .26 and 9.45. Clearly either of these confidence limits makes the same point, i.e., that we are almost completely ignorant about the size of the true odds ratio.

Application to Matched Data. We now consider another example illustrating the use of the test-based procedure for confidence limits. For matched pair data arranged as in Table 5-7 and using $\hat{O}R(\text{MP})$ to represent the estimated odds ratio from matched pair data, the proper estimate of $OR(\text{MP})$ is g/h, as in Equation 5-18.

The M–H χ^2 test to evaluate whether $OR(\text{MP})$ is significantly different from unity depends on whether g is significantly different from $\frac{1}{2}(g + h)$. Under the condition that the test relates only to samples in which the total number of discordant pairs equals $g + h$, the number of discordant pairs actually observed, the M–H χ_1^2 is exactly equivalent to Equation 1-21 as applied to a binomial variable and uses

g as the number of successes observed in $g + h$ trials
$\frac{1}{2}(g + h)$ as the expected number of successes
$g + h$ as the number of trials
$(g + h)(\frac{1}{2})(\frac{1}{2})$ as the variance of the number of successes observed

Then

$$\chi_1^2 = \frac{(g - (g + h/2))^2}{(g + h)(\frac{1}{2})(\frac{1}{2})} = \frac{((g/2) - (h/2))^2 4}{g + h} = \frac{(g - h)^2}{g + h}$$

and using the continuity correction, the M–H χ_1^2 for testing if $\hat{O}R(\text{MP})$ is significantly different from unity is

$$\chi_1^2 = \frac{(|g - h| - 1)^2}{g + h} \tag{5-24}$$

For Table 5-6 data, this is

$$\chi_1^2 = \frac{(|13 - 11| - 1)^2}{13 + 11} = \frac{1}{24} = .042$$

clearly not a large departure from expectation under the null hypothesis.

Recalling that $\hat{OR}(MP)$ from Table 5-6 is 1.18, we can now use Equation 1-21 with $\ln \hat{OR}(MP)$ substituted for x and solve for $SE[\ln \hat{OR}(MP)]$:

$$\chi_1^2 = \frac{(\ln \hat{OR}(MP) - 0)^2}{\text{var}[\ln \hat{OR}(MP)]} = \frac{(.1655 - 0)^2}{\text{var}[\ln \hat{OR}(MP)]} = .042$$

$$\text{var}[\ln \hat{OR}(MP)] = .6521$$

$$SE[\ln \hat{OR}(MP)] = .8076$$

and the 95 percent confidence limits on $\ln OR(MP)$ are

$$\ln \hat{OR}(MP) \pm 1.96(.8076) = .1655 \pm 1.5829 = -1.4174 \text{ and } 1.7484$$

The corresponding antilogs, $e^{-1.4174}$ and $e^{1.7484}$, are .24 and 5.75. These are the 95 percent confidence limits on the $OR(MP)$ derived from Table 5-6.

Validity of Mantel–Haenszel Summary χ^2

A prescription for evaluating the validity of the M–H χ^2 calculation has been suggested by Mantel and Fleiss [1980]. We will use the data of Table 5-5 to describe it. First, with all marginal totals considered as fixed, we need to determine the largest and smallest *possible* values for the number of MI cases with $SBP \geqslant 140$ in each stratum (a_i).

a. The number of MI cases with $SBP \geqslant 140$ can *never be larger* than the smaller of the two marginal totals for (i) MI cases and (ii) persons with $SBP \geqslant 140$.

b. The number of MI cases with $SBP \geqslant 140$ can *never be smaller* than the larger of (i) zero or (ii) the total number of MI cases minus the total number of persons with $SBP < 140$. (If this is not immediately self-evident, simply recognize that the total with $SBP < 140$ includes MI cases with $SBP < 140$.)

Applying these rules for maxima and minima to a_i in Table 5-5 we have:

	Maximum	Minimum
a_1	15	0
a_2	41	0
Total	56	0

The remaining value required for this computation has previously been calculated. It is the sum of the expected values of a_i that we found to be 23.13. The Mantel–Fleiss prescription for satisfactory interpretation of the Mantel–Haenszel χ^2 is that the sum of the maximum values be 5 or more larger and the sum of the minimum values be 5 or more smaller than the sum of the expected values for a_i. For Table 5-5 these conditions are met since $56 - 23.13 \geqslant 5$ and $23.13 - 0 \geqslant 5$.

MULTIPLE MATCHED CONTROLS
Estimating Odds Ratios

Matching K controls to each case, where K may be 2, 3, or possibly even larger, is sometimes done when controls are available at much lower cost than cases. This procedure is also sometimes used in an effort to obtain the maximum information possible from a case-control comparison when only a small number of cases are available. If we cross-classify each set consisting of a case and its K matched controls, as in Table 5-13, we can consider each set as a separate stratum and calculate the odds ratio using Equation 5-17. In Table 5-13 we use the a_i, b_i, c_i, d_i, t_i designations previously described. However, we have used total row and column symbols appropriate to matching K controls per case. Thus, $a_i + c_i - 1$, $b_i + d_i = K$, and $t_i = 1 + K$. We again use the M–H procedure to combine sets and to estimate the overall odds ratio as $\dfrac{\Sigma\,(a_i d_i)/t_i}{\Sigma\,(b_i c_i)/t_i}$. Comparable to the case of one-to-one matching, zero will be added to $\Sigma\,(a_i d_i)/t_i$ and to $\Sigma\,(b_i c_i)/t_i$ if the case and all controls are all factor-positive or all factor-negative. Either $a_i d_i/t_i$ or $b_i c_i/t_i$ will have nonzero values whenever case and controls show disagreement as to proportion with the factor positive, e.g., case is factor positive and at least one control is factor negative.

Returning to the 56 myocardial infarction cases from our sample from the Israeli Ischemic Heart Disease Study population, we randomly matched each case with two controls and calculated the odds ratio. The data consist of 11 triplets as in Table 5-14, 9 triplets as in Table 5-15, 11 triplets as in Table 5-16, and 5 triplets as in Table 5-17. Eight triplets

Table 5-13. Notation for Matched Case and K Controls (ith Set)

	Case	Controls	Total
Risk factor $+$	a_i	b_i	$a_i + b_i$
Risk factor $-$	c_i	d_i	$1 + K - a_i - b_i$
Total	1	K	$1 + K(t_i)$

Table 5-14. Data Summary in 2×2 Table for Each Set of Two Controls and One Case with Case Positive and Both Controls Negative[a,b]

	MI case	Control	Total
SBP $\geqslant 140$	1	0	1
SBP < 140	0	2	2
Total	1	2	3

$K = 2, \ ad = 2, \ bc = 0, \ Ka - b = 2, \ (a + b)(1 + K - a - b) = 2, \ ad/t = 2/3$

[a] Eleven sets of this type; see text.
[b] See Table 5-13 for explanation of notation.
Source: unpublished data from the Israeli Ischemic Heart Disease Study.

Table 5-15. Data Summary in 2×2 Table for Each Set of Two Controls and One Case with Case Positive and One Control Positive, One Negative[a,b]

	MI case	Control	Total
SBP $\geqslant 140$	1	1	2
SBP < 140	0	1	1
Total	1	2	3

$K = 2, \ ad = 1, \ bc = 0, \ Ka - b = 1, \ (a + b)(1 + K - a - b) = 2, \ ad/t = 1/3$

[a] Nine sets of this type; see text.
[b] See Table 5-13 for explanation of notation.
Source: unpublished data from the Israeli Ischemic Heart Disease Study.

Table 5-16. Data Summary in 2×2 Table for Each Set of Two Controls and One Case with Case Negative and One Control Positive, One Negative[a,b]

	MI Case	Control	Total
SBP $\geqslant 140$	0	1	1
SBP < 140	1	1	2
Total	1	2	3

$K = 2, \ ad = 0, \ bc = 1, \ Ka - b = -1, \ (a + b)(1 + K - a - b) = 2, \ bc/t = 1/3$

[a] Eleven sets of this type; see text.
[b] See Table 5-13 for explanation of notation.
Source: unpublished data from the Israeli Ischemic Heart Disease Study.

Table 5-17. Data Summary in 2 × 2 Table for Each Set of Two Controls and One Case with Case Negative and Both Controls Positive[a,b]

	MI case	Control	Total
SBP ⩾ 140	0	2	2
SBP < 140	1	0	1
Total	1	2	3

$K = 2$, $ad = 0$, $bc = 2$, $Ka - b = -2$, $(a + b)(1 + K - a - b) = 2$, $bc/t = 2/3$

[a] Five sets of this type; see text.
[b] See Table 5-13 for explanation of notation.
Source: unpublished data from the Israeli Ischemic Heart Disease Study.

were all factor-positive, and 12 were all factor-negative. These 20 triplets provided no information as to the odds ratio and are excluded from the calculations. In Tables 5-14 to 5-17 are also shown some derivative values needed for the significance test to be described.

The odds ratio based on data from Tables 5-14 through 5-17 computed using Equation 5-17 is

$$\hat{O}R(MK) = \frac{11(2/3) + 9(1/3)}{11(1/3) + 5(2/3)} = \frac{31/3}{21/3} = 1.48$$

with $\hat{O}R(MK)$ used to indicate an estimated odds ratio based on matching K controls per case.

Significance Test and Confidence Limits

A significance test comparing cases and controls that are factor-positive, in matched data with K controls for each case, is given by Miettinen [1969] as

$$z = \sum_i (Ka_i - b_i) \Big/ \left[\sum_i (a_i + b_i)(1 + K - a_i - b_i) \right]^{1/2} \qquad (5\text{-}25)$$

where z is a standardized normal deviate if the null hypothesis, that $\hat{O}R(MK) = 1$, is true.

Although different in appearance, Equation 5-25 is derived in a manner similar to that used to derive the M–H summary χ_1^2. We begin by establishing the statistic for testing departure from expectation if there is no difference between cases and controls in the proportion positive for the risk factor under study. As with the M–H χ_1^2, we shall focus upon the number of cases positive for the risk factor in each set (stratum), i.e., a_i in Table 5-13. In this matched design, a_i is either 1 or 0. Under the null hypothesis, a_i is *not* expected to equal b_i, which is the number of controls positive for the risk factor, because our design calls for K controls per case. Thus, with no relationship between disease and risk factor, we do not expect a_i to be as large as b_i. On the average, however, we would expect Ka_i to be as large as b_i. Our test statistic is then $Ka_i - b_i$, which has an expected value of zero under the null hypothesis. The next step is to derive the standard error of the test statistic, and we do so under the condition that, in each set, row and column totals are fixed and not subject to sampling variation. The statistic to be tested for significance contains two variables, a_i and b_i, and because their total is a constant, it is easy enough to convert this to a form with just one variable:

$$Ka_i - b_i = Ka_i + (a_i + b_i) - b_i - (a_i + b_i) = (K + 1)a_i - (a_i + b_i)$$

Since $a_i + b_i$ is a constant, its sampling variance is zero and

$$\text{var}(Ka_i - b_i) = \text{var}[(K + 1)a_i] = (K + 1)^2 \, \text{var}(a_i)$$

If we consider a_i in Table 5-13 as a binomial sum with estimated variance of $np(1 - p)$, as in Equation 1-18, or as $np(1 - p)(N - n)/(N - 1)$ if we include the finite sampling factor, then the equivalent notation from Table 5-13 is

$$n = 1 \quad p = \frac{a_i + b_i}{1 + K} \quad 1 - p = \frac{1 + K - a_i - b_i}{1 + K} \quad N = 1 + K$$

$$\hat{\text{var}}(Ka_i - b_i) = (K + 1)^2\left[1\left(\frac{a_i + b_i}{1 + K}\right)\frac{(1 + K - a_i - b_i)}{1 + K}\right]\left(\frac{1 + K - 1}{1 + K - 1}\right)$$

$$= (a_i + b_i)(1 + K - a_i - b_i)$$

Since the sets are independent, the estimated variance of $\sum (Ka_i - b_i)$ is $\sum (a_i + b_i)(1 + K - a_i - b_i)$ and dividing $\sum (Ka_i - b_i)$ by the square root of its variance leads to Equation 5-25 for a standardized normal deviate, as given by Miettinen [1969].

Using data from Tables 5-14 through 5-17[†] and Equation 5-25,

$$z = \frac{11(2) + 9(1) + 11(-1) + 5(-2)}{[11(2) + 9(2) + 11(2) + 5(2)]^{1/2}} = \frac{10}{8.49} = 1.18$$

Since z is a standardized normal deviate, we use z^2 as equivalent to χ_1^2 in Miettinen's method for estimating a variance that might be difficult to estimate directly. Thus, under the null hypothesis

$$\frac{[\ln \hat{OR}(MK) - 0]^2}{\text{var}[\ln \hat{OR}(MK)]} = z^2 = \chi_1^2$$

We have inserted zero for the expectation of ln $\hat{OR}(MK)$ in this equation because, if $OR(MK) = 1$, then ln $OR(MK) = 0$. Inserting the values calculated for $\hat{OR}(MK)$ and z^2 for the Israeli sample data relating hypertension to myocardial infarction prevalence results in

$$\frac{(.3920 - 0)^2}{\text{var}[\ln \hat{OR}(MK)]} = (1.18)^2 = 1.39$$

$$\text{var}[\ln \hat{OR}(MK)] = .1105$$

$$\text{SE}[\ln \hat{OR}(MK)] = .3324$$

and 95 percent confidence limits for ln $OR(MK)$ are

$$(.3920) \pm 1.96(.3324) = .3920 \pm .6515 = -.2595 \text{ and } 1.0435$$

with $e^{-.2595}$ and $e^{1.0435}$, or .77 and 2.84, as the 95 percent confidence limits for $OR(MK)$. As expected, these limits are narrower than the limits based on one control per case, which we earlier found to be .24 and 5.75.

Alternative Methods for Confidence Limits

These results are close to those we could have obtained by using the M–H χ^2 (Equation 5-23) for these data. If we omit the reduction by $\frac{1}{2}$ in the numerator of Equation 5-23 before it is squared, the results using Equation 5-23 are identical to those using Equation 5-25. The M–H χ^2 for matched data with more than one control per case or a varying number of controls per case can be computed in the same way as illustrated on pages 117–19 for unmatched data. For example, beginning with Table 5-14 but remembering that we have 11 sets (i.e., 11 tables) with identical data to Table 5-14:

$$\sum (a) = 11(1) = 11.000$$

$$\sum E(a) = 11(1)(1/3) = 3.667$$

$$\sum \text{var}(a) = 11(1)(1/3)(2/3)(3 - 1)/(3 - 1) = 2.444$$

Adding to these the $\sum (a)$, $\sum E(a)$, and $\sum \text{var}(a)$ values from Tables 5-15, 5-16, and 5-17 we get the totals

$$\sum (a) = 20.00$$

$$\sum E(a) = 16.67$$

$$\sum \text{var}(a) = 8.00$$

Calculating the M–H χ^2 but without the $\frac{1}{2}$ correction we have

$$\chi^2 = (20 - 16.67)^2/8 = 1.39$$

This corresponds exactly to $z = 1.18$ or $z^2 = 1.39$ as on page 127. If we use the $\frac{1}{2}$ reduction recommended by M–H the results are different.

When the data include varying numbers of controls per case, the method of test-based limits using the M–H χ^2 compares favorably with alternatives that are either more difficult to compute or more difficult to explain. Confidence limits on the odds ratio for odds of endometrial cancer, comparing those exposed to conjugated estrogen to those not exposed, are reported by Fleiss [1984]. He analyzes data on matched controls with 4 matched sets having 3 controls per case and 55 sets having 4 controls per case. The M–H summary odds ratio for these data is 5.75. Estimated 95% confidence limits reported by Fleiss together with test-based limits using the M–H χ^2 are:

	.95 Confidence limits
Method proposed by Fleiss	2.73–12.1
Method of maximum likelihood	2.76–11.1
Test-based limits using M–H	2.94–11.2

The test-based limits using the M–H χ^2 are in close agreement with the maximum likelihood procedure [Murphy 1982] which can be considered a "gold standard." We have not discussed it in this text because it is difficult to explain in elementary terms. Simpler methods often provide excellent approximations, as in this instance.

Efficiency of Multiple Controls

In considering the value of multiple controls per case, it is useful to keep in mind that the essential component of a case-control study is the comparison of cases to controls with respect to the proportion having the risk factor. How effective multiple controls are in increasing the precision of this comparison is suggested by the following discussion.

Under the null hypothesis the proportion of cases with the risk factor equals the proportion of controls with the risk factor. If this proportion is P_0, the variance of the difference between cases and controls is

$$\frac{P_0 Q_0}{n_{cases}} + \frac{P_0 Q_0}{n_{controls}}$$

Table 5-18. Ratio of Standard Error of Difference Between p_{case} and $p_{control}$, Comparing n Cases and nk Controls with n Cases and n Controls

Controls per case (k)	$\dfrac{\text{SE}(p_{n\ cases} - p_{nk\ controls})}{\text{SE}(p_{n\ cases} - p_{n\ controls})}$
1	1.00
2	.87
3	.82
4	.79
5	.77

Suppose that the sample size for controls is K times as large as that for cases, so that

$$\text{var}(p_{cases} - p_{controls}) = \frac{P_0 Q_0}{n} + \frac{P_0 Q_0}{Kn} = \frac{(K+1)}{K}\left(\frac{P_0 Q_0}{n}\right)$$

and

$$\text{SE}(p_{cases} - p_{controls}) = \left[\frac{K+1}{K}\left(\frac{P_0 Q_0}{n}\right)\right]^{1/2}$$

If we use the standard error of the difference in p between cases and controls as a basis for comparison and compute the ratio

$$\frac{\text{SE based on } K \text{ controls per case}}{\text{SE based on one control per case}}$$

we can see how much the standard error is decreased with increasing number of controls ($2n$, $3n$, etc.). This is shown in Table 5-18. It is obvious that there is little gain in precision, i.e., reduction of $\text{SE}(p_{cases} - p_{controls})$, after $K = 2$. Values of K larger than 2 are probably not warranted unless control data are available at essentially no cost.

AN ADDITIONAL ODDS RATIO ADVANTAGE

In Chapter 3 we stated that, unlike the relative risk, the odds ratio was equally informative whether the analysis was based on events or nonevents. We now identify an additional advantage and begin by quoting Nathan Mantel. "Unless risks are sufficiently small, it may not be meaningful to speak of a *common relative risk*" (personal communication, October 4, 1987). Suppose that data have been classified into several strata with a common relative risk of 2.50. This common relative risk could apply to strata with risks of .02 and .05, or .10 and .25. But for a stratum with a risk of .45 for those without the risk factor, an *RR* of 2.50 is necessarily imaginary. Any odds ratio, even one as large as 100/1, can be doubled, but risk is limited to certainty which is numerically 1.00. If risks are low, the odds ratio provides a good estimate of the relative risk, but whether or not risks are low, it is possible for a common odds ratio to exist and the sample summary odds ratio adjusted for confounding estimates the population odds ratio.

APPLICATION TO FRAMINGHAM HEART STUDY DATA

In this chapter we continue applying the methods described on Appendix data to estimate the association of systolic blood pressure with the risk of developing coronary heart disease. We will estimate this association after adjusting for, i.e., after removing or reducing, the confounding effects of age and sex. In Chapter 9, which will provide an overall comparison of methods taught in this book, we will also remove (1) the confounding effects of sex and blood pressure on the association of age with coronary disease and (2) the confounding effects of age and blood pressure on the association of sex with coronary disease. At the start it is important to investigate whether these variables are, in fact, confounders of each other's relationship to coronary heart disease. As stated earlier in this chapter, for all practical purposes a confounder must be related to the disease *and* to the risk factor under study after adjustment for all other risk factors under consideration. The Appendix data with regard to these relationships are summarized in Tables 5-19 to 5-22 inclusive for the population at risk.

Table 5-19. Eighteen-Year Risk of Coronary Heart Disease by Age and Sex

Sex	Age			
	45–49	50–54	55–59	60–62
Men	.22	.24	.30	.32
Women	.09	.14	.21	.19

Table 5-20. Average Systolic Blood Pressure at Exam 1 by Age and Sex

Sex	Age			
	45–49	50–54	55–59	60–62
Men	140	143	147	149
Women	143	153	157	158

Table 5-21. Percentage Distribution of Age by Sex

Sex	Total	Age			
		45–49	50–54	55–59	60–62
Men	100.0	32.5	31.2	27.4	8.9
Women	100.0	32.1	31.8	28.7	7.4

Table 5-22. Percentage Distribution of Age–Sex Categories by Blood Pressure Group

Blood pressure	Total	Age of men				Age of women			
		45–49	50–54	55–59	60–62	45–49	50–54	55–59	60–62
SBP $\geq$ 165	100.0	8.8	11.8	11.8	3.4	14.2	20.6	23.3	6.1
SBP < 165	100.0	17.2	15.6	13.2	4.4	17.7	15.7	12.9	3.3

Table 5-19 demonstrates that age is related to risk independently of sex and that sex is related to risk independently of age. Table 5-20 shows that age and sex are related to systolic blood pressure independently of each other. However, as shown by Table 5-21, in these data the age distribution is almost identical for each sex. If we were to adjust the crude risk factor estimates by sex for age differences or the crude risk factor estimates by age for sex differences we would expect essentially no change.

Adjustment for age and sex on the association of blood pressure with disease will change the crude results to the extent that the age–sex distribution is different in the two blood pressure groups being compared. Table 5-22 shows a modest difference in age–sex distribution between those with systolic blood pressure of 165 or higher and those with systolic pressure under 165.

Adjustment for potential confounding by age and sex of the association between systolic blood pressure measured on examination 1 ($\geq$165/ <165) and 18-year risk of coronary heart disease can be based upon the data in Table 5-23.

Direct and Indirect Standardization

The summary data in Table 5-24 were obtained as follows. The unadjusted risks are taken directly from the total line of Table 5-23 and their ratio is the relative risk. If the crude risks for each blood pressure category are designated as p_1 and p_2, then the odds ratio is $(p_1/1 - p_1)/(p_2/1 - p_2)$

The direct adjustment risks for each blood pressure category are $\sum w_i p_i / \sum w_i$ where p_i is the age–sex specific risk and w_i is the age–sex specific standard population. From Table 5-23 we see that for the

Table 5-23. Worksheet for Direct Adjustment for Age and Sex

| Age–sex category | | Coronary heart disease 18-year incidence rates | | Standard population | |
		SBP $\geqslant$ 165 (x_1/n_1)	SBP $<$ 165 (x_2/n_2)	Combined $(n_1 + n_2)$	Inversely proportional to variance $(n_1 n_2)/(n_1 + n_2)$
Men	45–49	9/26(.346)	36/183(.197)	209	(26)(183)/(26 + 183) = 22.8
	50–54	14/35(.400)	35/166(.211)	201	(35)(166)/(35 + 166) = 28.9
	55–59	16/35(.457)	36/141(.255)	176	(35)(141)/(35 + 141) = 28.0
	60–62	5/10(.500)	13/47(.277)	57	(10)(47)/(10 + 47) = 8.2
Women	45–49	7/42(.167)	13/189(.069)	231	(42)(189)/(42 + 189) = 34.4
	50–54	16/61(.262)	15/168(.089)	229	(61)(168)/(61 + 168) = 44.8
	55–59	25/69(.362)	18/138(.130)	207	(69)(138)/(69 + 138) = 46.0
	60–62	3/18(.167)	7/35(.200)	53	(18)(35)/(18 + 35) = 11.9
Total (crude)		95/296(.321)	173/1067(.162)	1363	Sum of weights = 225.0

combined standard $w_i = 209, 201 \ldots 53$ and for the standard inversely proportional to variance, $w_i = 22.8, 28.9 \ldots 11.9$.

The combined rates used in indirect adjustment are $(9 + 36)/209$ for men aged 45–49, $(14 + 35)/201$ for men aged 50–54 etc. For each blood pressure category and age–sex group, multiplying the combined rate by the number at risk provides the expected number of cases. Dividing the total observed cases by the total expected cases we get the standardized morbidity ratio ($S\hat{M}R$) for each blood pressure group. Multiplying the SMRs by the crude rate in the standard population produces the indirect standardized rate. As stated previously, it is not correct to compare these rates, but as can be seen in Table 5-24 the relative risks and odds ratios obtained from indirectly adjusted rates are quite similar to those found using direct adjustment.

Table 5-24. Comparing Risk or Odds of Disease for SBP of 165 or More to Risk or Odds of Disease for SBP of Less than 165 Using Different Methods of Adjustment

Based on	Relative risk	Odds ratio
Crude rates	(.321/.162) = 1.98	(.321/.679)/(.162/.838) = 2.45
Direct adjustment		
Combined standard	(.326/.160) = 2.04	(.326/.674)/(.160/.840) = 2.54
Standard proportional		
to inverse variance	(.322/.154) = 2.09	(.322/.678)/(.154/.846) = 2.61
Indirect adjustment		
Using combined rates	(.327/.162) = 2.02	(.327/.673)/(.162/.838) = 2.51

Table 5-25.[a] Systolic Blood Pressure and Coronary Heart Disease

Age–sex category	Systolic blood pressure	Cases	Negatives	Total
Men 45–49	SBP ⩾ 165	9(a)	**17(b)**	26
	SBP < 165	36(c)	**147(d)**	183
Total				209
Men 50–54	SBP ⩾ 165	14(a)	**21(b)**	35
	SBP < 165	35(c)	**131(d)**	166
Total				201

[a] Derived from Table 5-23.

Mantel–Haenszel Procedure

The coronary heart disease incidence data on each line of Table 5-23 can be expressed as a 2×2 table as shown in Table 5-25 for the first two lines of Table 5-23. The boldface numbers in Table 5-25 are not reported in Table 5-23 but are easily derived by subtraction. The a–b–c–d labels are the ones we have used throughout this chapter. The Mantel–Haenszel odds ratio for Table 5-23 data is equal to $(\sum a_i d_i / t_i)/(\sum b_i c_i / t_i)$. Using the arrangement of data in Table 5-25 this is $[(9)(147)/209 + (14)(131)/201 + \cdots]/[(17)(36)/209 + (21)(35)/201 + \cdots] = 2.69$.

Woolf's Method

The 2×2 tables outlined in Table 5-25 for the Mantel–Haenszel procedure can be summarized in terms of $\ln \hat{OR}_i$. Each $\ln \hat{OR}_i$ can then be weighted by the inverse of its estimated variance, which is $(1/a_i + 1/b_i + 1/c_i + 1/d_i)^{-1}$. Then $\ln \hat{OR} = \sum w_i \ln OR_i / \sum w_i$ and $\hat{OR} = e^{\ln \hat{OR}}$. For Table 5-23 data, $\hat{OR}$ by Woolf's method $= 2.71$. Testing the $\ln \hat{OR}_i$ for homogeneity (i.e., absence of interaction) we get a homogeneity χ^2 of 4.36 with 7 degrees of freedom ($p > .5$). Thus, there is nothing unusual in the variation among the eight $\ln \hat{OR}_i$ for age–sex categories and we lack evidence of interaction.

As is not uncommon, the adjustments shown in Table 5-26 have not produced any major changes. However, all slightly increase the estimated relative risk or odds ratio associated with comparing SBP ⩾ 165 to SBP < 165.

EXERCISES

Ex. 5-1. Using the age–sex specific rates for the two blood pressure categories in Table 5-23, select a standard population other than (a) the

Table 5-26. Association of Systolic Blood Pressure with Coronary Heart Disease after Adjustment for Age and Sex, Overview of Results Using Chapter 5 Methods

Method of adjustment	RR	OR
	(SBP $\geq$ 165/SBP $<$ 165)	
Unadjusted	1.98	2.45
Direct adjustment (combined population)	2.04	2.54
Direct adjustment (population inversely $\propto$ to variance)	2.09	2.61
Indirect adjustment (combined rate as standard)[a]	2.02	2.51
Mantel–Haenszel procedure	—	2.69
Woolf's method	—	2.71

[a] Technically incorrect to compare blood pressure categories. See text.

combined population or (b) the population inversely proportional to the variance between specific rates. Use census data, Appendix Table A-3, or any alternative source of population data available to you. Although this book recommends that the standard population be reasonably related to the study group, for purposes of this exercise do not restrict your choice in any way. For example you might choose the United States population in 1940 or the population of England and Wales in 1900. Calculate a relative risk for the two blood pressure categories after direct adjustment using the standard population selected. Are the results fairly close to those in Table 5-24? If so, why? If not, why not? If the standard population selected gives more weight to women aged 60–62 than does either of the weighting systems in Table 5-23, what result might be expected? Why?

Ex. 5-2. The data in Table 5-23 can be rearranged as follows:

Pressure–age category		Coronary heart disease 18-year incidence rates		Standard population	
		Men (x_1/n_1)	Women (x_2/n_2)	Combined $(n_1 + n_2)$	Inversely proportional to variance $(n_1 n_2)/(n_1 + n_2)$
SBP $<$ 165	45–49	36/183(.197)	13/189(.069)	372	$(183)(189)/(183 + 189) = 93.0$
	50–54	35/166(.211)	15/168(.089)	334	$(166)(168)/(166 + 168) = 83.5$
	55–69	36/141(.255)	18/138(.130)	279	$(141)(138)/(141 + 138) = 69.7$
	60–62	13/47(.277)	7/35(.200)	82	$(47)(35)/(47 + 35) = 20.1$
SBP $\geq$ 165	45–49	9/26(.346)	7/42(.167)	68	$(26)(42)/(26 + 42) = 16.1$
	50–54	14/35(.400)	16/61(.262)	96	$(35)(61)/(35 + 61) = 22.2$
	55–59	16/35(.457)	25/69(.362)	104	$(35)(69)/(35 + 69) = 23.2$
	60–62	5/10(.500)	3/18(.167)	28	$(10)(18)/(10 + 18) = 6.4$
Total (crude)		164/643(.255)	104/720(.144)	1363	Sum of weights = 334.2

Calculate the relative risk and or odds ratio (of disease) comparing men to women and using:

a. Unadjusted data
b. Direct standardization—combined population
c. Direct standardization—population inversely $\propto$ to variance
d. Indirect standardization—using combined rates
e. Mantel–Haenszel procedure
f. Woolf's method

Do the adjusted comparisons differ from the crude comparison? Do the different methods of adjustment show important differences in results?

Ex. 5-3. The following summary compares risk of coronary disease among those aged 55 and over to those under age 50. It was obtained from Table 5-23 by combining ages 55–59 and 60–62 and omitting individuals age 50–54.

Sex–pressure category	Coronary heart disease 18-year incidence rates		Standard population	
	Age ≥ 55 (x_1/n_1)	Age < 50 (x_2/n_2)	Combined $(n_1 + n_2)$	Inversely proportional to variance $(n_1 n_2)/(n_1 + n_2)$
Men				
SBP < 165	49/188(.261)	36/183(.197)	371	$(188)(183)/(188 + 183) = 92.7$
SBP ≥ 165	21/45(.467)	9/26(.346)	71	$(45)(26)/(45 + 26) = 16.5$
Women				
SBP < 165	25/173(.145)	13/189(.069)	362	$(173)(189)/(173 + 189) = 90.3$
SBP ≥ 165	28/87(.322)	7/42(.167)	129	$(87)(42)/(87 + 42) = 28.3$
Total (crude)	123/493(.249)	65/440(.148)	933	Sum of weights = 227.8

Comparing age 55 and over to under age 50, calculate (a) to (f) as outlined for Exercise 5-2. Comment on the change from crude comparison to adjusted comparison and on the degree of equivalence among various methods of adjustment.

Ex. 5-4. Use the Appendix listing to count the number in each cell of the following 2×2 tables for men aged 55–59. The Appendix summaries can help reduce the labor of counting.

	Incidence cases			Incidence cases	
SBP ≥ 165	+	−	SBP < 165	+	+
FRW ≥ 120	——	——	FRW ≥ 120	——	——
FRW < 120	——	——	FRW < 120	——	——

a. calculate the M–H summary odds ratio comparing FRW ≥ 120 to FRW < 120 as to the development of coronary disease after adjustment for the possible confounding effect of systolic blood pressure. Use the M–H χ^2 and Miettinen's test-based procedure to estimate .95 confidence limits on *OR*.

b. Estimate the summary odds ratio using Woolf's method for the estimate of *OR* and .95 confidence limits on it.

c. Compare your results from (a) and (b) and comment on them.

NOTES

* Matching can also be accomplished by considering age within ±x years, where the value of x depends upon the judgment of the investigator, i.e., matching within an age group.

† Those sets with the case and both controls alike as to presence of the risk factor contribute nothing to the value of z. They simply add zero to both numerator and denominator. The constant value of $(a_i + b_i)(1 + K - a_i - b_i) = 2$ for all relevant case-control sets is a peculiarity of Equation 5-25 for $K = 2$.

6

Adjustment Using Multiple Linear Regression and Multiple Logistic Functions

REVIEW OF SIMPLE LINEAR REGRESSION

The notation throughout this chapter refers to sample data and sample statistics unless specifically stated otherwise.

The simple linear regression equation

$$\hat{y} = a + bx \tag{6-1}$$

describes a linear relationship between x and y in which, for each unit increase in x, the estimated value of y increases on the average by b units and in which $\hat{y} = a$ when $x = 0$. For relevance to epidemiologic investigation, we shall assume that values of x and y are derived from a sample of individuals.

The specific numeric values of a and b are derived from the data by the method of least squares. The least-squares a and b values are those for which $\sum (y_j - \hat{y}_j)^2$ is a minimum, where $\hat{y}_j$ is the computed value of $a + bx_j$ for the jth individual and y_j is the actual value of y for the jth individual. Discussion of simple and multiple linear regression as well as formulas for regression coefficients and their standard error is available in most statistics texts [Draper and Smith 1981, Snedecor and Cochran 1980].

MULTIPLE LINEAR REGRESSION COEFFICIENTS

Because b relates to the association of change in y with change in x, epidemiologists are usually more interested in b than in a, and we now investigate the meaning of b_1 and b_2 in a multiple regression equation in which coefficients have been determined by the method of least squares:

$$\hat{y} = a + b_1 x_1 + b_2 x_2 \tag{6-2}$$

It is often stated that b_1 reflects the relationship between x_1 and y when x_2 is "held constant." We have always felt this to be somewhat lacking in clarity, and we hope the following explanation will be an improvement. To clearly distinguish that a and b in the simple regression equations below are not necessarily the same as the a, b_1, and b_2 in Equation 6-2, we shall use $a'b'$, $a''b''$, etc., to distinguish them.

We can calculate simple linear least-squares regression coefficients between y and x_2 and then estimate y as follows:

$$\hat{y} = a' + b'x_2 \tag{6-3}$$

We can similarly calculate simple linear least-squares regression coefficients between x_1 and x_2 and then estimate x_1 as follows:

$$\hat{x}_1 = a'' + b''x_2 \tag{6-4}$$

Using Equation 6-3, we can then calculate, for each individual, the discrepancy between the observed value of y and the value of $\hat{y}$ computed on the basis of the linear relationship with x_2. Using Equation 6-4, we can also calculate, for each individual, the discrepancy between the observed value of x_1 and the value of $\hat{x}_1$ computed on the basis of the linear relationship with x_2. For the jth individual, these two discrepancies are

$$y_j - \hat{y}_{j(x_2)}$$
$$x_{1j} - \hat{x}_{1j(x_2)}$$

where $\hat{y}_{j(x_2)}$ represents an estimated value for y_j derived from the linear regression of y on x_2 and $\hat{x}_{1j(x_2)}$ represents an estimated value for x_{1j} derived from the linear regression of x_1 on x_2. Now, if we compute simple linear regression coefficients between the portion of y *not* linearly related to x_2 and the portion of x_1 *not* linearly related to x_2, i.e., between

$$y - \hat{y}_{(x_2)} \quad \text{and} \quad x_1 - \hat{x}_{1(x_2)}$$

we obtain least-squares simple regression coefficients a''' and b''' for the equation:

$$y - \hat{y}_{(x_2)} = a''' + b'''[x_1 - \hat{x}_{1(x_2)}] \tag{6-5}$$

Understanding of the meaning of coefficients in multiple regression equations is improved by realizing that b''' in Equation 6-5 is *exactly* equal to b_1 in Equation 6-2. the point to be emphasized is that in an equation such as

$$\hat{y} = a + b_1 x_1 + b_2 x_2 + b_2 x_3 \tag{6-6}$$

b_1 indicates the average increase in y for a unit change in x_1 *after* the linear association with x_2 and x_3 has been removed from *both* x_1 and y. Similarly, b_2 indicates the average increase in y for a unit change in x_2 *after* linear association with x_1 and x_3 has been removed from *both* x_2 and y, etc. Thus, this method can be used to adjust for several confounding factors simultaneously. More generally, in multiple linear regression equations, the regression coefficient for x_i indicates an average change in y for a unit change in x_i after their linear association with all other x variables has been removed from both y and x_i.

Note that Equation 6-6 implies the absence of interaction among the x variables. If in fact interaction is important—for example, the change in y for a unit change in x_1 is quite different depending on whether x_2 is large or small—the agreement, or fit, of Equation 6-6 with the data is necessarily adversely affected. Under these conditions, the fit of the model (equation) to the data could be improved by adding a cross-product term, $b_4 x_1 x_2$, to Equation 6-6. When interaction is present it is better to present stratified calculations rather than coefficients of cross-product terms. If a cross-product term improved the fit of the data to the model, e.g., if the blood pressure relationship to coronary disease was different for young and for old, it would be easy to comprehend in terms of regression coefficients for blood pressure that were separately calculated for young and for old and seen to be different. Reporting that the coefficient of the variable age times blood pressure was large or significant or both does not convey nearly as much information.

Table 6-1 presents data for the systolic blood pressures, ages, and weights of 15 individuals taken from a large epidemiologic study. These will be used to illustrate the relationship between simple and multiple linear regression.

Table 6-2 presents, for each of the 15 individuals listed in Table 6-1, (a) estimates of weight based on a simple linear regression with age, (b) estimates of systolic blood pressure based on a simple linear regression with age, and (c) estimates of systolic blood pressure based on multiple linear regression with age and weight. Alongside each of the estimated values in Table 6-2 is the discrepancy between the estimate and the actual value.

If we now calculate the simple regression between weight after removal of a component linearly related to age (column 2 in Table 6-2) as the independent variable and systolic blood pressure after removal of a component linearly related to age (column 4) as the dependent variable, we get

$$SBP - \hat{SBP} = 0.005 + 0.248(\text{weight} - \hat{\text{weight}})$$

Table 6-1. Data Fragment from a Large Epidemiologic Study

Individual	Systolic blood pressure (mm Hg)	Age (years)	Weight (lb)
1	132	49	145
2	155	56	216
3	130	52	115
4	142	46	170
5	150	57	172
6	128	42	166
7	126	43	164
8	118	45	152
9	180	56	275
10	124	52	221
11	150	42	175
12	134	57	132
13	140	56	188
14	142	56	178
15	128	53	168
Total	2079	762	2637

The important point is that the coefficient of the weight discrepancy in this *simple* regression is identical to the coefficient for weight shown in the *multiple* regression equation at the top of columns 5 and 6 in Table 6-2.

ASSUMPTIONS UNDERLYING MULTIPLE REGRESSION METHODS

To simplify exposition, we summarize the assumptions underlying least squares estimation of multiple regression parameters in terms of the specific model for two X variables:

$$Y = A + B_1 X_1 + B_2 X_2 + e \qquad (6\text{-}7)$$

where A, B_1, and B_2 are population parameters, X_1, X_2, and Y are variables in the population, and e is the difference between the actual Y and that predicted by the model.

Related to the Model Fitting the Data

The first two assumptions to be made are

1. *Linearity* For every pair of X_1 and X_2 values, the mean of the corresponding Y values lies on a flat surface.
2. *No interaction* The effect of changes in X_1 on Y is independent of the level of X_2.

Table 6-2. Simple and Multiple Linear Regression Computations Derived from Table 6-1

Individual	Weight = 80.859 + 1.869(age) (simple regression)		SBP = 81.900 + 1.116(age) (simple regression)		SBP = 61.844 + 0.653 (age) + 0.248 (weight) (multiple regression)	
	Weight estimated from age = $\hat{w}$ (1)	Actual weight − weight estimated from age = $w - \hat{w}$ (2)	SBP estimated from age = $\hat{SBP}$ (3)	Actual SBP − SBP estimated from age = $SBP - \hat{SBP}$ (4)	SBP estimated from age *and* weight = $\hat{SBP}'$ (5)	Actual SBP − SBP estimated from age and weight = $SBP - \hat{SBP}'$ (6)
1	172.4	−27.4	136.6	−4.6	129.8	2.2
2	185.5	30.5	144.4	10.6	152.0	3.0
3	178.0	−63.0	139.9	−9.9	124.3	5.7
4	166.8	3.2	133.2	8.8	134.0	8.0
5	187.4	−15.4	145.5	4.5	141.7	8.3
6	159.4	6.6	128.8	−0.8	130.4	−2.4
7	161.2	2.8	129.9	−3.9	130.6	−4.6
8	165.0	−13.0	132.1	−14.1	128.9	−10.9
9	185.5	89.5	144.4	35.6	166.6	13.4
10	178.0	43.0	139.9	−15.9	150.6	−26.6
11	159.4	15.6	128.8	21.2	132.7	17.3
12	187.4	−55.4	145.5	−11.5	131.8	2.2
13	185.5	2.5	144.4	−4.4	145.0	−5.0
14	185.5	−7.5	144.4	−2.4	142.5	−0.5
15	179.9	−11.9	141.1	−13.1	138.1	−10.1
Total	2636.9	0.1	2078.9	0.1	2079.0	0

Both these assumptions relate to how well the model fits the sample data at hand. The basic method for testing whether they hold (at least approximately) is to examine the error in fit $(y_i - \hat{y}_i)$ for various categories of observed values. Fitting the coefficients by the method of least squares will ensure that $\sum (y_i - \hat{y}_i) = 0$. The question of satisfactory fit relates to whether or not this sum is approximately zero for various subgroups of x values. Systematic errors suggest that the model is inadequate.

For example, suppose that observed x_1 values are grouped in quartiles and that corresponding $y_i - \hat{y}_i$ values are averaged for each quartile. There should be a similar average for each quartile of x_1. Also, $y_i - \hat{y}_i$ differences can be averaged in association with quartiles of all other x variables and with simple cross-classification of x variables. If, for example, the average value of $y_i - \hat{y}_i$ associated with x_1 and x_2 both high is much different from the average when x_1 is high and x_2 low, perhaps the model requires a term for interaction. All that follows in this text with respect to multivariate methods presumes that the model is a reasonably adequate description of the data in the sense that the mean values of the $y_i - \hat{y}_i$ discrepancies are approximately equal (i.e., not far from zero) for various subgroups. Thus, $\sum (y_i - \hat{y}_i)/n$ computed for each of several subgroups representing cross-classifications of the x variables reflects the extent to which the model fits the data within subgroups.

To illustrate this concept, we return to column 6 of Table 6-2, in which are shown $y_i - \hat{y}_i$ values calculated for each individual using a multiple linear regression model. (Table 6-2 uses the specific notation SBP $-$ SBP rather than $y_i - \hat{y}_i$.) As required by the model, the sum of these discrepancies over all individuals equals zero. However, this overall total of zero might be the consequence of large positive discrepancies in most subgroups balanced by very large negative discrepancies in a few others. Under those circumstances we are unlikely to consider the fit adequate.

To investigate this possibility we look at the average of the discrepancies between the model values and the actual values in four subgroups, as shown in Table 6-3. Recalling that actual systolic blood

Table 6-3. Agreement Between Data and Prediction from Multiple Linear Regression Model in Four Age–Weight Subclasses (Based on Tables 6-1 and 6-2)

Age	Weight	n	$\sum (\text{SBP} - \text{SBP}')/n$
<53	<172	6	−0.3
<53	≥172	2	−4.6
≥53	<172	2	−4.0
≥53	≥172	5	+3.8

pressure values ranged from 118 to 180 and considering the substantive meaning of an average systolic blood pressure difference of 4 to 5 mm Hg, we can conclude that the model, in some sense, is similar to the data. Of course, to permit easy verification of the numbers, this trivial example is based on fewer cases than would be included in any real study. However, the principal point being made is that, in addition to appropriate tests of significance, you should look at the average agreement in major subsets of the data and, based on substantive considerations, make a judgment as to adequacy of fit.

At times, the observation of $\sum (y_i - \hat{y}_i)/n$ in various groups suggests ways of improving the model (e.g., adding cross-product terms, such as $x_1 x_2$, or squared terms, such as x_1^2), but if the end result shows one or more major subcategories of data with poor fit, the model is suspect.

Note that the preceding discussion deals exclusively with the extent of the discrepancy between model and data and not with any statistical significance testing to determine whether the decrease in residual error of, say, a four parameter model over a three-parameter model is any greater than what could reasonably be expected by chance alone. This latter point is fully discussed in standard texts [Draper and Smith 1981].

Related to Estimates of Variance and Significance Tests

Adding to our list of assumptions, we have

3. *Independence of observations* Knowledge of the Y value for any individual provides no information about the Y value for any other individual.
4. *Homoscedasticity* For every pair of X_1 and X_2 values, the variance of Y (var e) is a constant.
5. *Normality* For every pair of X_1 and X_2 values, Y is normally distributed.

In epidemiologic studies, assumption 3 is almost always true. If variances are not constant as required by assumption 4, there are methods for weighting the observations so that coefficients and variances can be properly estimated. As the sample statistics b_1 and b_2 are essentially sums, their sampling distribution tends toward normality even when the Y values are not normally distributed as required by assumption 5.

It is beyond the scope of this book to provide the reader with the details of the calculation of least-squares regression coefficients, their estimated standard error, and the many other specifics required for data analysis. Epidemiologists require a general understanding of some multivariate methods, but most need statistical assistance in carrying out the specific analyses required by particular studies.

MULTIPLE REGRESSION FOR CATEGORICAL VARIABLES

Multiple regression methods for categorical data have been described by Feldstein [1966]. They are analogous to directly standardized rates but include the possibility of adjusting for many variables at one time. We begin by assuming that y and all x variables are attributes, i.e., they are dichotomous variables that have the value 1 if the attribute they represent is *present* and the value 0 if it is *absent*. It should be noted that measurement variables can be transformed to attributes, e.g., age $<45 = 0$ and age $\geq 45 = 1$. Thus, the method described here applies both to attributes and to measurement variables that have been transformed to attributes.

If we also assume that each x variable adds a constant amount to y, independent of other x values, the following model might suitably describe the relationship between y_j predicted and a set of x_i values:

$$\hat{y}_j = b_0 + b_1 x_{1j} - b_2 x_{2j} + b_3 + x_{3j} \tag{6-8}$$

For each individual, this does not make too much sense since all the x are either 1 or 0. However, after replacing x with the 1 and 0 values appropriate to each individual and then summing Equation 6-8 over all n individuals, we get

$$\sum_{j=1}^{n} \hat{y}_j = nb_0 + b_1 \sum_{j=1}^{n} x_{1j} + b_2 \sum_{j=1}^{n} x_{2j} + b_3 \sum_{j=1}^{n} x_{3j}$$

If the b are determined by the method of least squares, then $\sum \hat{y}_j = \sum y_j$, that is, the sum of all predicted y_j values equals the sum of all actual y_j values. Substituting $\sum y_j$ for $\sum \hat{y}_j$ and dividing both sides of the equation by n, we get

$$\bar{y} = b_0 + b_1 \bar{x}_1 + b_2 \bar{x}_2 + b_3 \bar{x}_3 \tag{6-9}$$

At this point, it will simplify our discussion of multiple regression for categorical data if we assign to the variables in Equation 6-9 the following meanings from the Israeli Ischemic Heart Disease study sample data used previously:

$y = 1$ if myocardial infarction is present

$y = 0$ if myocardial infarction is absent

$x_1 = 1$ if SBP ≥ 140

$x_1 = 0$ if SBP < 140

$x_2 = 1$ if the individual is aged 40 through 49

$x_2 = 0$ if the individual is not aged 40 through 49

$x_3 = 1$ if the individual is aged 50 through 59

$x_3 = 0$ if the individual is not aged 50 through 59

Recalling that data were presented for individuals age $\geqslant 60$ in the study sample, it may appear that we have neglected to assign a code to this age group, but we have in fact assigned such a code, however. The code for age $\geqslant 60$ is $x_2 = 0$ and $x_3 = 0$, i.e., not 40 to 49 and not 50 to 59. Binary data can be used in this way to code data classified into any number of groups. Because complications arise in solving the regression equations whenever they include perfectly correlated variables, it is necessary to code classification data using one fewer variable than the number of categories. To illustrate with blood pressure, two categories (SBP $\geqslant 140$ and SBP < 140) are coded into one variable, x_1, as shown above. The three age categories require two variables (x_2 and x_3). If we use another variable (x_4) to define age $\geqslant 60$, perfect correlation would exist, in that values for x_2 and x_3 would determine x_4. For example, if x_2 and x_3 were both 0, x_4 would necessarily $= 1$. This perfect correlation is exactly the type referred to above as interfering with the solution to the equations for regression coefficients. Since such a variable would cause trouble and provides no additional information we avoid using it.

Returning to Equation 6-9 with variables as defined, $\bar{y}$ can be interpreted as the crude rate for myocardial infarction prevalence. We can modify this crude rate into various adjusted rates or differences between adjusted rates as follows. Suppose we use the least-squares regression coefficients to determine the prevalence rate for myocardial infarction *if* everyone in the population had SBP $\geqslant 140$, with all other variables unchanged. This would mean that x_1 for every individual is 1 and that the summation of Equation 6-8 over all individuals divided by n would equal

$$\bar{y}_{adj} \text{ (if all SBP} \geqslant 140) = b_0 + b_1 + b_2\bar{x}_2 + b_3\bar{x}_3 \qquad (6\text{-}10)$$

This is identical to Equation 6-9 except that $b_1\bar{x}_1$ has been changed to b_1 (with each individual having $x_1 = 1$, $\bar{x}_1$ will equal 1 and thus $b_1\bar{x}_1$ simply equals b_1). The $\bar{y}_{adj}$ of Equation 6-10 could be compared with another $\bar{y}_{adj}$ in which everyone had SBP < 140 but was otherwise unchanged. The adjusted prevalence rate for SBP < 140 requires that all values of x_1 equal zero. In that event $\bar{x}_1$ would equal 0 and thus $b_1\bar{x}_1$ must also equal 0. Thus, the adjusted prevalence for SBP < 140 is

$$\bar{y}_{adj} \text{ (if all SBP} < 140) = b_0 + 0 + b_2\bar{x}_2 + b_3\bar{x}_3 \qquad (6\text{-}11)$$

Note that the difference between adjusted rates for those with SBP $\geqslant 140$ and SBP < 140 is exactly b_1 and that the effect of possible age differences between those with higher SBP and lower SBP has been eliminated by using the identical age distribution in the estimation of both adjusted rates.

Thus, b_1 is the difference between prevalence rates for myocardial infarction comparing SBP $\geqslant 140$ ($x_1 = 1$) with SBP < 140 ($x_1 = 0$), adjusted for possible age differences between those with higher or lower blood pressure. *In general, b_i may be interpreted as the difference in adjusted rates comparing persons for whom $x_i = 1$ with persons in the reference class for that variable.* For dichotomous variables, the reference class is represented by those for whom $x = 0$. For the age variable with three categories, the reference class is represented by those individuals age $\geqslant 60$ who are included in the equation not explicitly but only indirectly through x_2 and x_3. Those who are *not* 40 to 49 and *not* 50 to 59, i.e., $x_2 = 0$ *and* $x_3 = 0$, are in the reference class for age. Thus, in Equation 6-9, b_2 is the difference in MI prevalence between those 40 to 49 and those 60 and over, adjusted for SBP differences between the two age groups. Similarly, b_3 is the difference in MI prevalence between those 50 to 59 and those 60 and over, adjusted for possible SBP differences between the two groups.

Should we wish to compare adjusted rates for those age 40 to 49 ($x_2 = 1$) and those age 50 to 59 ($x_3 = 1$), i.e., a comparison not involving the reference class age 60 to 69 ($x_2 = 0$ *and* $x_3 = 0$), only $b_2 - b_3$ need be computed. Since b_2 is the difference between age 40 to 49 and the reference age and b_3 is the difference between age 50 to 59 and the reference age, $b_2 - b_3$ is the difference in adjusted rates between age 40 to 49 and age 50 to 59.

Adjusted rates can be calculated for any binary variable in relation to its reference class. This can be done whether the other variables are binary or continuous. If x_1, the variable for SBP in the preceding example, were a continuous variable, the difference in MI prevalence rates between age 40 to 49 and age 60 to 69, adjusted so that the difference in prevalence rates is unaffected by blood pressure differences, would still be exactly equal to b_2. Although the special computational convenience of having differences in adjusted rates represented by regression coefficients applies only to variables expressed in binary form, in other respects multiple regression using continuous variables and binary multiple regression are alike. In either case, the regression coefficient b_i represents the average change in y associated with a unit change in x_i, after adjusting for the linear relationships between all other x variables and x_i and between all other x variables and y. If x_i is a binary variable, then a unit change in x_i represents a change from x_i present to x_i absent (or vice versa). If x_i is a continuous variable, then a unit change in x_i may represent only 1 mm Hg of blood pressure or 1 mg% of serum cholesterol, etc. No matter how x_i is expressed, however, b_i represents the average change in y associated with a unit change in x_i, adjusted for all other x variables included in the regression.

An advantage of the categorization approach is that it avoids assuming any particular form of regression for the variable categorized. For example, if age is categorized into three classes, the middle class coefficient may indicate that middle age adds, on the average, .15 to the rate for the young but the coefficient for the older class may indicate that older age adds nothing to the rate for the young.

DISCRIMINANT FUNCTIONS

Related to multiple linear regression but derived differently is the linear discriminant function. Given two groups, for example, sick (s) and well (w), with several x variables measured in each, we might wish to use the x variables to discriminate between the two groups. For each individual in each group we could form a score $z = b_1 x_1 + b_2 x_2 + b_3 x_3 + \cdots$.

The b values would be the same for every individual in the two groups and would provide a weighted sum of the x values. If more weight is given to those x variables that discriminate well and less weight to those that discriminate poorly, we have a discriminant function. Fisher [1936] solved this problem by finding the b values that maximize the function

$$\frac{|\bar{z}_s - \bar{z}_w|}{\mathrm{var}(\bar{z}_s - \bar{z}_w)} \qquad (6\text{-}12)$$

where $\bar{z}_s$ is the average value of $\sum b_i x_i$ in the sick population and $\bar{z}_w$ its average value in the well population. By choosing the b values that made the difference in average scores as large as possible in relation to the variance of the difference, Fisher obtained the linear discriminant function.

Discrimination using the x variables is generally accomplished by designating some value of z as a separation point, with individuals having values that large or larger classified as belonging to one population and all those with smaller z values classified as belonging to the other population. Obviously, the error in the first classification can be made as small as desired. Simply designate all individuals having the smallest z score obtained, or larger, as members of the sick population. Not a single member of the actual sick population would be missed by this classification rule. However, none of the well individuals would have scores below this cutoff point and the error in classifying well persons would be 100 percent. If the two populations are multivariate normal with the same variance–covariance matrix, for any specific size of error in classifying one category, the discriminant function minimizes the error classifying the other category.

Epidemiologists are usually less interested in actual discrimination between two populations than in interpreting the discriminant function coefficients, e.g., for evaluating the importance of risk factors. Knowledge of the fact that discriminant function coefficients are essentially similar to multiple regression coefficients is helpful in this regard. If the identical data set (with y as a binary variable) is tabulated to obtain multiple regression coefficients a, b_1, b_2, b_3, etc., and also to obtain discriminant function coefficients which, for convenience, we label β_1, β_2, β_3, etc., then the ratio of any two discriminant function coefficients β_i/β_j is exactly equal to the b_i/b_j ratio of the corresponding regression coefficients. This equality shows that discriminant function coefficients reflect the relationship between a particular x variable and y after adjustment for all other variables, as discussed earlier for multiple regression coefficients.

This presentation of multiple regression, including binary variable multiple regression and discriminant functions, is intended to provide some general understanding of these procedures. Techniques for computing coefficients, their estimated standard error, and related matters are outside the scope of this book, and statistical assistance regarding them is recommended [Draper and Smith 1981, Snedecor and Cochran 1980].

MULTIPLE LOGISTIC FUNCTIONS
Original Development

Whenever y is a binary variable, nothing in the method of multiple regression prevents an estimate of y from being less than zero or more than unity. Since the estimated value of y is not defined as a probability, values outside the 0 to 1 range are not impossible or wrong, but neither are they entirely satisfactory as an estimate of a variable that equals zero if the condition is absent and unity if it is present. Although this is an undesirable feature of multiple regression methods applied to dependent binary variables (y), it does not invalidate the method. The key to the usefulness of multiple regression methods is whether the model fits the data. Nevertheless, it clearly would be an improvement in interpreting regression coefficients if estimates of y (when it is a binary variable) would be expressed as probabilities.

This, in addition to other benefits in analysis and interpretation, results if the data are fitted to a multiple logistic function. This function was first used by Cornfield et al [1961] as an estimator of risk when the joint distribution of all the independent variables (i.e., the "x" variables) was multivariate normal with the same variance–covariance matrix for both sick and well populations. For two x variables, the function has the form

$$\hat{y} = \frac{1}{1 + e^{-(\alpha + \beta_1 x_1 + \beta_2 x_2)}} \tag{6-13}$$

Cornfield used this function to estimate the risk of developing coronary heart disease (y) from a knowledge of systolic blood pressure (x_1) and serum cholesterol (x_2). By logarithmic transformation of x_1 and x_2, approximate bivariate normality was achieved for the joint distribution of

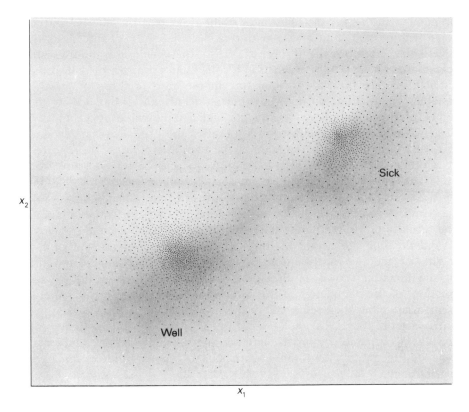

Figure 6-1. Number of persons at each x_1, x_2 point in sick and well populations. Number is indicated as a third dimension rising vertically from the plane of the page.

x_1 and x_2 separately among those developing and those not developing heart disease. The transformed variables also demonstrated approximate equality of the two variance–covariance matrices. The approximately bivariate normal distribution for these two groups is as shown in Figure 6-1, where the height of the distribution above the paper at any "point" represents the number of individuals in the distribution having x_1 and x_2 values intersecting at that point. Although it is not possible to show this clearly in the diagram because both joint distributions are bivariate normal (i.e., for every value of x_1, x_2 is normally distributed and vice versa), all points within the range of x_1 and x_2 values shown in the figure have some representation from each distribution. The risk of developing heart disease for an individual with a specific x_1 and x_2 value can then be expressed as the number in the sick distribution at point x_1, x_2 divided by the total number in both distributions at point x_1, x_2. This total equals the number in the sick distribution at point x_1, x_2 *plus* the number in the well distribution at point x_1, x_2. With this basic definition of risk and with x variables transformed, if necessary, so that they are multivariate normal, the multiple logistic function results as an estimator of risk. If the distributions are bivariate normal (or, in the case of three or more x variables, multivariate normal), it is not a difficult matter to calculate the height of the distribution for any particular joint value of x_1 and x_2. Clearly, this height of the distribution (called the ordinate) is a function of x_1 and x_2 and of the parameters of the two distributions. As reported by Cornfield et al [1961], for relating systolic blood pressure and cholesterol to risk, the parameters for each population, sick and well, are the mean and variance of systolic blood pressure and serum cholesterol, the correlation coefficient between them, and the size of each population. The result obtained by finding the height of each distribution at point x_1, x_2 and dividing the height of the sick distribution by the sum of the heights of the two distributions is what would be obtained from the logistic function shown as Equation 6-13, where α, β_1, and β_2 are functions of the parameters of the two distributions. Since in the general multivariate case, the coefficients of the multiple logistic function require matrix algebra for their complete description, we shall refer to them only as values computable from the number of cases, the mean values and variances of the x_i, and the covariances of the x_i and x_j for each distribution.

It is interesting to note that β_1 and β_2 are exactly equal to the linear discriminant function coefficients that would have resulted from relating x_1 and x_2 to binary y in a linear discriminant function analysis. The parameter α has no parallel in the discriminant analysis and is related to the general level of risk. Particular values of $\sum \beta_i x_i$ for specific individuals raise or lower that general level. The discriminant scores, on the other hand, have no intrinsic meaning as to risk or anything else. Their only interpretation is with reference to being larger or smaller than other scores in the study. Individuals with the largest scores are judged to belong to one group and those with the smallest scores to another.

Cornfield's original derivation of the logistic function as an estimator of risk depended on multivariate normality of the x variables within both sick and well populations, together with equal variances and covariances in the two populations. This latter point is necessary or else the logistic function would have to contain terms involving products of x variables such as $\beta_3 x_1 x_2$. The need for product terms to obtain a satisfactory fit between model and data suggests the presence of interaction. In practice, logistic functions are usually calculated without these product terms and the terms are added only if the model fits the data significantly better with their addition. Of course, whenever a priori knowledge points to the presence of interaction between variables, product terms should be included.

Range Equals the Range for Probability

Because this function is one that increases only with increasing values of $\alpha + \sum \beta_i x_i$, we can demonstrate that the y_i values computed from the logistic function have the property required of probabilities. To show that they are limited to the range zero to unity inclusive, we can substitute $+\infty$ and $-\infty$ for $\alpha + \sum \beta_i x_i$ in Equation 6-13. Since $\alpha + \sum \beta_i x_i$ cannot be larger or smaller than these limits, the resultant values of the function are

for $\alpha + \sum \beta_i x_i = +\infty$:

$$\hat{y} = \frac{1}{1 + e^{-\infty}} = \frac{1}{1 + 0} = 1$$

for $\alpha + \sum \beta_i x_i = -\infty$:

$$\hat{y} = \frac{1}{1 + e^{\infty}} = 0$$

To complement these calculations, we also solve for $\hat{y}$ if $\alpha + \sum \beta_i x_i = 0$. In that case,

$$\hat{y} = \frac{1}{1 + e^{-0}} = \frac{1}{1 + 1} = \frac{1}{2}$$

Thus, if the exponent of e is very large and positive the risk is close to unity, if the exponent of e is zero the risk is $\frac{1}{2}$, and if the exponent of e is very large and negative the risk is close to zero.

Evaluating Fit of Model to the Data

Up to this point, the multiple logistic function has been derived from the multivariate normal distribution of the x variables in both sick and well populations. However, the real world is rarely multivariate normal, nor is it always possible to transform variables so that multivariate normality results. For example, binary variables cannot possibly be transformed to normal. Nevertheless, it has been found that the logistic function fits the data in a variety of circumstances in which the distribution of the x variables is surely not multivariate normal [Truett et al 1967, Halperin et al 1971, Kahn et al 1971]. The fit of the logistic function to the data can be assessed rather simply in accord with the principles* outlined earlier in this chapter and illustrated in the following procedure for a function with three x variables.

1. Calculate $\hat{y}_j$ for each individual in the study by using α and the β_1, β_2, and β_3 values from the multiple logistic function for every individual,

together with the specific values of x_1, x_2, and x_3 relevant to each individual.

2. Array the $\hat{y}_j$ values in order of size.
3. Divide the array of step 2 into quartiles, quintiles, deciles, or some other grouping.
4. Add up the $\hat{y}_j$ values within each group and compare the sum with the sum of the actual y_j values in that group. The sum of the $\hat{y}_j$ equals the number of cases expected according to the model, and the sum of the y_j equals the number of cases actually observed.

For technical reasons these observed and expected values cannot always be summarized ($\sum [(O - E)^2/E]$) into the ordinary goodness-of-fit χ^2 value [Tsiatis 1980], but a good sense of agreement or lack of it can usually be obtained by inspection. An illustration of this procedure for checking fit using data from Kahn et al [1971] is shown as Table 6-4. In this instance the $\hat{y}_j$ values (probability of becoming diabetic) were arrayed in order from smallest to largest and then grouped into quartiles. The agreement between observed cases and expected cases (i.e., the sum of the probabilities of becoming a case) is quite satisfactory. For a review of methods to evaluate goodness of fit, see Lemeshow and Hosmer [1982].

The observation that the multiple logistic risk function often fits rather well to data that are obviously not normal has an explanation. Although the distribution of the x variables in multivariate normal fashion is sufficient to define risk according to the multiple logistic function, it is not necessary. Univariate normality of the sum $\alpha + \sum \beta_i x_i$ also leads to definition of risk according to the multiple logistic function [Truett et al 1967].

Table 6-4. Evaluating Fit of Multiple Logistic Risk Function to Data by Comparing Diabetes Cases Observed with Cases Predicted by Risk Function[a]

Percentile of risk function array	Diabetes incidence cases	
	Number of observed ($\sum y_i$)	Number expected according to multiple logistic risk function ($\sum \hat{y}_j$)
0–24	10	10.5
25–49	23	19.5
50–74	28	31.3
75–100	70	72.1

[a] Kahn et al [1971].

Current Approach for Obtaining Coefficients

An alternative approach with respect to fittng the multiple logistic function, which is the one in current use, is to assume that the risk function is multiple logistic and to determine the coefficients by methods analogous to the least-squares fit of a nonlinear function [Walker and Duncan 1967]. The assumption that multiple logistic is the correct form of the risk function is in some way equivalent to the assumptions about the form of the multivariate distribution of the x variables. The least-squares regression approach does lead to different estimates of the coefficients, although these are frequently quite similar to the discriminant approach [Halperin et al 1971, Kahn et al 1971].

Interpreting Coefficients as Odds Ratios

In addition to providing an estimate of y_i that is interpretable as a probability, another desirable feature of the multiple logistic function is that each of the β_i can be interpreted as the logarithm of an odds ratio relating disease to the variable x_i, after adjustment for all other x variables. We demonstrate this first for a binary variable, $x_1 = 1$ or 0, in a function with three x variables:

$$\hat{y} = \text{estimated probability of event} = 1/(1 + e^{-(\alpha + \beta_1 x_1 + \beta_2 x_2 + \beta_3 x_3)})$$

$$1 - \hat{y} = \text{estimated probability of no event}$$

$$= 1 - [1/(1 + e^{-(\alpha + \beta_1 x_1 + \beta_2 x_2 + \beta_3 x_3)})]$$

$$= \frac{1 + e^{-(\alpha + \beta_1 x_1 + \beta_2 x_2 + \beta_3 x_3)}}{1 + e^{-(\alpha + \beta_1 x_1 + \beta_2 x_2 + \beta_3 x_3)}} - \frac{1}{1 + e^{-(\alpha + \beta_1 x_1 + \beta_2 x_2 + \beta_3 x_3)}}$$

$$= \frac{e^{-(\alpha + \beta_1 x_1 + \beta_2 x_2 + \beta_3 x_3)}}{1 + e^{-(\alpha + \beta_1 x_1 + \beta_2 x_2 + \beta_3 x_3)}}$$

By dividing the probability of an event by the probability of no event, we get the odds of the event. To illustrate this with numeric data, suppose that the probability of an event is 3 out of 10 and the probability of its not happening is 7 out of 10. If we divide the probability of occurrence (3/10) by the probability of nonoccurrence (7/10), we get 3/7. This is the odds that the event will occur. Returning to the logistic function, the estimated odds of an event are

$$\frac{\hat{y}}{1 - \hat{y}} = \frac{1}{e^{-(\alpha + \beta_1 x_1 + \beta_2 x_2 + \beta_3 x_3)}} = e^{\alpha + \beta_1 x_1 + \beta_2 x_2 + \beta_3 x_3} \qquad (6\text{-}14)$$

The relative odds of an event (odds ratio), which compares those for whom x_1 is present ($x_1 = 1$) with those for whom x_1 is absent ($x_1 = 0$) is

$$\text{odds ratio} = \frac{e^{\alpha + \beta_1 + \beta_2 x_2 + \beta_3 x_3}}{e^{(\alpha + 0 + \beta_2 x_2 + \beta_3 x_3)}}$$

$$= e^{(\alpha + \beta_1 + \beta_2 x_2 + \beta_3 x_3) - (\alpha + 0 + \beta_2 x_2 + \beta_3 x_3)}$$

$$= e^{\beta_1}$$

Thus,

$$\ln \text{ odds ratio} = \beta_1 \qquad (6\text{-}15)$$

If, for example, x_1 relates to the presence or absence of diabetes and y to the probability of developing a myocardial infarction, then e^{β_1}, the antilog of β_1, provides the ratio of odds of myocardial infarction for those with diabetes present to the odds for those with diabetes absent. As in the case of multiple linear regression, β_1 is adjusted for linear association with other x variables. However, keep in mind that the function $\alpha + \beta_1 x_1 + \beta_2 x_2 + \beta_3 x_3$ is linear not in probabilities but in the natural logarithm of the odds that an event will occur.

If x_1 were a continuous variable, the derivation shown above for x_1 as a binary variable would lead to β_1 as the natural logarithm of the odds ratio relating the odds of developing the disease to a one-unit increase in x_1 (e.g., comparing $x_1 = 150$ to $x_1 = 149$). If we wanted an odds ratio related to a 10- or 20-unit increase in x_1, we would begin the derivation with Equation 6-14:

$$\text{odds of event to no event} = e^{\alpha + \beta_1 x_1 + \beta_2 x_2 + \beta_3 x_3}$$

odds ratio comparing those with $x_1 = K + 10$ to those with $x_1 = K$

$$= \frac{e^{\alpha + \beta_1(10 + K) + \beta_2 x_2 + \beta_3 x_3}}{e^{\alpha + \beta_1 K + \beta_2 x_2 + \beta_3 x_3}}$$

$$= e^{\alpha + 10\beta_1 + \beta_1 K + \beta_2 x_2 + \beta_3 x_3 - (\alpha + \beta_1 K + \beta_2 x_2 + \beta_3 x_3)}$$

$$= e^{10\beta_1}$$

$$\ln \text{ odds ratio} = 10\beta_1$$

Thus, we see that the natural logarithm of the odds ratio comparing two different values of x_1 equals β_1 multiplied by the difference in those x_1 values.

In all cases, the natural logarithm of the odds ratio (β_i) relating x_i to odds of disease has been adjusted for linear relationships as discussed in the section on multiple linear regression. Although the multiple logistic function coefficients are nonlinear with respect to *probability* of risk, the *ln odds* equation is exactly analogous to multiple linear regression:

$$\text{ln odds} = \ln\left(\frac{\hat{y}}{1-\hat{y}}\right) = \alpha + \beta_1 x_1 + \beta_2 x_2 + \beta_3 x_3 \qquad (6\text{-}16)$$

Comparison to Mantel–Haenszel Summary Odds Ratio

To illustrate the essential equivalence between adjusted odds ratios computed using the multiple logistic function and those computed using the M–H procedure, we refer to Table 6-5. These data are from a study of serologic markers of hepatitis B among Italian navy recruits [Pasquini et al 1983]. Only two of the nine variables in Table 6-5 show adjusted odds ratio differences of any consequence. These are region of residence, 1.67 versus 1.42, and multiple injection scars, 3.51 versus 2.99. In each of these instances, the odds ratio derived from multiple logistic analysis is larger. The fit of the data to the logistic model, determined as in Table 6-4, is entirely satisfactory. However, failure to find a difference between the actual data and the data predicted by a model does not, of course, establish the model as correct, and the calculation of the multiple logistic coefficients depends upon the correctness of the model as a reflection of risk. The M–H results, however, depend only on a reasonable implicit

Table 6-5. Adjusted Odds Ratios for Presence of Serologic Markers of Hepatitis B among Italian Navy Recruits[a]

Variable	Adjustment by multiple logistic analysis[b]	Adjustment by M–H procedure
Age (>19/≤19)	.77	.79
Number of siblings (>3/≤3)	1.58	1.62
Region of birth $\left(\dfrac{\text{southern Italy or islands}}{\text{northern or central Italy}}\right)$	1.50	1.40
Region of residence $\left(\dfrac{\text{southern Italy or islands}}{\text{northern or central Italy}}\right)$	1.67	1.42
Education level (above elementary/elementary)	.62	.62
Altitude of residence $\left(\dfrac{\text{hills or mountains}}{\text{lowlands}}\right)$	.77	.78
History of jaundice (yes/no)	1.71	1.66
History of intravenous injection (yes/no)	1.45	1.47
Multiple injection scars noted (yes/no)	3.51	2.99

[a] The odds ratio for each variable is adjusted for possible confounding by all other variables in the table.
[b] No assumption of multivariate normality among those with and without positive serologic markers of hepatitis B. Coefficients estimated by methods similar to those described in Walker and Duncan [1967].
Source: Pasquini et al 1983.

weighting of the estimated odds ratios for each stratum. Thus, when the two methods differ for equivalent calculations (i.e., all variables are attributes), we would choose the M–H result. When they are not different, as in seven of nine instances in Table 6-5, the comparison is a valuable reenforcement of the findings and a useful check on all aspects of the computations. When a method is as simple and free of assumptions as the M–H procedure, it deserves to receive a strong recommendation, and we do not hesitate to give it.

Variable with Most Effect on Risk

Often there is interest in knowing which of the x variables has the most effect on risk (y). This is a distinctly different question from which x variable is the most "significant" (i.e., most unusual under the null hypothesis). The largest β_i in terms of absolute value (disregarding sign) is not necessarily the one with the most effect, since the size of β_i depends on the units of x_i. If x_i is weight, it might be measured in grams or in kilograms. The β_i for x_i measured in kilograms would be 1000 times larger than the β_i for x_i measured in grams. Obviously, then, the largest β_i is in part determined by the accident of choice of units. A simple procedure permitting comparison of how β_i values affect y, free of distortion due to differences in units, is to compare $\beta_i \sigma_i$ values. Note first that σ_i refers to the standard deviation of the x_i values. It is *not* the standard error of β_i that is wanted here but something that will remove the effect of arbitrary choice of units. Analogous to our previous derivation of $10\beta_1$ as the natural logarithm of the odds ratio comparing those with an x_1 value of $K + 10$ with those with an x_1 value of K, $\beta_i \sigma_i$ represents the natural logarithm of the odds ratio related to one standard deviation change in x_i. If x_i is a weight variable measured in grams, β_i would be $1/1000$ as large and σ_i would be 1000 times as large as the comparable values for x_i measured in kilograms. Thus, $\beta_i \sigma_i$ is independent of the choice of units and comparing $\beta_1 \sigma_1$ with $\beta_2 \sigma_2$, etc., to find the largest absolute value is an excellent way of determining which x variable has the most effect on the natural logarithm of the odds ratio.

$\beta_i \sigma_i$ is often referred to as a standardized regression coefficient. Its use, as recommended herein, is entirely appropriate in order to compare the effects of *different independent variables within the same population.* Using standardized regression coefficients to compare effects of the *same variable in studies of different populations* may not be correct [Greenland et al 1986]. Consider the same actual variable, which we will call the ith, in each of two different populations, a and b. Even if β_{ia} were identical to β_{ib}, the standardized coefficients $\beta_{ia}\sigma_{ia}$ and $\beta_{ib}\sigma_{ib}$ might differ appreciably because σ_{ia} is not equal to σ_{ib}.

In Cross-Sectional and Retrospective Studies

Although originally developed for use in an incidence study, the multiple logistic function can also be used for relating x variables to prevalence of existing disease [Seigel and Greenhouse 1973] and even for investigating difference in exposure between cases and controls in a retrospective study [Seigel and Greenhouse 1973, Prentice 1976]. In the latter case, it should be obvious that α has no intrinsic meaning since the general level of risk in a case-control study is arbitrarily determined by the selected number of controls per case.

Analyzing Matched Pair Data

Matched pair data can also be analyzed this way provided no meaning is attached to the β_i for those variables that are matched if they are represented in the function. The β_i for variables not matched should be interpreted as adjusted for association with all matched variables as well as all other variables in the study. The nature of the adjustment for *matched* variables is not limited, as previously outlined, to linear relationships but is more comprehensive.

There is a method of applying multiple logistic procedures to matched pair case-control data that emphasizes the paired data [Holford et al 1978]. In this method, they y variable is the *difference* in disease status between case and control. This is always $1 - 0 = 1$. Similarly, each x variable for each pair is the difference between case and control for that variable.

Comparison to Multiple Regression

Although it is certainly a valuable tool, multiple logistic analysis is unlikely to identify a different set of variables, as related to outcome, than would be identified by multiple linear regression. An example of this similarity can be found in a report on the Coronary Drug Project [1974] in which the data were analyzed by both methods.

SIGNIFICANCE TESTING AND CONFIDENCE LIMITS

We outline below the essential similarities between hypothesis testing or finding confidence limits for univariate or multivariate regression coefficients and these same procedures for simpler statistics. Fuller discussion of appropriate methods can be found in Draper and Smith [1981] for linear regression, in Schlesselman [1982] and Kleinbaum et al [1982] for logistic regression, and in Lee [1980] for Cox regression (see Chapter 7).

Statistical significance of a coefficient β can be judged if the difference between the value of the coefficient and its expected value under the hypothesis being tested is divided by the standard error of the coefficient as in Equation 1-24.

$$z = \frac{\hat{\beta} - E(\beta)}{SE(\beta)}$$

This presumes that the distribution of all possible sample values of $\hat{\beta}$ is approximately normal. Because regression coefficients are analogous to sums, this assumption is reasonable for large size samples. If under the hypothesis being tested $E(\beta)$ is zero, z is frequently written as $[\hat{\beta}/SE(\beta)]$. Again if the normality assumption is appropriate, 95 percent confidence limits for β are

$$\hat{\beta} \pm 1.96 \, SE(\beta)$$

as in Equation 1-19.

If the coefficient $\hat{\beta}$ comes from a logistic regression model, $\hat{\beta}$ is an estimate of $\ln OR$ and $\hat{\beta} \pm 1.96 \, SE(\beta)$ will provide .95 confidence limits on $\ln OR$. The corresponding .95 confidence limits on OR are

$$e^{[\hat{\beta} \pm 1.96 \, SE(\beta)]}$$

We prefer confidence limits to significance tests because they provide much more information. Significance tests indicate whether a statistic is or is not unusual as a sample result from a hypothesized population. Confidence limits include this information in terms of whether or not the limits include the hypothesized parameter. In addition, they indicate how precise an estimate of the unknown parameter is provided by the sample data. Consider the following Framingham data from the logistic regression relating systolic blood pressure greater than or equal to 165 mm Hg to risk of coronary heart disease, with adjustment for sex and age in four classes.

$$\hat{\beta} = 1.0004, \qquad \hat{SE}(\beta) = .1571$$

If SBP $\geqslant 165$ is unrelated to CHD then the odds ratio for odds of developing CHD comparing SBP $\geqslant 165$ to SBP < 165 would equal one and $\ln OR = 0$. Since $\hat{\beta}$ is an estimator of $\ln OR$, the hypothesis that SBP $\geqslant 165$ is unrelated to risk of CHD implies that $E(\beta)$ is really 0. To test whether $\hat{\beta}$ is significantly different from 0 we calculate

$$z = \frac{\hat{\beta} - E(\beta)}{\hat{SE}(\beta)} = \frac{1.0004 - 0}{.1571} = 6.37$$

With a z value this large we reject the hypothesis that $\hat{\beta}$ is a sample from a population in which systolic blood pressure is unrelated to coronary heart disease. Instead of doing a significance test we can use these data to calculate confidence limits as in Equation 1-19. Remembering that $\hat{\beta}$ estimates $\ln OR$ we get

$$.95 \text{ CL for } \ln OR = 1.0004 \pm 1.96(.1571) = .6925 \text{ and } 1.3083$$
$$.95 \text{ CL for } OR = e^{.6925} \text{ and } e^{1.3083} = 2.00 \text{ and } 3.70$$

Since the confidence limits for $\ln OR$ do not include zero and the corresponding limits for OR do not include one they indicate that SBP ≥ 165 is significantly related to risk of CHD. They also tell us that the true odds ratio is probably between 2.00 and 3.70. If we had different data and had estimated that the true odds ratio was probably between 1.05 and 1.35 it would have been a much different finding. Nevertheless, in both instances a test of significance would only find that our logistic regression coefficient was significantly different from zero.

CONSTRUCTION OF STRATA USING A MULTIVARIATE FUNCTION

Epidemiologists generally encounter multivariate methods used directly to reduce or eliminate confounding. However, such methods may also be used to establish strata within which the association of prime interest can be examined essentially free of confounding [Miettinen 1976b]. We can illustrate this approach by first assuming that we have the necessary data and have calculated a discriminant function relating age, blood pressure, serum cholesterol, cigarette smoking, and abdominal skinfold to the risk of myocardial infarction in men. Although it is somewhat artificial to consider one of these variables as the one of major interest and the others as just potential confounders, such considerations do arise. For the moment, imagine that we want to investigate the association of abdominal skinfold with risk of myocardial infarction free of possible confounding by the other variables. After calculating discriminant function coefficients for abdominal skinfold and for each of the other variables in the usual way, we do not compute the ordinary discriminant function score for each individual. Instead we compute a discriminant function score for each individual after fixing the abdominal skinfold coefficient at zero. The resultant scores represent the tendency of each individual to a higher or lower score with respect to development of myocardial infarction based solely on the potential confounding variables. These scores can, for example, be divided into quartiles, and then within each quartile the relationship of skinfold to myocardial infarction risk could be studied. The persons in each quartile would be roughly homogeneous as to myocardial infarction risk related to the nonskinfold variables, at least insofar as a linear combination of the potential confounders is able to discriminate risk. Thus, comparisons in myocardial infarction risk between those with large abdominal skinfolds and those lacking this particular badge of overeating are free of the confounding that might result because those with large skinfolds tend to smoke more, have higher blood pressure, etc.

If skinfold is dichotomized within each quartile, we could summarize the relevant data in a 2×2 table. The individual 2×2 tables could then be combined by means of the Mantel–Haenszel procedure [Mantel and Haenszel 1959].

The use of the discriminant function is not essential for this procedure. Multiple linear regression or multiple logistic functions serve equally well. Remember, however, that multivariate functions used this way are not exempt from the basic requirement that they fit the data.

APPLICATION TO FRAMINGHAM HEART STUDY DATA
Multiple Linear Regression

The multiple linear regression equation relating the presence or absence of categorical variables on examination 1 to 18-year risk of coronary heart disease is

$$\hat{y} = .0613 + .0277x_1 + .0826x_2 + .0845x_3 + .1273x_4 + .1680x_5$$

where

$x_1 = 1$ if age 50–54, otherwise $x_1 = 0$ $(\bar{x}_1 = .315)$

$x_2 = 1$ if age 55–59, otherwise $x_2 = 0$ $(\bar{x}_2 = .281)$

$x_3 = 1$ if age 60–62, otherwise $x_3 = 0$ $(\bar{x}_3 = .081)$

$x_4 = 1$ if male,   otherwise $x_3 = 0$ $(\bar{x}_4 = .472)$

$x_5 = 1$ if SBP $\geqslant 165$, otherwise $x_4 = 0$ $(\bar{x}_5 = .217)$

$\hat{y} =$ estimate of CHD variable

The 18-year incidence rates for SBP $\geqslant 165$ and SBP < 165 adjusted for potential confounding by age and sex are estimated from the above coefficients by substituting for x_1 to x_4 inclusive the average value of the variable and "1" or "0" for x_5 according to the blood pressure category, as follows:

$\hat{y}$ for SBP $\geqslant 165 = .328 = [.0613 + .0277(.315) + .0826(.281)$
$$+ .0845(.081) + .1273(.472) + .1680(1)]$$

$\hat{y}$ for SBP $< 165 = .160 = [.0613 + .0277(.315) + .0826(.281)$
$$+ .0845(.081) + .1273(.472) + .1680(0)]$$

Based on these adjusted incidence rates of .328 and .160, the estimated relative risks and odds ratios adjusted for potential confounding by age and sex are

$$\text{for } SBP \geq 165 \text{ compared to } SBP < 165$$
$$\hat{R}R = (.328/.160) = 2.05$$
$$\hat{O}R = (.328/.672)/(.160/.840) = 2.56$$

Multiple Logistic Regression

The multiple logistic regression equation relating age, sex, and systolic blood pressure to 18-year risk of coronary heart disease is

$$\hat{y} = 1/[1 + e^{-(-7.254+.0519x_1+.0173x_2+.917x_3)}]$$

where

$x_1 = $ age in years

$x_2 = $ systolic blood pressure in mm Hg

$x_3 = 1$ if male, otherwise $x_3 = 0$

$\hat{y} = $ estimated 18-year risk of CHD

The average blood pressure for those with systolic values of 165 or more is 188.4. The average for those with values under 165 is 136.5. The difference between these averages is 51.9. *According to the above (continuous variable) model* the adjusted odds ratio for SBP $\geq$ 165/SBP $<$ 165 is estimated as

$$\hat{O}R = e^{.0173(51.9)} = 2.45$$

To get a sense of how well this continuous variable model fits the data, we use the estimated logistic regression coefficients to calculate the probability of CHD for each individual, array these risks in order of increasing size, and then split the array into parts. For the examples herein, we divide the array into quintiles. Within each quintile we sum the predicted probability of disease for each individual. We also sum the "1" or "0" values indicating actual presence or absence of disease for each individual. The results are then assembled as in Table 6-6. Table 6-6 shows that many more cases are observed in the middle quintile than are expected under the model and makes it reasonable to doubt that the model adequately reflects the actual data.

We now consider blood pressure and age as categorical variables with blood pressure in two classes ($<$165, $\geq$165) and age in four (45–49, 50–54, 55–59, 60–62). The corresponding logistic regression coefficients

Table 6-6. Evaluating Fit of Multiple Logistic Risk Function to Framingham Data, 18-Year CHD Incidence Cases Observed and Predicted, Age and Systolic Blood Pressure as Continuous Variables

Quintile of risk function probability	Coronary heart disease incidence cases		
	Observed	Expected according to logistic model	O/E
1	16	21.3	.75
2	30	34.5	.87
3	67	47.6	1.41
4	60	63.5	.94
5	95	101.1	.94

are

$$.862x_1, \text{ where } x_1 = 1 \text{ if male,} \qquad \text{otherwise } x_1 = 0$$
$$.219x_2, \text{ where } x_2 = 1 \text{ if age 50–54,} \quad \text{otherwise } x_2 = 0$$
$$.564x_3, \text{ where } x_3 = 1 \text{ if age 55–59,} \quad \text{otherwise } x_3 = 0$$
$$.572x_4, \text{ where } x_4 = 1 \text{ if age 60–62,} \quad \text{otherwise } x_4 = 0$$
$$1.000x_5, \text{ where } x_5 = 1 \text{ if SBP} \geqslant 165, \quad \text{otherwise } x_5 = 0$$
$$\text{constant} = -2.418$$

According to this categorical variable model with five variables,[†] the adjusted odds ratio corresponding to that given for the continuous variable model is

$$\text{for SBP} \geqslant 165/ < 165 \qquad \hat{OR} = e^{1.000} = 2.72$$

To see whether this model with age and blood pressure as categorical variables fits the data any better than the continuous variable model, we repeat in Table 6-7 the calculations outlined above for Table 6-6, but this time for the categorical variable model.

This model is clearly more in keeping with the actual data than the continuous variable model. With no quintile as much as 10% discrepant from prediction, this model fits the data reasonably well.

We now consider a further illustration of the difference that can occur in estimating the effect of a risk factor using a multiple logistic function. To this end we reexamine the model for categorical variables but with blood pressure in six classes instead of two. These logistic regression coefficients are

$.892x_1$, where $x_1 = 1$ if male,	otherwise $x_1 = 0$
$.200x_2$, where $x_2 = 1$ if age 50–54,	otherwise $x_2 = 0$
$.528x_3$, where $x_3 = 1$ if age 55–59,	otherwise $x_3 = 0$
$.484x_4$, where $x_4 = 1$ if age 60–62,	otherwise $x_4 = 0$
$.404x_5$, where $x_5 = 1$ if SBP is 140–149,	otherwise $x_5 = 0$
$.620x_6$, where $x_6 = 1$ if SBP is 150–159,	otherwise $x_6 = 0$
$.837x_7$, where $x_7 = 1$ if SBP is 160–169,	otherwise $x_7 = 0$
$1.236x_8$, where $x_8 = 1$ if SBP is 170–179,	otherwise $x_8 = 0$
$1.380x_9$, where $x_9 = 1$ if SBP is 180 or more,	otherwise $x_9 = 0$
constant $= -2.691$	

For this categorical variable model with nine variables, the estimated adjusted odds ratios are

$$\text{for SBP } 150–159/140–149 \quad \hat{O}R = e^{.620-.404} = 1.24$$
$$\text{for SBP } 170–179/160–169 \quad \hat{O}R = e^{1.236-.837} = 1.49$$

Look at the two odds ratios comparing blood pressure groups. Note that the odds ratio comparing 170–179 to 160–169 is greater than the odds ratio comparing 150–159 to 140–149. The difference in mean blood pressure values is almost identical for these two comparisons. The 170–179 group average is 10.2 mm Hg higher than the 160–169 group. The 150–159 group average is 10.3 mm Hg higher than the 140–149 group. The continuous variable model that assumes that blood pressure is

Table 6-7. Evaluating Fit of Multiple Logistic Risk Function to Framingham Data, 18-Year CHD Incidence Cases Observed and Predicted, Age and Systolic Blood Pressure as Categorical Variables

Quintile of risk function probability	Coronary heart disease incidence cases		
	Observed	Expected according to logistic model	O/E
1	23	23.8	.97
2	33	34.4	.96
3	33	30.6	1.00
4	63	64.8	.97
5	94	94.4	1.00

linearly related to log odds ratio necessarily reflects the same odds ratio for the same amount of change in blood pressure. In fact the continuous variable model estimates an odds ratio of 1.19 for any 10 mm Hg increase. The designation of specific blood pressure groups as distinct categorical variables allows the estimated odds ratio relating to 10 mm Hg increases in blood pressure to be more dependent on the data and less on the assumed model.

Stratification Based on Multivariate Function

We first use a multiple linear regression equation to estimate the relationship between 18-year risk of CHD and Framingham Heart Study measurements made on examination 1. The equation with age and blood pressure as continuous variables and specifying the estimated coefficients is

$$\hat{y}_{(CHD)} = -.6752 + .00737 \text{ (age in years)}$$
$$+ .1329 \text{ (sex with male} = 1 \text{ and female} = 0)$$
$$+ .00286 \text{ (SBP in mm Hg)}$$

To evaluate each person's potential risk of CHD from their age and sex independently of systolic blood pressure, we compute $\hat{y}_{(CHD)}$ for each individual *after substituting zero for the coefficient of SBP.* The resultant confounding score for each person in the study can be used to assess the independent association of SBP to coronary heart disease risk. We array these scores from smallest to largest and divide them into groups split at relevant percentile points. For this illustrative calculation we use the

Table 6-8. Estimated Odds Ratios for Systolic Blood Pressure Compared to Risk of CHD, Chapter 6 Methods, 18-Year Framingham Heart Study Data

	Adjustment method					
	Multiple linear regression					
	Categorical variables		Stratification (confounder score)	Multiple logistic regression		
SBP groups being compared	4 Ages 2 SBPs and sex	4 Ages 6 SBPs and sex	Age cont. SBP cont. and sex	4 Ages 2 SBPs and sex	4 Ages 6 SBPs and sex	Age cont. SBP cont. and sex
≥165/<165	2.56	—	2.66	2.72	—	2.45
150–159/140–149	—	1.24	—	—	1.24	1.20
170–179/160–169	—	1.48	—	—	1.49	1.19
any +10 mm Hg	—	—	—	—	—	1.19

25th, 50th, and 75th percentiles to form four groups. All individuals falling into the same group will be approximately equal in the degree to which their age and sex are related to risk, independently of systolic blood pressure. The next step is to assemble the data within each group into a 2×2 table relating CHD incidence to a dichotomized SBP. For this example we classify SBP as <165 or ≥ 165. The remaining step in this procedure is to use the data from all four tables to calculate a Mantel–Haenszel summary odds ratio using Equation 5-17. The result, quite similar to the odds ratios computed directly from categorical multiple linear regression or multiple logistic regression, is

$$\hat{OR} = 2.66$$

Calculations using Chapter 6 methods to estimate odds ratios related to different blood pressure groups are summarized for convenient comparison in Table 6-8. Our comments on this table are:

1. There is good agreement between multiple regression and multiple logistic methods when both are applied to the same categorical variables.
2. Estimated odds ratios using the multiple continuous variable model are in some instances fairly close to and in others definitely different from comparable odds ratios estimated by either of the categorical methods. The assumption that a variable such as systolic blood pressure is linearly related to the log odds for developing coronary heart disease is not required if blood pressure is subdivided into categories. We have a definite preference for methods requiring fewer assumptions.

EXERCISES

Ex. 6-1. The multiple linear regression equation relating development of coronary disease during 18-year follow-up to age and systolic blood pressure in categories and to sex is

$$\hat{y} = .056 + .024x_1 + .083x_2 + .084x_3 + .129x_4 + .151x_5$$

where $x_1 = 1$ if aged 50–54, otherwise $x_1 = 0$ $(\bar{x}_1 = .315)$

           $x_2 = 1$ if aged 55–59, otherwise $x_2 = 0$ $(\bar{x}_2 = .281)$

           $x_3 = 1$ if aged 60–62, otherwise $x_3 = 0$ $(\bar{x}_3 = .081)$

           $x_4 = 1$ if male, otherwise $x_4 = 0$ $(\bar{x}_4 = .472)$

           $x_5 = 1$ if SBP ≥ 160, otherwise $x_5 = 0$ $(\bar{x}_5 = .281)$

a. What is the estimated proportion developing CHD within 18 years?
b. What are the estimated 18-year risks for men and women each standardized for age and blood pressure differences?
c. What is the estimated odds ratio for CHD in 18 years comparing:
    i.   men to women (adjusted for age and SBP)
    ii. SBP $\geqslant 160$ to SBP < 160 (adjusted for age and sex)
    iii. aged 55–59 to aged 45–49 (adjusted for sex and SBP)
    iv. aged 55–59 to aged 50–54 (adjusted for sex and SBP)

Ex. 6-2. The coefficients for the multiple logistic equation relating probability of CHD in 18 years to serum cholesterol in categories, sex, and age are

$$-.754x_1, \text{ where } x_1 = 1 \text{ if female, otherwise } x_1 = 0$$

$$.066x_2, \text{ where } x_2 = \text{age in years}$$

$$.214x_3, \text{ where } x_3 = 1 \text{ if cholesterol} \geqslant 220, \text{ otherwise } x_3 = 0$$

$$\text{constant} = -4.664$$

a. According to this multiple logistic model, what are the estimated probabilities of developing coronary heart disease in 18 years for:
    i. 55-year-old males with serum cholesterol level of 240
    ii. 45-year-old females with serum cholesterol level of 215
b. What are the adjusted odds ratios for coronary disease within 18 years for:
    i.   female/male (adjusted for age and cholesterol)
    ii. cholesterol $\geqslant 220$/cholesterol < 220 (adjusted for age and sex)
    iii. age 60/age 50 (adjusted for sex and cholesterol)

Ex. 6-3. Changing the cholesterol categories from $\geqslant 220/<220$ to $\geqslant 260/<260$ changes the coefficients in Exercise 6-2 above to the following:

$$-.802x_1, \text{ where } x_1 = 1 \text{ if female, otherwise } x_1 = 0$$

$$.065x_2, \text{ where } x_2 = \text{age in years}$$

$$.464x_3, \text{ where } x_3 = 1 \text{ if cholesterol} \geqslant 260, \text{ otherwise } x_3 = 0$$

$$\text{constant} = -4.611$$

Repeat the calculations outlined in Exercise 6-2 [except (b)ii] and compare and comment on the differences or similarities found.

NOTES

* Selecting these with high, medium, or low risk under the model is equivalent to selecting the cross-classification categories for which risk is high, medium, or low.

† We used three variables for four age classes, one variable for two blood pressure classes, and one variable for sex.

7
Follow-up Studies: Life Tables

INTRODUCTION

The remark attributed to John Maynard Keynes that "in the long run we are all dead" [Pigou 1947] indicates why it is often insufficient to compare percentage mortality among those given treatment A with percentage mortality among those given treatment B. Obviously, if the period for observation of mortality is very long, Lord Keynes' dictum can be controlling. Forty years after a middle-aged or elderly population is treated, there can be little distinction in percentage dead among those given one treatment or another. Shorter investigations can avoid the more obvious consequences of our common mortality. Whether the investigation covers a long period or a short one, however, the difference between dying one year and dying ten years after treatment is of great importance not only to the individual but to the epidemiologic analyst wishing to evaluate the two treatments.

The types of studies encountered by epidemiologists in which these problems arise include randomized, controlled clinical trials with moderately long to long observation time after treatment [Diabetic Retinopathy Study 1976]; evaluation of differential mortality in different population groups, such as smokers and nonsmokers [Rogot 1974]; summarization of mortality risk for groups, such as radiologists, hypothesized to be at greater than average risk [Matanoski et al 1975]; and evaluation of survival after the diagnosis of specific types of cancer [Axtell et al 1976]. In all of these investigations, the end point is not necessarily mortality; it may be onset of disease or disability, for example, in accordance with study interests and objectives.

NOTATION

If longitudinal studies include data on persons observed for long periods or for varying lengths of time, some systematic procedure is required for summarizing the observations. The life table [Chiang 1968, Cutler and Ederer 1958] provides one way of handling such data, and we begin by describing a simple example. Assume that 300 persons have received cardiac transplants and that we wish to estimate the probability of surviving the surgery by one year. The data might be as shown in Table 7-1. The probability of dying during each interval is the number dying in the interval divided by the number alive at the beginning of the interval. More precisely, this quotient is the probability of dying during an interval for those alive at its beginning. Standard notation for this probability is $_nq_x$, read as "the probability of dying during the interval x to $x+n$ for those alive at time x." Other useful symbols are

x time at beginning of interval
O_x number under observation at exact time x
n length of interval
$_nd_x$ number dying in interval x to $x+n$
$_np_x$ probability of surviving from time x to time $x+n = 1 - _nq_x$

Table 7-2 restates the data from Table 7-1, incorporating the above notation and also columns for $_2q_x$ and $_2p_x$. Although n(equal to 2) is constant in this example, it does not have to be.

SURVIVAL OVER SEVERAL INTERVALS

Usually, the primary interest in data of this type is not in the probability of surviving through any particular interval but in the probability of surviving 6 months or 12 months or some other specific period from time 0, the time of surgery. To symbolize this cumulative, or overall, survival

Table 7-1. Basic Data Summarization for Survival after Cardiac Transplant

Postoperative interval (months)	Under observation at start of interval	Died during interval
0–1.99	300	195
2–3.99	105	27
4–5.99	78	15
6–7.99	63	12
8–9.99	51	9
10–11.99	42	12
12–13.99	30	

Table 7-2. Data from Table 7-1 with Life Table Calculations and Notation

Time at beginning of interval (months)	Under observation at time x	Died during interval	Probability of	
			Dying during interval	Surviving through interval
x	O_x	$_2d_x$	$_2q_x$	$_2P_x$
0	300	195	.65	.35
2	105	27	.26	.74
4	78	15	.19	.81
6	63	12	.19	.81
8	51	9	.18	.82
10	42	12	.29	.71
12	30			

spanning several periods, we use a slightly different notation: $_nP_x$ symbolizes the probability of surviving from time x to time $x + n$ with the capital letter P signifying a period longer than a single interval. The $_nP_x$ is derived from the product of several $_np_x$ values as outlined below.

Suppose we wish to estimate the 12-month probability of survival after surgery. Obviously, to survive for 12 months one must survive the 2-month period beginning with $x = 0$ *and* the period beginning with $x = 2$ *and* the period beginning with $x = 4$ *and* . . . . Using notation analogous to the summation notation reviewed in Chapter 1 but with $\prod$ to represent the product of terms, we have*

$$_{12}P_0 = \prod_{i=0}^{5} {}_2P_{2i} = ({}_2p_0)({}_2p_2)({}_2p_4)({}_2p_6)({}_2p_8)({}_2p_{10})$$

For the data in Table 7-2, this is

$$_{12}P_0 = (.35)(.74)(.81)(.81)(.82)(.71) = .10$$

The probability of surviving 12 months from the date of cardiac transplant (.10) corresponds to the number surviving to that date (30) divided by the number receiving transplants (300), Why, then, do we bother with the product of probabilities for surviving several periods when the desired statistic seems readily at hand, i.e., the number surviving to 12 months divided by the number given transplants? We do this because the number surviving to the time we wish to evaluate is almost always affected by cases withdrawn from the study or lost to observation before the evaluation time is reached. In Table 7-2, there happened to be no withdrawals or cases lost to observation and so the simple calculation is satisfactory.

WITHDRAWALS

The term *withdrawals* is used to describe persons still alive who must be dropped from a study because the length of time they have been in the study is shorter than the interval for which survival is being calculated. For example, in a calculation of five-year survival, someone who received initial treatment (and entered the study) three and a half years ago and was a survivor would have to be withdrawn before the start of the 4–4.99-year interval.

To illustrate how withdrawals come about, let us consider a survival study following a specific type of surgery for breast cancer. The study begins on January 1, 1970, and the data are analyzed as of December 31, 1978, using all information collected to that date. A woman treated on January 1, 1970, might contribute to data on survival from the seventh year after treatment to the eighth anniversary. However, a woman treated on July 1, 1975, and added to the study on that date, cannot possibly provide any information about survival from the seventh to the eighth year after treatment. If the person treated on July 1, 1975, has survived until December 31, 1978, she must be treated as a subject who has been withdrawn during the fourth year of observation. For this individual, year 1 runs from July 1, 1975 to June 30, 1976, year 2 from July 1, 1976 to June 30, 1977, year 3 from July 1, 1977 to June 30, 1978, and year 4 from July 1 1978 to June 30, 1979. However, since the study cutoff date is December 31, 1978, it is impossible for her to complete the fourth year of observation before the cutoff. If she has survived to the cutoff date, she must be withdrawn in the year that includes it.

Cases lost to observation are also considered as having been withdrawn alive, but the reason for their withdrawal is that the follow-up procedures failed to determine their status rather than that they had reached the limits of time for observation. Because withdrawals and losses to observation can have different effects on the estimated probability of survival, we use distinct terminology for them. We shall emphasize these differences again later, but for the present we group them together under the label *withdrawals* and use $_nw_x$ as the symbol for the number of cases withdrawn alive (necessarily or otherwise) between time x and time $x + n$.

Assumptions

We now examine how cases withdrawn from a study *at the beginning of each interval* affect our original data. For this illustration we also assume that those withdrawn experience the same probability of death after withdrawal as those remaining under observation. These assumptions are reflected in Table 7-3. A column is also provided for a new cumulative survival function, "probability of surviving from time 0 to time $x + 2$."

Table 7-3. Data from Table 7-1 in Life Table Format Modified for Withdrawals at Beginning of Interval

Time at beginning of interval x	Under observation at exact time x O_x	Number of deaths observed between x and $x+2$ $_2d_x$	Number withdrawn between x and $x+2$ $_2w_x$	Adjusted O_x $(O_x - {_2w_x})$ O'_x	Probability of		
					Dying during interval $(_2d_x/O'_x)$ $_2q_x$	Surviving through interval $(1 - {_2q_x})$ $_2p_x$	Surviving from time 0 to time $x+2$ $\left(\prod_{i=0}^{x/2} {_2p_{2i}}\right)$ $_{x+2}p_0$
0	300	191	6	294	.65	.35	.35
2	103	25	8	95	.26	.74	.26
4	70	11	10	60	.18	.82	.21
6	49	7	11	38	.18	.82	.17
8	31	4	10	21	.19	.81	.14
10	17	2	10	7	.29	.71	.10
12	5						

Note that in Table 7-3 the number of deaths observed in each interval has been reduced in keeping with the assumption that those withdrawn have the same probability of death after withdrawal as those remaining under observation. Thus, in the period beginning at $x = 0$ and having a probability of death during the interval of about 2/3, we presume that four of the six withdrawals died following withdrawal and subtract these four deaths from the 195 reported in Table 7-1 as the total deaths for this interval. Among those kept under observation, 191 deaths were observed. An additional four deaths occurred among the six withdrawals, and these were not observed. Combining observed and unobserved deaths, we have the same total (195) as in Table 7-1. The column for cumulative probability of survival relates to survival from time 0 to time $x + 2$. Thus, if 12-month survival is desired, the product $\prod_{i=0}^{x/2} {_2}p_{2i}$ uses $x = 10$.

The index then relates to $i = 0, 1, 2, \ldots, 10/2$, with corresponding values of ${_2}p_{2i}$ of ${_2}p_0, {_2}p_2, {_2}p_4, \ldots, {_2}p_{10}$. The calculation for ${_2}q_x$ in Table 7-3 has been modified to reflect the assumption that the ${_n}w_x$ are lost to observation at the *beginning of each interval*. Thus, in the first interval, the probability of death is calculated as 191/294 rather than 191/300. If ${_2}w_0$ of the individuals given transplants withdrew from the study immediately following surgery and thus from *any* possibility of being recorded among the ${_2}d_0$, we calculate the probability of dying among those remaining under observation as ${_2}d_0/(O_0 - {_2}w_0)$. The data presented in Table 7-3 reflect almost (because ${_2}d_x$ and ${_2}w_x$ are restricted to integer values) the same probability of dying $({_2}q_x)$ for those under observation as for the total group defined in Table 7-2. In summary, some individuals withdrew alive, but both those who withdrew and those who remained under observation had the same probability of death as experienced by the total group in Table 7-2.

The existence of withdrawals is very much in keeping with real experience and real data. Our stipulation that the withdrawals and those remaining under observation have the same probability of death and that withdrawals all take place exactly at the beginning of an interval are less realistic, but they are included to permit step-by-step explanation of the elements involved in calculating summary statistics.

Note in Table 7-3 that the number observed to be alive at 12 months divided by the number given transplants is 5/300, or .017, not the .10 that was calculated from Table 7-2 as the probability of survival for the entire group. However, the ${_2}q_x$ probabilities in Table 7-3 are almost identical with those in Table 7-2. By first calculating $1 - {_2}q_x = {_2}p_x$ and then forming the product ${_{12}}P_0 = \prod_{i=0}^{5} {_2}p_{2i}$, we arrive at .10 as the probability of surviving from surgery to the first anniversary, exactly as in Table 7-2. In this illustration, which includes some withdrawals, it is clear that the product of survival probabilities for individual intervals provides a good estimate of overall survival whereas the number observed to have survived divided by the number given transplants does not. Studies without withdrawals, while deserving of high praise, are extremely rare, and so we concentrate only on the use of the product of interval probabilities of survival to estimate overall survival.

The calculation of each interval probability of death is affected by assumptions regarding withdrawals. Suppose we consider data relating to a one-year interval x to $x + 1$ as O_x, $_1d_x$, and $_1w_x$, with $O_x - _1w_x - _1d_x = O_{x+1}$. When $n = 1$, it is customary to omit it from the notation used, and we shall adopt this convention. Possible assumptions about the w_x individuals are

1. All have died by time $x + 1$
2. None has died by time $x + 1$
3. They experience the same probability of death after withdrawal as those who remain under observation

The first two assumptions tend to be unrealistic, but they permit calculation of limits within which the truth lies. The calculation of q_x under the assumption that all withdrawals died before the end of the interval in which they withdrew (assumption 1) is

$$q_x = \frac{d_x + w_x}{O_x}$$

Under the assumption that none died before the end of the interval in which they withdrew (assumption 2), it is

$$q_x = \frac{d_x}{O_x}$$

Assumption 3 is commonly adopted but much less commonly justified by evidence. If all withdrawals are due to the termination of the observation period and if no change in patient selection or treatment occurs over the study period, assumption 3 is probably justified. In most studies, however, we really do not know how withdrawals differ from those remaining under observation, and the very best studies exert considerable effort to keep withdrawals to a minimum.

We now investigate the effect of assumption 3 on the calculation of q_x. Consider a single individual, included among the w_x, who moved from the area and was thus lost to observation at time $x + 3/4$. If this individual had died at time $x + \frac{1}{4}$ or $x + \frac{1}{2}$, she or he would have been recorded among the d_x. She or he was, in fact, under observation and at risk of being included among the d_x from time x to time $x + \frac{3}{4}$. It is only the time following $x + \frac{3}{4}$ that is lost to observation. If we now shift to consideration of all individuals in w_x and make the assumption that withdrawals occur *uniformly* throughout the interval x to $x + 1$, it follows that, on the average, members of w_x are under observation for half of the interval, and it is necessary to use this fact in calculating q_x.

Under the assumptions that withdrawals are uniformly distributed within the interval with respect to time of withdrawal and that the subsequent experience of withdrawals is the same as those remaining under observation, the applicable formula is

$$q_x = \frac{d_x}{O_x - w_x/2} \tag{7-1}$$

This method of calculating q_x removes, from the O_x at risk, only half of the w_x, thus effectively counting half of the w_x as being under observation. Of course, it is not half of the w_x individuals who were at risk of being included among the d_x but rather all of the w_x individuals, each for an average of half an interval.

Equation 7-1 for q_x adjusted for withdrawals can also be derived by estimating the number of deaths among withdrawals and adding this to the observed d_x. Under the assumptions of uniform withdrawal and equal risk for withdrawals and those remaining under observation, the number of deaths occurring among the w_x would be $(w_x/2)q_x$. Risk in the entire O_x group can then be estimated by combining deaths among the w_x with the d_x actually observed. Under the assumptions of uniform withdrawal and equal risk, the number of deaths occurring in the w_x is

$$\frac{w_x}{2}\left(\frac{d_x}{O_x - w_x/2}\right)$$

and our alternative estimate of risk is

$$q_x' = \frac{d_x + \dfrac{w_x}{2}\left(\dfrac{d_x}{O_x - w_x/2}\right)}{O_x} \tag{7-2}$$

By multiplying the first term in the numerator by

$$\frac{O_x - (w_x/2)}{O_x - (w_x/2)}$$

q'_x in Equation 7-2 can be shown to be identical to q_x in Equation 7-1:

$$q'_x = \frac{\dfrac{d_x(O_x - w_x/2)}{O_x - w_x/2} + \dfrac{d_x}{O_x - w_x/2}\left(\dfrac{w_x}{2}\right)}{O_x} = \frac{d_x O_x - \dfrac{d_x w_x}{2} + \dfrac{d_x w_x}{2}}{\left(O_x - \dfrac{w_x}{2}\right)O_x}$$

$$= \frac{d_x O_x}{\left(O_x - \dfrac{w_x}{2}\right)O_x} = \frac{d_x}{O_x - \dfrac{w_x}{2}} = q_x$$

Both equations assume equal probability of death for those withdrawn and those still under observation. Thus

$$q_x = \frac{d_x}{O_x - (w_x/2)}$$

is the probability of death during the interval x to $x+1$ for those withdrawn, for those remaining under observation, and, consequently, for the total group alive and under observation at the beginning of the interval.

Whenever there is reason to believe that the stipulated assumptions do not apply, the adjustments for withdrawals given in Equations 7-1 and 7-2 are not to be used. The extreme assumptions of all w_x dying or none dying are always possible, although not too often helpful. If you have specific data about time of withdrawals or risk after withdrawal, substitute such data for the "standard" assumptions.

We now repeat the data of Table 7-2 with q_x calculated according to the standard assumptions. This is shown in Table 7-4. As in prior modifications, the original data presented in Table 7-1 have been adjusted in Table 7-4 to fit the assumptions used. For example, in Table 7-4 the six withdrawals in the first interval are now presumed to have been under observation for half the interval. Thus, the approximately $\frac{2}{3}$ probability of death reported for this interval in Table 7-1 results in (6) $\left(\frac{1}{2}\right)\left(\frac{2}{3}\right) = 2$ deaths among the $_2 w_0$. The total of 195 deaths reported for $_2 d_0$ in Table 7-1 has accordingly been reduced to 193 in Table 7-4. The number of withdrawals has been changed slightly from Table 7-3 to 7-4. Under the assumption that withdrawals have the same experience as those remaining under observation, calculations of q_x are not affected.

Although different methods of calculating $_2 q_x$ are used in Tables 7-3 and 7-4, each method is in keeping with the assumptions relating to it. The overall results, to three digits, of .100 survival for one year in Table 7-3 and .093 in Table 7-4 differ because of the need to keep to integer values for the number of deaths and not because of any fundamental discrepancy. Withdrawals occurring immediately at the beginning of each

Table 7-4. Data from Table 7-1 in Life Table Format Modified for Uniform Withdrawals during an Interval

Time at beginning of interval x	Under observation at exact time x C_x	Number of deaths observed between x and $x+2$ $_2d_x$	Number withdrawn between x and $x+2$ $_2w_x$	Adjusted O_x $\left(O_x - \dfrac{_2w_x}{2}\right)$ O'_x	Probability of — Dying during interval $\left(\dfrac{_2d_x}{O'_x}\right)$ $_2q_x$	Probability of — Surviving through interval $(1 - _2q_x)$ $_2p_x$	Probability of — Surviving from time 0 to time $x+2$ $\left(\prod\limits_{i=0}^{x/2} {}_2p_{2i}\right)$ $_{x+2}p_0$
0	300	193	6	297	.65	.35	.35
2	101	25	8	97	.26	.74	.26
4	68	12	10	63	.19	.81	.21
6	46	8	10	41	.20	.80	.17
8	28	4	10	23	.17	.83	.14
10	14	3	10	9	.33	.67	.09
12	1						

interval, as in Table 7-3, are unlikely in real data. They are used solely to introduce the subject of adjustment for withdrawals.

Our discussion on adjustment for withdrawals has been based on two unstated assumptions, which we now specify. The first is that the risk of death is fairly constant within the interval of analysis. For many investigations, this will be the case; in others, it may be possible to approximate this requirement by shortening the interval being analyzed. Note that the approximate constancy of risk within an interval is of concern only when adjustment is required for withdrawals. If no cases are withdrawn, the intervals of analysis can be of any length and there is no requirement of constant risk within them. If there are withdrawals, however, we need a basis for assuming that someone withdrawn for the last $1/k$ of the interval and subject to the same risk as those remaining under observation has $1/k$ the probability of an event applicable to an individual observed over the entire interval. Without this assumption, the use of Equations 7-1 and 7-2 is not justified. Of course, if the nature of the changing risk within the interval is known, alternative estimates of the risk of death among cases withdrawn may be possible. To illustrate the importance of constant risk, consider a life table calculation on survival incorporating birth to age 9.99 years as a single interval. The risk of death during this interval is very heavily concentrated between birth and age one. We further assume a large number of withdrawals exactly at age five; thus, the withdrawals were present for the first half of the 0 to 9.99 interval but not for the second half. By using Equations 7-1 and 7-2, we would be incorporating into our estimate of $_{10}q_0$ the idea that the risk during the period lost to observation among the $_{10}w_0$ individuals is proportional to that actually observed over the whole period. This is false, however, and thus Equations 7-1 and 7-2 are not appropriate. This problem can be avoided easily by subdividing the intervals into periods having approximately constant risk.

The second assumption that has been unstated to this point relates to combining data from different calendar periods. For any specific interval of analysis x to $x + n$, if data come from different calendar periods, we must assume that there is no secular trend in risk. The life table method can, and does, distinguish between risks in various time periods following entry. There is no requirement to assume anything as to the nature of risk changes with time after entry. However, if several different calendar periods contribute data on the risk in the *same time interval after entry,* it is necessary to assume that the risk for this interval is not changing over time. If it is, the life table statistics are difficult or impossible to interpret.

In summary, if the study contains cases withdrawn from observation, Equations 7-1 and 7-2 may provide satisfactory estimates if it is reasonable to assume that

1. Those withdrawn do not differ from those continued under observa-

tion as to expected mortality both in the interval of withdrawal and in later intervals

2. Within an interval, the risk of death for subintervals of equal length is approximately constant
3. Withdrawals occur uniformly within an interval
4. If data for several different *calendar periods* are being combined into a single interval x to $x + n$, there is no secular trend in risk

Withdrawals Compared to Losses from Observation

We now return to the distinction between withdrawals and losses from observation. Because withdrawals, which occur because of cutoff date for analysis, represent more recent cases, their survival rates may conceivably differ from those of nonwithdrawals, which may represent older patients treated many years ago (see assumption 4 above). However, they are less subject to the myriad biases potentially affecting losses to observation. Although most investigators feel comfortable about the assumption that the future experiences of withdrawals are similar to those of subjects remaining under observation, the only way to feel secure about losses from observation is to have very few of them. The fewer the losses, the less distortion possible in using assumptions that may or may not be justified. If data are available on some characteristics of the lost cases, they can then be compared with cases remaining under observation. Although the prime variable of interest—outcome—remains unknown, comparison of auxiliary variables provides some sense of whether or not lost cases are similar to others. Exactly the same procedure may be followed in comparing withdrawals and cases remaining under observation.

LIFE TABLES FOR SPECIFIC CAUSES

At times the investigator wishes to calculate the probability of death from a particular cause, either with or without adjustment for competing causes. Suppose we are investigating the probability of dying from cancer among those diagnosed as having cancer of a particular type. Persons in the study who are killed in traffic accidents no longer have the possibility of dying from cancer. It is in this sense that the deaths due to traffic and all other noncancer deaths are "competing" with the principal study outcome, i.e., mortality from cancer.

Crude and Net Probabilities

We shall call probabilities adjusted for competing causes, net probabilities of death and those not adjusted for competing causes *crude probabilities of death* [Chiang 1961a]. We illustrate these calculations by returning to the data of Table 7-4, but with a subdivision of $_2d_x$ data into

Table 7-5. Data from Table 7-4 with Subdivision of $_2d_x$ and Calculation of *Crude* Probability for Death from Heart Disease

x	O_x	$_2d_x$ Total	$_2d_x$ Heart disease	$_2d_x$ Other	$_2w_x$	O'_x	$_2q_x$ Total	$_2q_x$ Heart disease	$_2q_x$ Other
0	300	193	24	169	6	297	.650	.081	.569
2	101	25	7	18	8	97	.258	.072	.186
4	68	12	6	6	10	63	.190	.095	.095
6	46	8	1	7	10	41	.195	.024	.171
8	28	4	2	2	10	23	.174	.087	.087
10	14	3	1	2	10	9	.333	.111	.222
12	3								

deaths from heart disease and deaths from all other causes. These subdivided data are shown in Table 7-5. Life table symbols x, O_x, $_nd_x$, $_nw_x$, and $_nq_x$, which have been used several times previously, are used in Table 7-5 without additional labeling. Readers who are doubtful about any of these symbols should refer to Table 7-3.

In Table 7-5 the ratios of heart disease deaths to total deaths for the six intervals beginning with $x = 0$ are .124, .280, .500, .125, .500, and .333. Applying these proportions to the corresponding total $_2q_x$ values results in .081, .072, .095, .024, .087, and .111 as the *crude* probabilities of death from heart disease.

A *net* probability of death from heart disease can be calculated by treating patients who died from all the other causes as if they had been withdrawn alive. By this method, the actual deaths from other causes are

Table 7-6. Data from Table 7-4 with Subdivision of $_2d_x$ and Calculation of *Net* Probability of Death from Heart Disease

x	O_x	$_2d_x$ Heart disease	$_2d_x$ Other	$_2w_x$	O_x adjusted for net probability from heart disease $\left[O_x - \frac{_2w_x}{2} - \frac{_2d_x(\text{other})}{2}\right]$ O'_x	Net probability of death from heart disease $[_2d_x(\text{h.d.})/O'_x]$ $_2q_x(\text{h.d.})$
0	300	24	169	6	212.5	.113
2	101	7	18	8	88.0	.080
4	68	6	6	10	60.0	.100
6	46	1	7	10	37.5	.027
8	28	2	2	10	22.0	.091
10	14	1	2	10	8.0	.125
12	3					

"permitted" to die, in the future, of the net cause under the standard assumption that withdrawals are subject to the same risks after withdrawal as those remaining under observation. The assumption that, had they remained alive, patients dying of other causes would have been at no different risk for heart disease than the surviving population is necessary if this procedure is to yield sensible results. Whenever a competing cause is correlated with the net cause—for example, suicide (competing) with cancer mortality (net)—the use of this method becomes questionable. The calculation of net probability of death from heart disease (all other causes not operating) is illustrated in Table 7-6. The net probability of death from heart disease (Table 7-6) is higher in every interval than the crude probability of death from heart disease (Table 7-5). Of course, this is due to the artificial canceling of other causes of death and to the applying of the risk of dying from heart disease both to the living *and* to those dead of other causes.

COMPARISON TO MORE RIGOROUS METHODS

In his excellent book *Introduction to Stochastic Processes in Biostatistics*, Chiang [1968] derives life table functions based on the force of mortality operating over infinitesimal intervals. These same functions are defined herein from the viewpoint of simplicity rather than rigor. We shall use the data reported by Chiang relating to survival following diagnosis of breast cancer to compare calculations described herein with those described by Chiang. These comparisons are shown in Table 7-7. The statistic we use for comparison is the probability of surviving to the tenth anniversary after entry into the study, with respect to three specifically

Table 7-7. Computed Probability of Surviving Specific Risks: Comparison of Procedures in This Book with Those of Chiang

Risk	Probability of surviving to tenth anniversary with respect to specified risk	
	Chiang[a]	This book
Net probability of death from breast cancer		.488
Net probability of death from breast cancer acting alone	.486	
Crude probability of death from breast cancer		.493
Partial crude probability of death from breast cancer when risk of being lost is eliminated	.491	
Death from any cause		.363
Net probability of death when risk of being lost is eliminated	.361	

[a] Data from Chiang [1968] (p. 292).

identified risks. The terminology used in this book is slightly different from that used by Chiang, and we report both labelings in Table 7-7.

All calculations of probability of surviving to the tenth anniversary were derived from Chiang's data. The appropriate values of q_x were converted to p_x and then survival to the tenth anniversary was computed as $\prod_{x=0}^{9} p_x$. It is comforting to know that the methods described herein for calculating P_x lead to results that are in substantial agreement with the more precise methods described by Chiang.

Note that for either method of calculation the probability of *surviving* a net risk of death from breast cancer is less than the probability of *surviving* a crude risk of death from breast cancer. This is in agreement with our previous observation that the net probability of *dying* from a specific cause is larger than the crude probability. Note also the very small change from crude to net risk. Unless the competing risks are very large, crude and net risks will be similar.

Kuzma [1967] has reported on extensive comparisons of Chiang's method and the Cutler-Ederer [1958] method, which is equivalent to the life table calculations reported herein. After investigating various rates of withdrawal and various risks of death, Kuzma concluded, "The discrepancy of the two methods was found to be negligible for survival rates and standard errors when the withdrawing rates were ≤30 percent and the lost to follow-up rate <40 percent."

SAMPLING ERROR AND SIGNIFICANCE TESTS

Life table functions, as any other statistics, are subject to sampling error. Consider $_x\hat{P}_0$, the estimated probability of surviving several intervals from time 0 to time x. Had different individuals been included in our sample data, we very likely would have different results. In calculating the standard error of $_x\hat{P}_0$, we are estimating the standard deviation of the distribution of all possible $_x\hat{P}_0$ values resulting from all possible samples of 300 from the universe[†] of individuals given cardiac transplants.

We will shortly describe how the standard error of $_x\hat{P}_0$ can be, and historically was, calculated. Before doing that we wish to point out that this calculation is not currently of major importance to epidemiologists who are more often interested in *comparing* survival of different groups. An insurance company could be interested in a specific survival probability such as "What is the 20-year survival for nonsmoking white males age 55?" In that case the survival probability and its standard error are obviously useful. Epidemiologists are more likely to be interested in questions such as "How does 20 year survival for nonsmoking white males aged 55 compare to 20 year survival for cigarette smoking white males aged 55?" If your principal interest relates to the survival contrast between groups you can (with a clear conscience) skip to "Comparison of Complete Survival Curves" on page 185.

We are now ready to consider Greenwood's formula for the standard error of $_{x+1}P_0$ [Greenwood 1926] which is

$$\hat{SE}(_{x+1}P_0) = {}_{x+1}\hat{P}_0\sqrt{\sum_{i=0}^{x}\frac{q_i}{O_i' - d_i}} \tag{7-3}$$

As written, Equation 7-3 relates to $_{x+1}\hat{P}_0$ calculated from p_x values for one-year (or one-month) intervals. We can rewrite it to fit the data in Table 7-4 based on two-month intervals:

$$\hat{SE}(_{x+2}P_0) = {}_{x+2}\hat{P}_0\sqrt{\sum_{i=0}^{x/2}\frac{_2q_{2i}}{O_{2i}' - {}_2d_{2i}}} \tag{7-4}$$

Since the form of Equations 7-3 and 7-4 is a bit confusing, the following attempt to verbalize these equations may be helpful: SE $_kP_0 = {}_kP_0$ multiplied by the square root of [sum of $\lfloor q_i/(O_i' - d_i)\rfloor$] over all intervals used to compute $_kP_0$]. Note that Equation 7-3 pertains to survival from time 0 to time $x + 1$ and Equation 7-4 pertains to survival from time 0 to time $x + 2$. Select the value of x appropriate for the period you wish to analyze. Applying Equation 7-4 to the data in Table 7-4, we get

$$\hat{SE}(_2P_0) = .35\sqrt{\frac{.65}{297 - 193}} = .0277$$

$$\hat{SE}(_4P_0) = .26\sqrt{\frac{.65}{297 - 193} + \frac{.26}{97 - 25}} = .0258$$

$$\hat{SE}(_6P_0) = .21\sqrt{\frac{.65}{297 - 193} + \frac{.26}{97 - 25} + \frac{.19}{63 - 12}} = .0245$$

$$\hat{SE}(_8P_0) = .17\sqrt{\frac{.65}{297 - 193} + \frac{.26}{97 - 25} + \frac{.19}{63 - 12} + \frac{.20}{41 - 8}} = .0238$$

$$\hat{SE}(_{10}P_0) = .14\sqrt{\frac{.65}{297 - 193} + \frac{.26}{97 - 25} + \frac{.19}{63 - 12} + \frac{.20}{41 - 8} + \frac{.17}{23 - 4}}$$

$$= .0237$$

$$\hat{SE}(_{12}P_0) =$$

$$.09\sqrt{\frac{.65}{297 - 193} + \frac{.26}{97 - 25} + \frac{.19}{63 - 12} + \frac{.20}{41 - 8} + \frac{.17}{23 - 4} + \frac{.33}{9 - 3}} = .0260$$

When

$$\frac{\hat{SE}(_{x+n}P_0)}{_{x+n}\hat{P}_0}$$

is $\frac{1}{3}$ or less and $_nd_x$ is 10 or greater, the assumption that the sampling distribution of $_{x+n}\hat{P}_0$ is approximately normal is a reasonable one and $\hat{SE}(_{x+n}P_0)$ can be used to establish confidence limits on $_{x+n}P_0$ as was done with $\bar{x}$ in Equations 1–19 and 1–20:

$$_{x+n}\hat{P}_0 \pm 1.96\,\hat{SE}(_{x+n}P_0) = 95\%\text{ CL for }_{x+n}P_0$$

$$_{x+n}\hat{P}_0 \pm 2.58\,\hat{SE}(_{x+n}P_0) = 99\%\text{ CL for }_{x+n}P_0$$

where $_{x+n}P_0$ is the true value for survival from time 0 to time $x + n$ in the universe being sampled. If either or both of the conditions— $\hat{SE}(_{x+n}P_0)/_{x+n}\hat{P}_0 \leqslant 1/3$ and $_nd_x \geqslant 10$—are not met, then the assumption as to normality of the sampling distribution cannot be taken for granted.

Standard errors for $_{x+1}P_0$ can be used for establishing confidence limits as described above or can be used to test whether two groups differ significantly in proportion surviving for time 0 to time $x + 1$. The test makes use of Equation 1-9:

$$\text{var}(x - y) = \text{var}(x) + \text{var}(y)$$

if x and y are independent.

For our present interest in comparing $_{x+1}\hat{P}_0$ for groups a and b, which we designate $_{x+1}\hat{P}_{0a}$ and $_{x+1}\hat{P}_{0b}$, respectively, we have

$$\text{var}(_{x+1}P_{0a} - _{x+1}P_{0b}) = \text{var}(_{x+1}P_{0a}) + \text{var}(_{x+1}P_{0b})$$

Since $_{x+1}\hat{P}_{0a}$ and $_{x+1}\hat{P}_{0b}$ are derived from different populations, it is reasonable to assume that they are independent variables (e.g., if we know that our sample value of $_{x+1}\hat{P}_{0a}$ happens to be higher than the population parameter it estimates, this knowledge provides no basis for concluding that our sample value of $_{x+1}\hat{P}_{0b}$ is therefore likely to be higher, or lower, than the population parameter it is estimating).

Since the standard error of a statistic is the standard deviation of its sampling distribution (Chapter 1), the variance of that statistic is simply the square of its standard error:

$$\text{var}(_{x+1}P_{0a}) = [\text{SE}(_{x+1}P_{0a})]^2$$

Conversely, the standard error of a statistic is the square root of its variance. Therefore the difference minus the expected value of the difference (equal to zero under the null hypothesis) divided by the square root of the variance of the difference, under the null hypothesis and the usual constraints of adequate sample size, is distributed as a standardized normal deviate and can be tested as such:

$$\frac{(_{x+1}\hat{P}_{0a} - _{x+1}\hat{P}_{0b}) - 0}{\{[\hat{SE}(_{x+1}P_{0a})]^2 + [\hat{SE}(_{x+1}P_{0b})]^2\}^{1/2}} = z$$

COMPARISON OF COMPLETE SURVIVAL CURVES

Before discussing other methods for evaluating whether or not life tables differ significantly, let us outline the general characteristics of these alternative approaches. In contrast to the calculation of standard error for a specific survival time, both the Mantel–Haenszel procedure [Mantel and Haenszel 1959, Mantel 1966] and the logrank method [Mantel 1966, Peto et al 1977] compare the two survival curves over the entire period being analyzed. For example, consider the two survival curves labeled A and B in Figure 7-1. At the 12-month anniversary, the survival for group A is equal to that for group B, but this equal survival for A has just appeared. At two, four, six, eight, and ten months, B had better survival. Under these conditions, the simple comparison at 12 months misses a great deal of the information that is available and used by the two alternative methods we now discuss.

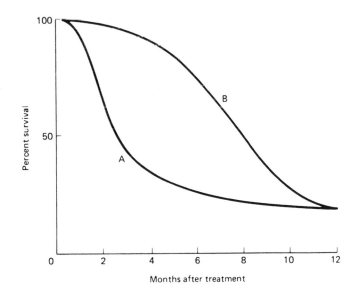

Figure 7-1. Survival curves that differ greatly prior to a point of equality.

Mantel–Haenszel Procedure

The M–H method for obtaining a summary χ^2 from a series of 2×2 tables is an excellent method for judging whether two life tables differ by more than can be reasonably attributed to chance. Theoretical justification for treating each life table interval as a separate stratum and comparing the two life tables within each stratum according to the M–H procedure is given by Mantel [1966]. For illustration, let us assume that we have life table data on two groups, m and n, as in Table 7-8. For each interval in Table 7-8, a 2×2 table can be constructed as shown in Table 7-9 for the interval beginning at $x = 0$. For each cell and marginal total in Table 7-9, there is shown in parentheses the notation used extensively in Chapter 5 on adjustment of data. The odds ratio calculation, as in the more general examples discussed earlier, is

$$\hat{OR} = \frac{\sum\limits_i a_i d_i / t_i}{\sum\limits_i b_i c_i / t_i}$$

In this case $\hat{OR}$ refers to the odds of dying for those in group m compared with those in group n. The summations extend over all intervals to be included in the comparison. This is usually the full set of data, but it is possible to compare life tables for only part of the full period (e.g., from $x = 2$ to $x = 6$).

The overall significance test comparing group m with group n with respect to risk of death is based on

$$\chi^2_{1df} = \frac{[|\sum a_i - \sum (Ea_i)| - \frac{1}{2}]^2}{\sum \text{var}(a_i)}$$

Table 7-8. Comparison of Life Table Data for Groups m and n

x	O'_x (no. at risk)		$_2d_x$ (deaths)		$O'_x - _2d_x$ (survivors)		$_{x+2}P_0$ (probability of surviving to $x + 2$)	
	m	n	m	n	m	n	m	n
0	297	297	193	165	104	132	.350	.444
2	97	132	25	30	72	102	.260	.343
4	63	102	12	15	51	87	.210	.293
6	41	87	8	15	33	72	.169	.242
8	23	72	4	11	19	61	.140	.205
10	9	61	3	17	6	44	.093	.148
Total			245	253				

Table 7-9. Basic Life Table Data Arranged in 2×2 Table Format[a]

Group	Died	Survived	Total at risk
m	193 (a)	104 (b)	297 (m_1)
n	165 (c)	132 (d)	297 (m_2)
Total	358 (n_1)	236 (n_2)	594 (t)

[a] Data are from Table 7-8 for the interval beginning at time $x = 0$.

as explained and illustrated in Chapter 5. Using Table 7-8 data to compute the overall odds ratio and the overall χ^2_{1df} according to the M–H procedure, we get

$$\hat{OR} = 1.37$$

$$\chi^2_1 = 5.66$$

Thus, group m is estimated to be about 1.4 times as risky as group n with respect to the odds of dying. Furthermore this estimated odds ratio is unlikely to result simply by chance because the probability of a χ^2 with one degree of freedom being as large as or larger than 5.66 when the null hypothesis of no difference between groups is true is less than .02.

Recalling that the M–H odds ratio estimates (a) the common odds ratio if there is one, or (b) a reasonably weighted average of the separate odds ratios in the different strata otherwise, this method, like all epidemiologic methods, needs to be applied with understanding. If the two survival curves have, as in Figure 7-1, no crossover or at most trivial amount of crossover, comparison according to the M–H summary chi square can be useful. But what of survival curves that cross over to the extent that, during the first half of the study, results are exactly the opposite of those during the second half? In this situation an M–H summary indicating little difference overall is obviously misleading. Averages are most useful and informative when derived from similar quantities, and like all other averages the M–H summary can be misleading if used thoughtlessly.

The M–H procedure can also be used to compare life tables after adjustment for confounding [Mantel 1966]. Table 7-9 compares groups m and n for the interval beginning at $x = 0$. If we wished to adjust this comparison for sex difference between groups m and n (assuming that sex confounds the survival-group relationship), Table 7-9 could have been separately prepared for men and women. We would then have two survival comparisons of group m with n (for the period 0–2). Of course, the M–H procedure can compare survival in groups m and n after adjustment for sex over the complete time period covered by Table 7-8 (six intervals). This requires summarizing 12 2×2 tables (six intervals for men and six for women) into an overall $\hat{OR}$ and χ^2. The principle is simple. Consider the life table time periods as if they were strata of a confounding variable. Prepare a 2×2 table for each combination of time period with a specific stratum of confounding variables for which adjustment is to be made. In the example just cited, if we wished to adjust for sex and two age classes, we would use 24 2×2 tables. Each would compare survival in groups m and n *specific for a single time period, sex, and age group*. The 24 2×2 tables can be summarized by the M–H procedure to obtain an overall odds ratio and χ^2 related to survival, adjusted for sex and age confounding. Confidence limits for this odds ratio can be derived using Miettinen's method for test-based confidence limits and the M–H χ^2.

Logrank Test

Another method for an overall statistical comparison of life tables is the logrank test. This was first reported by Mantel as a rank order statistic dependent only on the ranking of time of death of individuals in the two groups [Mantel 1966]. The name *logrank* and details of the computation of approximate χ^2 values for this test come from Peto et al [1977]. Although it is presented as a test arising from small intervals of analysis (such as single days or periods encompassing only one death), it is suitable for analyzing data in more common and somewhat longer intervals, provided that the proportion dying within any interval is small (less than 10 percent).

We shall describe the logrank method, illustrate its application to ordinary interval summary data, and then compare the logrank approximate χ^2 values with M–H χ^2 values. In order to demonstrate the conditions under which these two χ^2 values are very similar, we compare intervals in which the risk is high and intervals without high levels of risk.

As described by Peto et al [1977], the logrank method depends on the number at risk at the beginning of each interval. Thus, using Table 7-8 notation, O'_{xm} and O'_{xn} are at risk for the period beginning at time x in groups m and n, respectively. The expected number of deaths in each interval for each group is equal to the same proportion of the total deaths $(d_{xm} + d_{xn})$ as each group's proportion of the total number at risk $(O'_{xm} + O'_{xn})$. Therefore the expected number of deaths in group m for the period beginning at time x is

$$E(d_{xm}) = \frac{O'_{xm}}{O'_{xm} + O'_{xn}} (d_{xm} + d_{xn})$$

Similarly,

$$E(d_{xn}) = \frac{O'_{xn}}{O'_{xm} + O'_{xn}} (d_{xm} + d_{xn})$$

Under the null hypothesis of no difference in survival between groups m and n, the expectation that the group with the larger number of individuals at risk at the beginning of an interval will have the larger number of deaths in that interval is both simple and intuitively appealing. By this process, the expected number of deaths is derived for each interval of each life table. It is then an easy matter to compare the *total observed* number of deaths from each life table with the *total expected* number of deaths for the same life table. Totals are obtained from all intervals to be included in the analysis.

Under the null hypothesis (and the assumption of very small intervals of analysis or low interval risk), the square of the difference between total observed deaths and total expected deaths divided by the total expected deaths summed for two groups is approximately χ^2 with one degree of freedom. For groups m and n, this is

$$\chi_1^2 \simeq \frac{\left[\sum_x d_{xm} - \sum_x E(d_{xm})\right]^2}{\sum_x E(d_{xm})} + \frac{\left[\sum_x d_{xn} - \sum_x E(d_{xn})\right]^2}{\sum_x E(d_{xn})}$$

In general, if k life tables are being compared to see if they differ by more than can be readily attributed to chance, we can compute

$$\chi_{k-1}^2 \cong \sum_{i=1}^{k} \frac{\left(\begin{array}{cc}\text{total observed} & \text{total expected} \\ \text{deaths in } i & \text{deaths in } i\end{array}\right)^2}{\text{total expected deaths in } i} \qquad (7\text{-}5)$$

where i represents the ith life table and *total* refers to the total over the life table intervals being evaluated. Within each interval the expected number of deaths in group i is obtained by multiplying the total number of deaths $d_{x(\text{total})}$ by the ratio $U'_{xi}/U'_{x(\text{total})}$. The statistical significance of life table comparisons is then evaluated by referring to a table of chi square values to determine if the χ^2 calculated is or is not unusual (for the appropriate number of degrees of freedom).

A numeric illustration will clarify how the logrank method is used. To this end we compare life table data for two groups. In Table 7-10, columns 1 and 2 are taken from basic life table data for two groups, r and s. Column 3 expresses how the total at risk within each interval is proportionately distributed between groups r and s. Expected numbers of deaths are derived by multiplying the *total* number of deaths in column 2 by the proportionate distribution of the total number at risk in column 3. Thus, for the interval beginning at time 0, the expected number of deaths in group r is $45(.667) = 30.02$ and in group s is $45(.333) = 14.98$. To compare the two groups over the period from time 0 to time 6 requires

Table 7-10. Basic Life Table Data and Work Sheet for Logrank Comparison of Groups r and s

	(1)			(2)			(3)		(2 total) × (3)	
							Proportion of		Expected deaths under null	
	O'_x (no. at risk)			d_x (deaths)			O'_x total in		hypothesis	
x	r	s	Total	r	s	Total	r	s	r	s
0	300	150	450	25	20	45	.667	.333	30.02	14.98
1	275	130	405	4	3	7	.679	.321	4.75	2.25
2	271	127	398	3	2	5	.681	.319	3.40	1.60
3	268	125	393	1	1	2	,682	.318	1.36	.64
4	267	124	391	2	1	3	.683	.317	2.05	.95
5	265	123	388	1	1	2	.683	.317	1.37	.63
6	264	122	386	—	—	—	—	—	—	—
Total				36	28	64			42.95	21.05

summation of all deaths and expected deaths over this interval. These sums are shown in Table 7-10 on the "total" line. Note that deaths or expected deaths in the interval *beginning* at time 6 do not belong in the above comparison and are properly omitted. Using Table 7-10 data for this specific comparison of groups r and s, we get

$$\chi_1^2 \cong \frac{(36 - 42.95)^2}{42.95} + \frac{(28 - 21.05)^2}{21.05} \cong 3.42$$

To compare two life tables, the formal equation in accordance with Equation 7-5 with $k = 2$ is

$$\chi_1^2 \cong \sum_{i=1}^{2} \frac{\left[\sum_{j=1}^{t} O_{ij} - \sum_{j=1}^{t} E(d_{ij}) \right]^2}{\sum_{j=1}^{t} E(d_{ij})} \tag{7-6}$$

where

$$i = 1, 2 = \text{groups being compared}$$
$$j = 1, 2, \ldots, t = \text{life table intervals being evaluated}$$
$$O_{ij} = \text{observed deaths in } j\text{th interval of } i\text{th group}$$
$$E(d_{ij}) = \text{expected deaths in } j\text{th interval of } i\text{th group}$$

The logrank method (and the M–H method as well) can be used to compare survival curves over any interval of interest. All that is necessary is to set the index of summation to fit the interval to be evaluated:

$$\sum_{j=0}^{x} , \sum_{j=x}^{x+\Delta} , \text{ etc.}$$

Equivalence of Logrank χ^2 and Mantel–Haenszel χ^2

The logrank method is excellent, and an approximate summary χ^2 derived from it is easy to calculate, but this method can be misleading if the need to avoid intervals of high risk is forgotten. To demonstrate this, we shall compare summary χ^2 values obtained from logrank and from M–H procedures for different sets of data. We begin by considering the data in Table 7-8, which clearly violate the logrank requirement for low-risk intervals (e.g., in the interval beginning at time $x = 0$, $_2q_{0(m)} = 193/297 = .65$ and $_2q_{0(n)} = 165/297 = .56$. Table 7-11 presents the data from Table 7-8 in a form convenient for logrank calculations. Using Equation 7-6 and the total observed and total expected deaths in Table 7-11, we get a one degree of freedom, approximate summary χ^2 comparing groups m and n by logrank methods:

$$\chi_1^2 \, (\text{logrank}) \cong \frac{(245 - 226.20)^2}{226.20} + \frac{(253 - 271.80)^2}{271.80} = 2.86$$

We previously calculated a M–H χ^2 using the same data to compare groups m and n and found χ_1^2 (M–H) = 5.66. This discrepancy for χ^2 is substantial and can be attributed to an inappropriate use of the logrank method.

Table 7-11. Basic Life Table Data from Table 7-8 and Work Sheet for Logrank Comparison of Groups m and n

	(1)			(2)			(3)		(4)	
							Proportion of		Expected deaths under null	
	O_x' (no. at risk)			$_2d_x$ (deaths)			O_x' total in		hypothesis	
x	m	n	Total	m	n	Total	m	n	m	n
0	297	297	594	193	165	358	.500	.500	179.00	179.00
2	97	132	229	25	30	55	.424	.576	23.32	31.68
4	63	102	165	12	15	27	.382	.618	10.31	16.69
6	41	87	128	8	15	23	.320	.680	7.36	15.64
8	23	72	95	4	11	15	.242	.758	3.63	11.37
10	9	61	70	3	17	20	.129	.871	2.58	17.42
Total	—	—	—	245	253	498	—	—	226.20	271.80

Table 7-12. Basic Life Table Data from Table 7-10 Arranged for Mantel–Haenszel Computations

	Group "r"			Group "s"			Total		
i	Deaths (a_i)	Survivors (b_i)	At risk (m_{1i})	Deaths (c_i)	Survivors (d_i)	At risk (m_{2i})	Deaths (n_{1i})	Survivors (n_{2i})	At risk (t_i)
0	25	275	300	20	130	150	45	405	450
1	4	271	275	3	127	130	7	398	405
2	3	268	271	2	125	127	5	393	398
3	1	267	268	1	124	125	2	391	393
4	2	265	267	1	123	124	3	388	391
5	1	264	265	1	122	123	2	386	388

We now compare logrank and M–H calculations of summary χ^2 values using Table 7-10 data. For this purpose we show Table 7-12 with data derived from Table 7-10 and labeled to show cells a_i, b_i, c_i, d_i, etc., as follows:

	Deaths	Survivors	At risk
Group r	a_i	b_i	m_{1i}
Group s	c_i	d_i	m_{2i}
Total	n_{1i}	n_{2i}	t_i

Using Table 7-12 data and the M–H procedure, we get $\chi_1^2 = 3.16$. This is quite similar to the χ_1^2 value of 3.42 obtained with the logrank procedure on these same data. In fact, the values are so close that their relationship (i.e., which of the two is larger) is determined by the use or avoidance of the $\frac{1}{2}$ "continuity correction" used in the M–H calculation but not in the logrank method. Thus, in this instance, with no $_2q_x$ value greater than .133 (20/150 for group s in the period beginning at time $x = 0$) and most considerably lower, the logrank χ^2 computation is entirely satisfactory.

PRODUCT–LIMIT OR KAPLAN–MEIER METHOD

To this point we have considered life table methods with survival times grouped into convenient intervals. A special case of the life table method using arbitrarily small intervals that contain only persons with exactly equal survival times is called the Kaplan–Meier or product–limit method [Kaplan and Meier 1958]. Apart from using very small time intervals, it is not different from standard life tables. The essential distinction between the product–limit method and ordinary life tables is that an arbitrarily small interval eliminates the need for assumptions as to whether withdrawals or losses from observation occur uniformly throughout the interval or whether risk is constant over the interval. The only assumption required regarding losses and or withdrawals is that they have the same future experience as those remaining under observation. The product–limit method can be used for any sample size, but it is especially useful when the sample size is too small for satisfactory interval grouping. The standard life table may be more appropriate for large samples [Lee 1980].

To estimate the survival function $(_iP_0)$ using the product–limit method, first order the survival times (i) for each person from smallest to largest. List the lost and withdrawn cases after the deaths in the same interval. Then calculate for each survival time the number of events and the number who were at risk. Their ratio estimates q_i and $1 - q_i = p_i$. The probability of survival from time 0 to time n $(_nP_0)$ is estimated by the product of all p_i's for $i \leq n$. Each p_i represents the probability of surviving the ith interval. Their product, over a series of adjacent intervals, represents the probability of surviving all the intervals. The formula for the survival function $(_nP_0$ for survival from time 0 through time $n)$ is

$$_nP_0 = \prod_{i \leq n} (1 - d_i/O_i) \qquad (7\text{-}7)$$

where

$$i = \text{specific survival time}$$
$$O_i = \text{number at risk at time } i$$
$$d_i = \text{number of events at time } i$$

To illustrate the calculation, the following survival times after treatment were observed for 10 patients. Seven patients died at 2, 5, 6, 9, 9, 12, and 17 months, respectively. One patient was withdrawn alive at 12 months (study end) and two patients were lost to follow-up at 4 and 15 months. The data and the simple calculations to obtain an estimated survival function are shown in Table 7-13.

PROPORTIONAL HAZARDS MODEL (COX REGRESSION)

The life table methods discussed to this point permit us to calculate the risk that an event will occur during a specified time period, provided that the individual is at risk at the beginning of the period. In addition, using Mantel–Haenszel procedures, we can estimate the odds ratio for such conditional risk, comparing various categories of persons, e.g., those with and without high blood pressure. This comparison relates events in each time period to the individuals at risk during that time period separately

Table 7-13. Product–Limit or Kaplan–Meier Estimates of the Survival Function

| Time in months (i) | Number at risk (O_i) | Deaths (d_i) | Interval probability | | Survival function ($_iP_0$) |
			Of death (q_i)	Of survival (p_i)	
2	10	1	1/10	9/10	.900
4^a	9	0	0	1	.900(1) = .900
5	8	1	1/8	7/8	.900(7/8) = .788
6	7	1	1/7	6/7	.788(6/7) = .675
9	6	2	2/6	4/6	.675(4/6) = .450
12	4	1	1/4	3/4	.450(3/4) = .338
12^a	3	0	0	1	.338(1) = .338
15^a	2	0	0	1	.338(1) = .338
17	1	1	1	0	.338(0) = 0

^{a} Indicates lost or withdrawn alive.

for those with and without the risk factor present. Adjustment for confounding variables is achieved by stratification. An alternative to the Mantel–Haenszel procedure is the Cox proportional hazards model [Cox 1972]. This model relates events to the individuals at risk at the time of the event and in that respect is similar to the M–H procedure. The essential difference between the two methods is that the Cox procedure uses a mathematical model to adjust for covariables, whereas the M–H procedure simply uses stratification. The Cox model is currently in common use to report the results of longitudinal studies. We will first attempt to explain the rationale of this model and then compare the results obtained from its use with results for the same data using the M–H procedure.

Suppose the annual risk of dying at specific ages for a group of individuals such as United States white males could be represented by a curve as in Figure 7-2. It is at least imaginable that the annual risk of death for United States white males in a specific group (e.g., those who have systolic blood pressure of 160 or more and are regular cigarette smokers) could be approximated by a curve that is a constant multiple of the one in Figure 7-2. For example, if the general risk was .007 at age 50 and .018 at age 60, the risks at these ages for those who smoke and have elevated systolic blood pressure might be exactly double the general risk, i.e., .014 and .036 at ages 50 and 60, respectively. Plotting both curves on graph paper with a logarithmic scale for the vertical axis so that the constant ratio difference is shown as a fixed vertical difference, we could have something like Figure 7-3.[‡] Under this model the risks on a log scale do not have to be straight lines. Whatever the shape of the functions relating log risk to age, the model specifies only that there be a fixed *vertical* distance between them. The fixed vertical distance indicates a

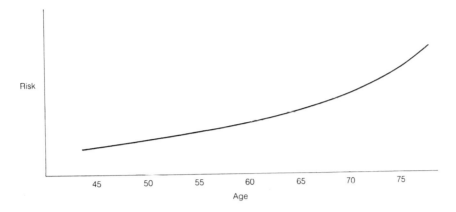

Figure 7-2. Indication of changing mortality risk by age. United States white males.

constant risk multiple at all ages. Of course the risk functions could relate to some other constant function of time such as time since treatment.

We now expand the foregoing idea as follows:

There exists a risk function (for instantaneous risks it is called a hazard function) applicable to the general population which, since it is clearly a function of time, we can label as $h_0(t)$. We can label the hazard function for a specific individual as $h_i(t)$. The ratio of the hazard functions, comparing that for an individual with that for the general population $[h_i(t)/h_0(t)]$, can be considered to be constant.

The value of this constant depends on the characteristics of the individual. Cox calls these characteristics explanatory variables. The notation we use is as follows: x_{1j} is the value of explanatory variable 1 for

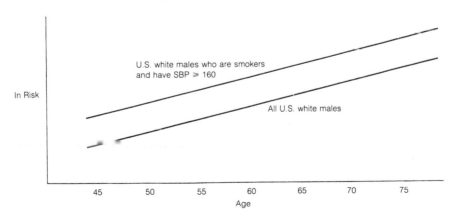

Figure 7-3. Natural logarithm of mortality risk by age illustrating a constant risk relationship between two groups. All United States white males and a subgroup of cigarette smokers with elevated blood pressure.

the jth individual, x_{2j} and x_{ij} are the values of the second and ith variables for the jth individual. Cox suggested that the fixed ratio of the two hazard functions be considered as an exponential function of the explanatory variables. In particular he suggested that

$$h_j(t)/h_0(t) = e^{\beta_1 x_{1j} + \beta_2 x_{2j} + \beta_3 x_{3j} + \cdots} \qquad (7\text{-}8)$$

By taking the logarithm of each side and recognizing that the hazard function ratio expresses relative risk, we get

$$\ln \text{ relative risk} = \beta_1 x_{1j} + \beta_2 x_{2j} + \beta_3 x_{3j} + \cdots \qquad (7\text{-}9)$$

It is plain from Equation 7-9 that the model assumes that the explanatory variables are linearly related to $\ln RR$. Equation 7-9 further assumes that the effects of the several explanatory variables are additive in the logarithmic scale, which is equivalent to multiplicative effects in the arithmetic scale

If the x_{ij}'s are deviations from $\bar{X}_i$, the population average, then $\ln RR$ for a person with average values for all variables would equal β_1 times zero $+ \beta_2$ times zero $+ \cdots = 0$. If $\ln RR$ equals 0, then the relative risk for someone with those average x values would equal 1.00, as seems reasonable.

The $\ln RR$ in Equation 7-9 refers to risk for the jth individual with the specific values x_{1j}, x_{2j}, and x_{3j} compared to risk for the general population. The corresponding relative risk for the jth person is $e^{\beta_1 x_{1j} + \beta_2 x_{2j} + \beta_3 x_{3j} + \cdots}$. To simplify explanation, let us assume that $x_{1j} = 1$, $x_{2j} = 0$, and $x_{3j} = 140$. Thus, RR (for the jth person) $= e^{\beta_1 + 140\beta_3}$. Consider the kth individual with $x_{1k} = 0$, $x_{2k} = 0$, and $x_{3k} = 140$ so that RR (for the kth person) $= e^{140\beta_3}$. If one individual had 5 times the average risk and another had 3 times the average risk it should be obvious that the first individual has $5/3$ times the risk of the latter. Treating the algebraic expressions for RR the same way,

$$RR \text{ (comparing person } j \text{ to } k) = e^{\beta_1 + 140\beta_3}/e^{140\beta_3} = e^{\beta_1}$$

If persons j and k differed with respect to additional variables, the relative risk comparing them would include other coefficients. In any event, the antilog of the regression coefficient estimates the relative risk. If the variable is dichotomous, the antilog of the regression coefficient estimates the relative risk, comparing the presence of that attribute to its absence. For continuous variables, the antilog of the regression coefficient estimates relative risk related to a one unit increase in the variable. The relative risk corresponding to a 20 unit increase in variable 3 would be $e^{20\beta_3}$.

Often major interest is directed toward the relative risk of morbidity or mortality of two groups, adjusted for potentially confounding variables. In this instance, one of the variables (say x_1) can be an indicator variable so that $x_{1j} = 1$ if the jth individual is in the specified group (perhaps given experimental treatment) and $x_{1j} = 0$ if not in that group. Under these conditions, the $\ln RR$ of an event comparing treated to untreated, and adjusted for various confounding variables $(x_2, x_3 \cdots)$, is β_1. If x_2 were also a dichotomous variable, the $\ln RR$ comparing treated persons with x_2 present to those untreated with x_2 absent would be $\beta_1 + \beta_2$. Interpreting Cox regression coefficients as relative risks closely parallels the interpretation of multiple logistic coefficients as odds ratios outlined in Chapter 6.

In this text we do not describe how the coefficients β_1, β_2, etc. are estimated from the observed data on survival and explanatory variables for each individual. However, the methods are analogous to those used for multiple regression and the results may be similarly interpreted. Thus, β_j represents the estimated change in $\ln RR$ for each unit change in x_j after removing from both x_j and $\ln RR$ their linear relationship with the other explanatory variables included in the analysis.

Cox regression is used in epidemiologic analyses to identify variables affecting disease, death or survival. The suggestion by Cox that proportional hazard might be represented by the function $e^{\beta_1 x_1 + \beta_2 x_2 + \cdots}$ has been widely adopted. Cox used this function to illustrate his idea for ignoring the complication of time in estimating the relationship of explanatory variables to risk. However, he did not suggest that proportional hazards are necessarily related to explanatory variables in this way and alternatives are surely possible. For the present Cox regression analyses seem to be restricted to the relationship: $\ln RR = \beta_1 x_1 + \beta_2 x_2 + \cdots$. Our comments and calculations on the Cox proportional hazards model are also limited to this model, which is the one you can expect to encounter in the current epidemiologic literature.

A recent report used the Cox proportional hazards model to study the association between several variables, including exogenous estrogen use, and mortality after diagnosis of endometrial cancer [Schwartzbaum et al 1987]. We will use some of the regression coefficients reported to illustrate their interpretation.

Variable	Coefficient	Variable codes (implied)
Estrogen use	−.7182	1 if used, 0 if not
Age	.0326	Age in years
Grade II	.6178	1 if grade II, 0 if not
Grade III	.7059	1 if grade III, 0 if not

(The model does not include any interaction, i.e., cross-product terms. The reference category for cancer grade is grade I.)

The coefficient for estrogen use estimates the ln RR corresponding to a one unit increase in the variable, i.e., comparing use (1) to no use (0). The estimated relative risk *comparing estrogen use to no use* is then $e^{-.7182}$, which equals .4876. The report does not present this relative risk but instead provides the relative risk *comparing no estrogen use to use*. This latter relative risk is exactly the reciprocal of the one derived directly from the regression coefficient and is reported as 2.05 which equals 1/.4876.

The regression coefficient for the continuous variable age is given as .0326 and the relative risk comparing age 68 to age 55 is reported as 1.53. The relationship between the coefficient .0326 and the estimated relative risk comparing age 68 to age 55 is

$$\hat{RR} \text{ (comparing age 68 to age 55)} = e^{(.0326)(68-55)} = 1.53$$

The estimated relative risks comparing grades II and III to grade I are as follows: $\hat{RR} = e^{.6178} = 1.85$ for grade II and $\hat{RR} = e^{.7059} = 2.03$ for grade III. Recall that those with cancer graded I will have both the grade II and grade III variables coded zero. Thus if all other variables are equal, the ln $\hat{RR}$ will be .6178 larger for grade II [.6178(1)] than for grade I [.6178(0)]. This increase in ln $\hat{RR}$ corresponds to an $\hat{RR}$ of $e^{.6178} = 1.85$. Similarly, if all other variables are equal, the ln $\hat{RR}$ will be .7059 larger for grade III than for grade I. This increase in ln $\hat{RR}$ corresponds to a $\hat{RR}$ of 2.03.

Finally, the estimated RR comparing those aged 68 *and* grade III to those aged 55 *and* grade I, after adjustment for the other variables in the analysis, is computed as

$$\hat{RR} = e^{(.0326)(68-55)+(.7059)(1-0)} = e^{.4328+.7059} = e^{1.1297} = 3.09$$

Notice that the ln $\hat{RR}$ are additive but the $\hat{RR}$ are multiplicative, i.e., (1.53)(2.03) = 3.11, which differs from 3.09 only because of rounding.

DEMOGRAPHIC LIFE TABLES

There are two major types of life tables: one is called medical, clinical, or cohort and the other demographic. All the description and discussion of life tables to this point relates to medical life tables derived from data on a real cohort. The demographic life table, computed on the basis of national (or regional) mortality data, is obtained by *applying the currently observed mortality risks at various ages to an imaginary cohort.* Thus the expectation of life at birth in the United States, which was 74.7 for 1985 [National Center for Health Statistics 1987] depends on the assumption that a group born in 1985 will be exposed to 1985 age-specific risks of mortality as they go through life (e.g., when this group is age 30 in the year 2015, they will experience the 1985 mortality risks for 30 year olds). Although taken literally this presumption is unrealistic, the demographic life table is an excellent way of summarizing current mortality risks. While epidemiologists in certain specialized areas may use demographic life tables extensively, the medical life table is the one that is more likely to be prepared and analyzed by most epidemiologists. The two types are essentially similar in concept, with national or regional demographic life tables almost always prepared by governmental statistical bureaus. The literature on demographic life tables is enormous and can be complicated. A good general reference is Shryock and Siegel [1975].

APPLICATION TO FRAMINGHAM HEART STUDY DATA

The years of observation regarding development of coronary heart disease are shown in the Appendix listings and Appendix summary tabulations under the label YRS_CHD. We remind you that the Framingham examinations were approximately two years apart and that incidence cases of coronary disease could be identified for the first time either on one of the periodic examinations (silent infarct, angina pectoris, coronary insufficiency) or during the interval between examinations (hospitalization for or death from coronary heart disease). We also remind you that the Appendix variable labeled CHD is coded 0 for those remaining free of coronary heart disease, 1 for those found to have the disease on examination 1 (prevalence cases) and 2–10 for those first diagnosed as incidence cases on examinations 2–10, respectively. For teaching purposes, we have approximated and simplified the time under observation as follows:

a. If coronary heart disease code is *negative*, i.e., CHD never diagnosed, YRS_CHD = 2 (number of the last examination taken −1). Cutting off observation at the time of the last examination reflects the fact that occurrence of some manifestations of coronary disease after the last examination is unlikely to come to the attention of the examiners.
b. If coronary heart disease code is ⩾2, i.e., *incidence cases*, YRS_ CHD = 2 (CHD − 1) − 1. In this instance we are using the CHD code to represent the number of the first examination on which diagnosis was made or the number of the first examination following interval diagnosis. This formulation presumes that disease onset was midway between the examination on which diagnosed and the preceding examination.[§]

Subjects are removed from the life table population at risk in the interval within which YRS_CHD falls.** These subjects are designated withdrawals (w_x) if CHD = 0. They are counted as events (d_x) if

CHD ≥ 2. We will first make the common assumption that withdrawals occur uniformly throughout the interval (although for these data we know it not to be true since under our calculation of observation time, all withdrawals will occur only at 2.01–4.01–6.01 etc. years observation). This provides us with the opportunity to investigate the extent to which summary statistics vary in changing from a four-year interval with withdrawals assumed to be uniformly distributed (when they are not) to a one-year interval with withdrawals treated as appropriate for this particular data set.

In Table 7-14 we group the data in four-year and two-year intervals and use the uniform withdrawal assumption.

Table 7-15 shows some of the data from Table 7-14 arranged in a convenient format for computing a Mantel–Haenszel odds ratio. After calculating the expected number of events for each entry in the "Positive" column, we then have the data needed for computing the logrank χ^2.

Summary statistics from Table 7-15:

Mantel–Haenszel odds ratio SBP ≥ 165/SBP $< 165 =$ 3.07

Mantel–Haenszel χ^2 (1 df) $= 10.47$

Logrank χ^2 (1 df) $= 10.65$

If Table 7-15 data were stratified by one-year instead of two- or four-year intervals and withdrawals were treated appropriately for this set of data,

Table 7-14. Life Tables for Men 55–59 Comparing SBP ≥ 165 with SBP $<$ 165: Probability of Developing Coronary Heart Disease (Assuming Withdrawals at Midpoint)

Time at beginning of interval (x)	Length of interval (n)	O_x	$_nw_x$	O'_x	$_nd_x$	$_nq_x$	$_nP_x$	$_{x+n}P_0$
Systolic blood pressure less than 165								
0	4	141	10	136.0	9	.066	.934	.934
4	4	122	7	118.5	9	.076	.924	.863
8	4	106	10	101.0	7	.069	.931	.803
12	4	89	10	84.0	8	.095	.905	.727
16	2	71	6	68.0	3	.044	.956	.695
Systolic blood pressure of 165 or more								
0	4	35	4	33.0	8	.242	.758	.758
4	4	23	1	22.5	5	.222	.778	.590
8	4	17	7	13.5	2	.148	.852	.440
12	4	8	0	8.0	1	.125	.875	.440
16	2	7	1	6.5	0	.000	1.000	.440

Table 7-15. 2 × 2 Tables for Each Life Table Interval Comparing SBP ≥ 165 with SBP < 165: Probability of Developing Coronary Heart Disease (Assuming Withdrawals at Midpoint)

Interval beginning	SBP	Adjusted number at risk	Positive $(_nd_x)$	Negative (by subtraction)
0	SBP ≥ 165	33.0	8 (a)	25.0 (b)
	SBP < 165	136.0	9 (c)	127.0 (d)
		169.0 (t)		
4	SBP ≥ 165	22.5	5	17.5
	SBP < 165	118.5	9	109.5
		141.0		
8	SBP ≥ 165	13.5	2	11.5
	SBP < 165	101.0	7	94.0
		114.5		
12	SBP ≥ 165	8.0	1	7.0
	SBP < 165	84.0	8	76.0
		92.0		
16	SBP ≥ 165	6.5	0	6.5
	SBP < 165	68.0	3	65.0
		74.5		

e.g., allowing no observation time in the interval 6.00–6.99 for withdrawals at six years, the above summary statistics would change to:

Mantel–Haenszel odds ratio SBP ≥ 165/SBP < 165 = 3.10

Mantel–Haenszel χ^2 (1 df)   = 11.66

Logrank χ^2 (1 df)   = 12.28

The similarity of these results, even though one summary is based on finer intervals and more appropriate treatment of the withdrawals than the other, is partly due to the fact that there are few withdrawals in these data. This is an important lesson. If the number of withdrawals is small, how you treat them will not cause a substantial difference. But if the number of withdrawals is great, substantial differences are possible and results may depend heavily on whether or not the assumptions are correct.

Using data for those with SBP < 165 from Table 7-14 and standard error formula 7-4 adjusted for four-year intervals, we have

$$SE(_{x+4}P_0) = {}_{x+4}P_0 \sqrt{\sum_{i=0}^{x/4} \frac{_4q_{4i}}{O'_{4i} - {}_4d_{4i}}}$$

for $x = 12$ this is

$$SE(_{16}P_0) = .727 \sqrt{\frac{.066}{136 - 9} + \frac{.076}{118.5 - 9} + \frac{.069}{101 - 7} + \frac{.095}{84 - 8}}$$

$$= .041$$

If you were to compare survival at 16 years between those with SBP $\geqslant 165$ and those with SBP < 165, using standard errors computed in the manner described above, it is essential to realize that the two survival distributions are being compared just at the 16-year point. Deriving a standardized normal deviate by using

$$\frac{[_{16}P_0 \text{ (for SBP} \geqslant 165) - {}_{16}P_0 \text{ (for SBP} < 165)] - 0}{\sqrt{[SE(_{16}P_0) \text{ for SBP} \geqslant 165]^2 + [SE(_{16}P_0) \text{ for SBP} < 165]^2}} = z$$

does not compare the two distributions as is done by the Mantel–Haenszel or logrank procedures.

Cox Regression

The estimated relative risk of developing coronary heart disease within 18 years, comparing SBP $\geqslant 165$ to SBP < 165 and adjusting for age (four classes) and sex is $e^{1.000} = 2.72$ according to the Cox proportional hazards model. The full equation is

$$\ln RR = .195x_1 + .573x_2 + .761x_3 - .884x_4 + 1.000x_5$$

where

$$x_1 = 1 \text{ if aged 50--54, otherwise } x_1 = 0$$
$$x_2 = 1 \text{ if aged 55--59, otherwise } x_2 = 0$$
$$x_3 = 1 \text{ if aged 60--62, otherwise } x_3 = 0$$
$$x_4 = 1 \text{ if male, otherwise } x_4 = 2$$
$$x_5 = 1 \text{ if SBP} \geqslant 165, \text{ otherwise } x_5 = 0$$

Note that in this particular computation the code for sex (x_4) is 1 for males and 2 for females. Other tabulations in this book have used code 1 for male and 0 for female. Had we used the usual code for sex in this instance, the coefficient of x_4 would have been $+.884$ instead of $-.884$ with all other coefficients unchanged.

EXERCISES

The approximate years of observation with respect to mortality are shown in the Appendix listings and Appendix summary tabulations under the label YRS_DTH. For our purposes we have simplified mortality observation time as follows:

For those not reported dead during the 18-year observation period

$$YRS\_DTH = 18$$

For those dying during the observation period

$$YRS\_DTH = 2 \text{ (exam number following date of death} - 1) - 1$$

For a death occurring between scheduled examinations 6 and 7

$$YRS\_DTH = 2(7 - 1) - 1 = 11$$

This assumes two years between all scheduled examination dates and that death occurs only midway between dates.

Table 7-16 summarizes survival data for men aged 55–59 dependent upon whether or not systolic blood pressure is less than 165. Observe that, in contrast to life table data on incidence of coronary disease, there

Table 7-16. Mortality Tables for Men 55–59 and Free of CHD on Exam 1 Comparing SBP ⩾ 165 with SBP < 165 (Assumes All Withdrawals at Exactly 18 Years)

Exact time at beginning of interval (x)	Length of interval (n)	O_x	$_nW_x$	O'_x	$_nd_x$
		Systolic blood pressure less than 165			
0	4	141	0	141	7
4	4	134	0	134	7
8	4	127	0	127	13
12	4	114	0	114	9
16	2	105	0	105	7
		Systolic blood pressure of 165 or more			
0	4	35	0	35	4
4	4	31	0	31	2
8	4	29	0	29	8
12	4	21	0	21	6
16	2	15	0	15	3

are no cases lost to follow-up before the cutoff date. The presumption is that survival status, unlike morbidity status, is known for all.

Answer Exercises 7-1 to 7-5 based on the data in Table 7-16.

Ex. 7-1. For each blood pressure group what is the 18-year probability of survival and its standard error?

Ex. 7-2. Use the 16-year survival probabilities and their standard errors computed in Exercise 7-1 to calculate a one degree of freedom X^2 for testing whether the probabilities are significantly different. The probabilities for the two blood pressure groups can be considered as independent.

Ex. 7-3. Compare the two survival distributions through year 18 with the Mantel–Haenszel procedure. What is the odds ratio for dying, relating SBP $\geqslant 165$ to SBP < 165? What is the χ^2 value corresponding to this odds ratio?

Ex. 7-4. Compute the χ^2 derived from a comparison of observed and expected deaths in the two blood pressure groups through year 16. How does this χ^2 compare to the "Greenwood χ^2" computed in Exercise 7-2 and the Mantel–Haenszel χ^2 computed in Exercise 7-3?

Ex. 7-5. For SBP $\geqslant 165$, what are the numeric values of

$$a. \ _4q_8 \qquad _4p_8 \qquad _{12}p_0$$
$$b. \ _2q_{16} \qquad _2p_{16} \qquad _{18}p_0$$

Ex. 7-6. Use the data in Table 7-17 to compute the crude and net probability of death from cancer within 18 years.

Table 7-17. Mortality from Cancer and Other Causes, Men Aged 55–62

Exact time at beginning of interval (x)	Length of interval (n)	O_x	$_nw_x$	$_nd_x$ Cancer	$_nd_x$ Other
0	4	246	0	4	13
4	4	229	0	3	15
8	4	211	0	7	26
12	4	178	0	6	19
16	2	153	0	4	12

Ex. 7-7. Use the Appendix listing for men aged 60–62 to complete the following table with respect to the risk of developing coronary heart disease among those considered negative for CHD on examination 1.

x	O_x	$_2w_x$	O'_x	$_2d_x$	$_2q_x$	$_{x+2}p_x$
0	—	—	—	—	—	—
2	—	—	—	—	—	—
4	—	—	—	—	—	—

NOTES

* The joint probability of surviving consecutive intervals uses the basic probability formula $P(AB) = P(A)P(B/A)$, where $P(A)$ represents the probability of surviving the first period, $P(B/A)$ represents the probability of surviving the second period *given* that the first was survived, and $P(AB)$ represents the probability of surviving both periods. If withdrawals do not complicate the calculations, this relationship can be illustrated with a simple example. If 100 are observed at time 0 and 80 of these survive to time 1, $P(A) = 80/100$. If, *of the 80 surviving to time 1*, 40 survive to time 2, $P(B/A) = 40/80$. The probability of surviving both periods is then the product: $(80/100)(40/80) = 40/100$. Since all the $_np_x$ values are conditional probabilities, the same calculations and logic apply to a chain of three or more intervals.

† Often the "universe" is poorly described or not described at all, leaving it unclear as to whether the sample at hand is a sample in time, in space, or of surgeons. All extrapolations from the universe sampled to other universes of interest are matters of scientific judgment and are not based on statistical considerations.

‡ On arithmetic graph paper the vertical distance between the two curves would widen as the constant multiplier was applied to the higher risks at older ages. The logarithm of a constant ratio is constant and this is reflected in the constant vertical difference between the two lines on the logarithmic scale. Using the risks specified for this illustration, the difference in the logarithm of the risk is (ln .014 − ln .007) for age 50 and (ln .036 − ln .018) for age 60. Each of these differences equals .6931, which is the natural logarithm of 2.00.

§ If the last examination before diagnosis was not the immediately preceding scheduled examination, the above formula was modified to place the event halfway between the last two examinations taken.

** The program we used for life table computations did this in a somewhat unconventional way. It created intervals such as 5.01–6.00 (actually greater than 5 but less than or equal to 6). Thus, an individual allocated six years of observation at the time of withdrawal from the study would be shown as a withdrawal in the interval 5.01–6.00. The life table arrangement taught in this book designates intervals as beginning at exact age x and our preferred groupings for this example would be 5.00–5.99 and 6.00–6.99. We achieved this, with the program at hand, by simply adding .01 to the years of observation for each individual with only a trivial effect on the basic data. The life table intervals can then be labeled as beginning at exact age x and someone withdrawn at six years of observation would be included in w_x in the interval 6.00–6.99.

8
Follow-up Studies: Person-Years

The life table method permits us to combine data on those observed for any length of time with data on those observed for longer or shorter periods. Such data can also be combined using the person-years method. We shall first describe this method and then indicate similarities and differences between it and the life table method and suggest how to choose between them.

COMPUTATIONS AND ASSUMPTIONS

Suppose we wish to estimate the annual incidence rate for disabling cataract and have observed two groups. In the first group, observed for one year, the number of persons varies from month to month but averages 500 persons at risk, with 13 developing cataract. In the second group, observed for two years, the size of the group averages 400 persons at risk, with 23 developing cataract. Although the average number of individuals at risk is 900, the number of person-years observed is $500 + 800 = 1300$. In order to combine the cataract incidence data from the two groups in a sensible way, two conditions must apply:

1. Risk must increase proportionately as length of observation increases.
2. Individuals in each group must be at similar risk.

These conditions are met in some studies, but if it is not reasonable to assume that they are, then the person-years method cannot be used.

   If cataract incidence is about 3 percent per year for persons at risk (those without cataract) at about age 70 and if all 900 individuals are age

69 to 71, then both conditions 1 and 2 are met and the person-year method is appropriate. If the individuals are all age 69 to 71 but one-year cataract incidence at age 70 is 60 percent of those at risk instead of 3 percent, person-years would not be appropriate because, at 60 percent risk for a single year, the two-year risk could obviously not be double that for one year. If the 500 individuals observed for one year are age 70 and the 400 observed for two years are age 17, again the person-year method would be inapplicable as cataract risk is known to increase with age. Thus, the two groups would not have a similar risk. In order to *pool* observations of different groups for varying periods of time, both conditions listed above must be satisfied.

Comparison of Rates and Probabilities

In our cataract example, the incidence rate of disabling cataract per person-year at risk can be estimated as

$$\frac{13 + 23}{500 + 800} = \frac{36}{1300} = .028 \text{ per person-year at risk}$$

Note that this is an incidence *rate* of acquiring cataract, not a probability. The distinction is simple. A probability, $q_x = d_x/O_x$, relates a number of events during an interval to the number *at risk at the beginning* of the interval. A rate, $m_x = d_x/P_x$, where P_x equals the *average population at risk* during the interval, is based on a different denominator. If the event being counted is death, the probability of death and the rate of death are usually unequal (the rate being greater) because the number under observation at the start of an interval (O_x) is reduced by deaths during the interval. This makes the average number under observation during the period, P_x, less than O_x.*

Similarly, for an event such as disabling cataract in either eye, the number under observation and at risk at the start of an interval is reduced during the interval by those developing cataract because these people are no longer at risk of becoming an incident case. For identical starting populations, the rate of a specified event is always larger than (or equal to) the probability of the same event. If we assume that the events are uniformly distributed during the interval, the relationship in a closed population, between $_nq_x$ (probability), $_nm_x$ (rate) and $d_x/_nL_x$ (rate per person year) is described in Equations 8-1 through 8-4. The symbol $_nL_x$ is used for person-years at risk between time x and $x + n$. $_nL_x$ can be estimated as the product of the length of the period and the number at risk at the beginning, then subtracting $n/2$ times the number of events in the period. In symbols $_nL_x = n(O_x - d_x/2)$.

The *probability per individual at risk* of an event in the interval x to

$x + n$ is

$$_nq_x = \frac{_nd_x(O_x - _nd_x/2)}{O_x(O_x - _nd_x/2)} = _nm_x \frac{(O_x - _nd_x/2)}{O_x}$$

$$= _nm_x \frac{n[O_x - (_nd_x/2)]}{nO_x} = _nm_x \frac{_nL_x}{_nL_x + n(_nd_x/2)} \tag{8-1}$$

Alternatively

$$_nq_x = \frac{_nd_x}{O_x} = \frac{_nd_x}{_nP_x + (_nd_x/2)} = \frac{_nd_x/_nP_x}{1 + (_nd_x/2_nP_x)}$$

$$= \frac{_nm_x}{1 + (_nm_x/2)} = \frac{2_nm_x}{2 + _nm_x} \tag{8-2}$$

The *rate per individual at risk* of an event in the interval x to $x + n$ is

$$_nm_x = \frac{[_nd_x]O_x}{[O_x - (_nd_x/2)]O_x} = _nq_x \frac{O_x}{O_x - _nd_x/2}$$

$$= _nq_x \frac{nO_x}{n[O_x - _nd_x/2]} = _nq_x \frac{[_nL_x + n_nd_x/2]}{_nL_x} \tag{8-3}$$

The *rate per person year at risk* of an event in the interval x to $x + n$ is

$$\frac{_nd_x}{_nL_x} = \frac{_nd_x}{n[O_x - _nd_x/2]} = \frac{_nm_x}{n} \tag{8-4}$$

Only in the case of events having very high risk (i.e., $d_x/2$ equals an appreciable fraction of O_x) do q_x and m_x differ to any practical extent. To illustrate, if the annual probability of death at age 70 is about .05 and at 80 about .12 and assuming uniform distribution of deaths during the year (possibly a questionable assumption at age 80), then

$$m_{70} = .05\left(\frac{100}{100 - 2.5}\right) = .051 \qquad \text{(compared to .050 for } q_{70})$$

$$m_{80} = .12\left(\frac{100}{100 - 6}\right) = .128 \qquad \text{(compared to .120 for } q_{80})$$

Thus, even for the high mortality risk associated with age 80 the distinction between rate and probability is not very great.

Similarity to Life Tables

The conditions stated above for using the person-years method made no reference to withdrawals, i.e., person lost from observation before occurrence of the event being studied. As discussed in Chapter 7 on life tables, these are of two kinds: (a) withdrawals from observation because the cutoff date for analysis is reached and (b) withdrawals from observation because the individual has moved from the study area or cannot be located or does not cooperate as required.

If there are withdrawals, the assumptions required for person-year calculations are the same as for the life table method. These are (a) withdrawals occur uniformly throughout the interval of analysis (so that simple estimates of average population at risk are possible) and (b) the experience of persons after withdrawal is the same as that of persons remaining under observation. As in the case of life table analysis, it is probably more correct to assume equivalent future experience for withdrawals due to cutoff date than for withdrawals lost to observation.

Two other assumptions required for life table calculations are also needed for person-year tabulations. Whether or not there are withdrawals, person-year tabulations require approximate uniformity of risk within the intervals in which data are summarized. The final assumption required for both life table and person-year analyses is that there be no secular trend in data pooled into a common interval.

A practical consequence of the assumption that, within intervals of analysis, the risk is directly proportional to the length of the interval is the need to avoid long intervals. Thus, if we consider the risk of lung cancer among cigarette smokers age 45 to 64, it is unreasonable to suppose that individuals observed for twenty years from age 45 to 64 are subject to only 20 times as much risk from lung cancer as individuals observed for one year beginning at age 45. Pooling such disparate risks into a person-year summary is likely to result in more confusion than enlightenment. If instead of using a twenty-year interval, these data were summarized into five-year intervals (45 to 49, 50 to 54, 55 to 59, and 60 to 64), the combining of person-years observation at the young end of the five-year interval with observation over the entire five-year interval or even only with observation at the old end of the five-year interval may not seriously contradict the requirement that, within intervals, risk be directly proportional to length of observation.

It is essential not to confuse the requirement for constant risk *within an interval* with the requirement for constant risk over the entire age range under study. For example, we may have observation on one individual from age 40 to 54 and on another from age 50 to 59. If the risks within the five-year intervals are approximately constant, pooling within these five-year periods is satisfactory. There is no requirement that risk be constant from age 40 to 59. It is only *within* intervals of analysis that pooling of person-year observation periods takes place, and thus it is only *within* intervals of analysis that the condition of constant risk applies. If there is constant risk within a short or moderately long interval of analysis, then the risk within any subinterval will be closely proportional to the length of observation.

Illustrative Computation

The typical study for which person-year analysis is appropriate concerns a group coming under observation at different ages and remaining under observation for varying periods of time. We first present detailed methods for calculating person-years of observation for age-specific periods, 35 to 44, 45 to 54, etc. This is useful for understanding the procedure and can also be the approach used if computer assistance is available. For illustrative purposes, we shall calculate age-specific risk of lung cancer mortality among six individuals who are regular cigarette smokers. The basic data are shown in Table 8-1. The first step is to convert date on which observation began to age at which observation began. We do this by subtracting date of birth from date observation began:

1. Subtraction when no "borrowing" required

Year	Month	Day	
1954	7	11	Date observation began
1897	1	4	Date of birth
57	6	7	Age observation began

2. Subtraction with "borrowing"

Year	Month	Day	
1954	8	3	Date observation began in original units
1953	19	33	Date observation began after subtraction of 1 year and addition of 11 months and 30 days
1884	9	5	Date of birth
69	10	28	Age observation began

By a similar process of subtracting date of birth from date on which observation terminated, we obtain the individual's age at the time observation terminated. Table 8-2 presents both beginning and terminating ages for all six individuals. Also in Table 8-2 are the lengths of

Table 8-1. Data for Calculation of Person-Years of Observation for Six Individuals

Individual	Date of birth	Date observation began	Date observation ended	Lung cancer mortality (0 = no, 1 = yes)
1	Jan. 4, 1897	July 11, 1954	Dec. 31, 1962	0
2	Sept. 5, 1884	Aug. 3, 1954	Nov. 25, 1960	1
3	Dec. 16, 1904	Oct. 25, 1954	Dec. 31, 1962	0
4	Jan. 16, 1899	Nov. 1, 1954	Dec. 31, 1962	0
5	Apr. 9, 1912	Feb. 19, 1957	Dec. 31, 1962	0
6	Feb. 22, 1910	Dec. 8, 1957	Aug. 18, 1959	1

observation periods allocated to the age-specific intervals for which data are being pooled. These are obtained by defining the beginning and ending ages of the intervals as 45 years, 0 months, 0 days and 54 years, 11 months, 30 days for age 45 to 54; 55 years, 0 months, 0 days and 64 years, 11 months, 30 days for age 55 to 64; and 65 years, 0 months, 0 days and 74 years, 11 months, 30 days for age 65 to 74 and subtracting as appropriate. The beginning date of observation for individual 1 completely avoids the 45 to 54 interval, but in the 55 to 64 interval we have

Year	Month	Day	
64	11	30	Ending age observed in interval
57	6	7	Beginning age observed in interval
7	5	23	Time in 55 to 64 interval for individual 1

and in the 65 to 74 interval we have

Year	Month	Day	
65	11	27	Ending age observed in interval
65	0	0	Beginning age observed in interval
0	11	27	Time in 65 to 74 interval for individual 1

Note that, in the 55 to 64 interval, individual 1 is observed until the terminal age for that interval. In the 65 to 74 interval, individual 1 is observed not to the ending age of the interval but to the terminal age of his or her observation in the study. The calculation of length of observation for each of the other five individuals is carried out in a similar way. The rather obvious rules for calculating the length of

Table 8-2. Conversion of Age Observation Began and Age Observation Terminated to Age-Specific Observation Periods

| | Age when observation | | | | | | Length of observation at age | | | | | | | | |
| | Began | | | Terminated | | | 45–54 | | | 55–64 | | | 65–74 | | |
Individual	Yr	Mo	Day	Yr	Mo	Day	Yr	Mo	Day	Yr	Mo	Day	Yr	Mo	Day
1	57	6	7	65	11	27	—	—	—	7	5	23	0	11	27
2	69	10	28	76	2	20	—	—	—	—	—	—	5	1	2
3	49	10	9	58	0	15	5	1	21	3	0	15	—	—	—
4	55	9	15	63	11	15	—	—	—	8	2	0	—	—	—
5	44	10	10	50	8	22	5	8	22	—	—	—	—	—	—
6	47	9	16	49	5	26	1	8	10	—	—	—	—	—	—
Total							11	17	53	18	7	38	5	12	29
Person-years[a]								12.56			18.69			6.08	

[a] One month = .08333 years; one day = .00274 years.

observation in terms of each age-specific period are

1. For observation beginning within an interval and extending beyond it, subtract the beginning age of observation from the age at the end of the interval.
2. For observation beginning at the start of an interval and ending within it, subtract the beginning age of the interval from the age at which observation is ended.
3. For observation beginning and ending within an interval, subtract the beginning age of observation from the ending age of observation.
4. For observation beginning at the start and continuing to the end of an interval, use the length of the interval.

Summing the years, months, and days contributed by each individual and then converting months and days to person-years, we obtain the total person-years of observation in each ten-year age class, as shown on the bottom line of Table 8-2.

While this detailed approach to calculating person-years of observation for each age class is always possible, and with the aid of computer processing is not unduly difficult, it is not always necessary. Various approximations and simplifications are possible. If the data set is not too large, the hand tally method illustrated in Table 8-3 is commonly used to summarize the age data given in Table 8-2. In Table 8-3, five-year age groupings for year observation began are cross-classified with five-year age groupings for year observation ended, with the number of individuals so classified tallied in each cell. If observation terminated because of death, the tally is in brackets. In the extreme right column of Table 8-3 are the total number of individuals whose observation started during the five-year periods beginning with x as specified. Thus, observation started on one individual during the five-year period beginning with $x = 40$ and on two individuals during the five-year period beginning with $x = 45$. In the bottom two rows are the cases withdrawn alive during each five-year period ($_5w_x$) and the cases dying during each five-year period ($_5d_x$). Those cells for which the age class for beginning observation is identical to the age class for ending observation are shaded for easy identification and later use. Approximate person-years of observation from x to $x + n$ are defined according to Equation 8-5:

$$_nL_x = nO_x + \frac{n}{2}(_na_x - _nw_x - _nd_x) + \frac{n}{4}(_naw_x + _nad_x) \qquad (8\text{-}5)$$

where

$_nL_x$ = approximate person-years of observation from age x to age $x + n$
n = length of interval under consideration
O_x = number of individuals under observation at exact age x

Table 8-3. Work Sheet for Summarizing Person-Year Data

Observation started during five-year period beginning with x equal to	Observation ended during five-year period beginning with x equal to								Additions[a] ($_5a_x$)
	40	45	50	55	60	65	70	75	
40			1						1
45		[1]		1					2
50									0
55					1				2
60						1			0
65								[1]	1
70									0
75									0
$_5w_x$	0	0	1	1	1	1	0	0	
$_5d_x$	0	1	0	0	0	0	0	1	

[a] Total number of individuals whose observation started during interval.

$_na_x$ = number of individuals added to those under observation in the age interval x to $x + n$; includes all such individuals whether or not withdrawn or died in the same age interval as added to observation

$_nw_x$ = number of individuals withdrawn alive (whether due to study cutoff date or to loss from observation) during age interval x to $x + n$; includes all such individuals whether or not added to observation in the same age interval as withdrawn

$_nd_x$ = number of deaths during age interval x to $x + n$; includes all such individuals, whether or not they died in the same age interval as added to observation

$_naw_x$ = number of individuals added and withdrawn in the same time interval

$_nad_x$ = number of individuals added and died in the same time interval

We shall first explain Equation 8-5 and then illustrate how the summary columns and rows of Table 8-3 provide the data required by the formula.

Equation 8-5 totals the person-years of observation from x to $x + n$ as follows. The first term, nO_x, counts n years of observation for each person under observation at exact age x. Since no one is *added* to the study *at exact age* x, it should be clear that these individuals are those who are continued under observation from the prior interval. The next term, $(n/2) (_na_x - _nw_x - _nd_x)$, adds $n/2$ years of observation for each individual added to observation during the age interval x to $x + n$ under the assumption that additions are uniformly distributed during the interval and subtracts $n/2$ years of observation for each individual withdrawn alive or dying during the age interval x to $x + n$ under the assumption that withdrawals and deaths are uniform during the interval.

The next term, $(n/4)(_naw_x + _nad_x)$, may seem somewhat mysterious. Recall that $n/2$ years have been added for each addition during the period x to $x + n$ and that $n/2$ years have been subtracted for each withdrawal or death during the same period. The first two terms thus do not include any observation time for individuals added *and* withdrawn or added *and* dying in the same interval. The third term in Equation 8-5 counts $n/4$ years of observation for each such case. Why $n/4$? If additions are uniformly distributed, then on the average additions will come under observation halfway through the interval. If withdrawals and deaths are uniformly distributed, the additions who have come under observation half way through the interval will leave halfway through the observation time remaining and thus will have been observed, on the average, for $n/4$ years. In other words, each such individual contributes $\frac{1}{4}$ of the length of the interval to the total observation time. Because it seems unlikely that individuals will be lost from observation *immediately* after becoming enrolled in a follow-up program, some investigators use $n/3$ instead of $n/4$.

We now return to Table 8-3 and use it to calculate successive values of O_x. According to Table 8-3, there were no additions to observation before age 40 to 44; therefore there was no one under observation at *exact* age 40. Thus $O_{40} = 0$. A necessary first step is to identify an O_x value preceding the youngest age of observation so that we know it equals zero. We can then begin with this starting O_x value and, by adding $_na_x$ values and subtracting $_nw_x$ and $_nd_x$ values, derive subsequent O_x values:

$$O_{40} + {}_5a_{40} - {}_5w_{40} - {}_5d_{40} = O_{45}$$
$$0 + 1 - 0 - 0 = 1$$
$$O_{45} + {}_5a_{45} - {}_5w_{45} - {}_5d_{45} = O_{50}$$
$$1 + 2 - 0 - 1 = 2$$

By this process we derive all of the O_x values for our six-person example:

$$O_{40} = 0 \qquad O_{65} = 1$$
$$O_{45} = 1 \qquad O_{70} = 1$$
$$O_{50} = 2 \qquad O_{75} = 1$$
$$O_{55} = 1 \qquad O_{80} = 0$$
$$O_{60} = 2$$

Recalling that tallies in brackets in Table 8-3 represent deaths (all other observations that terminate are withdrawals) and that shaded cells represent additions and withdrawals or additions and deaths in the *same age interval*, we are ready to use Equation 8-5:

$$_5L_{40} = 5(0) + \tfrac{5}{2}(1 - 0 - 0) + \tfrac{5}{4}(0 + 0) = 2.50$$
$$_5L_{45} = 5(1) + \tfrac{5}{2}(2 - 0 - 1) + \tfrac{5}{4}(0 + 1) = 8.75$$
$$_5L_{50} = 5(2) + \tfrac{5}{2}(0 - 1 - 0) + \tfrac{5}{4}(0 + 0) = 7.50$$
$$_5L_{55} = 5(1) + \tfrac{5}{2}(2 - 1 - 0) + \tfrac{5}{4}(0 + 0) = 7.50$$
$$_5L_{60} = 5(2) + \tfrac{5}{2}(0 - 1 - 0) + \tfrac{5}{4}(0 + 0) = 7.50$$
$$_5L_{65} = 5(1) + \tfrac{5}{2}(1 - 1 - 0) + \tfrac{5}{4}(0 + 0) = 5.00$$
$$_5L_{70} = 5(1) + \tfrac{5}{2}(0 - 0 - 0) + \tfrac{5}{4}(0 + 0) = 5.00$$
$$_5L_{75} = 5(1) + \tfrac{5}{2}(0 - 0 - 1) + \tfrac{5}{4}(0 + 0) = 2.50$$

Since our detailed calculation of person-years of observation is summarized in ten-year age classes, we combine the five-year age class data into ten-year classes for comparison:

$$_5L_{45} + {}_5L_{50} = 8.75 + 7.50 = 16.25 = {}_{10}L_{45}$$
$$_5L_{55} + {}_5L_{60} = 7.50 + 7.50 = 15.00 = {}_{10}L_{55}$$
$$_5L_{65} + {}_5L_{70} = 5.00 + 5.00 = 10.00 = {}_{10}L_{65}$$

The values 16.25, 15.00, and 10.00 correspond to the exact values 12.56, 18.69, and 6.08, respectively, derived previously and shown in Table 8-2. For as few as six cases, there is no particular reason to expect a close match between the exact computation of person-years of observation and the formula computation, which assumes uniform distribution of additions, withdrawals, and deaths. For large bodies of data, however, the two methods usually agree quite well. Agreement can almost always be improved by summarizing data into narrower intervals of analysis.

By either method of calculating person-years of observation, the death rate per person-year of observation is obtained by dividing the number of deaths in specific age classes by the number of person-years of observation for that age class.

SAMPLING ERROR AND CONFIDENCE LIMITS

As with all other types of statistics, person-year rates are subject to sampling error. Under the common assumption of uniform distribution of deaths within intervals of analysis, the standard error of a rate per person-year of observation can be estimated [Chiang 1961b] as

$$\hat{SE}(_nm_x) = \left[\frac{_nm_x(2 - n_nm_x)}{_nL_x(2 + n_nm_x)} \right]^{1/2} \tag{8-6}$$

where

$_nm_x$ = rate per person-year for the age interval x to $x + n$

$_nL_x$ = number of person-years observed in the interval x to $x + n$

n = length of age interval

To illustrate the use of Equation 8-6, we return to the example of 36 cataract cases developing during 1300 person-years of observation, cited earlier in this chapter. The rate per person-year of .028 was for individuals age 69 to 71, and thus the length of the age interval is three years and $n = 3$:

$$\hat{SE}(_{71}m_{69}) = \left\{ \frac{.028[2 - (3)(.028)]}{1300[2 + (3)(.028)]} \right\}^{1/2} = .00445$$

and 95 percent confidence limits are $.028 \pm 1.96(.00445) = .019$ and $.037$.

An alternative basis for estimating confidence limits for person-year rates is to assume the numerator of the rate to be a Poisson variable. If the rate is low (as it often is), this is not unreasonable. Recalling that for Poisson variables the square root of the parameter is the standard error of the statistic, we can define an upper limit to our 95 percent confidence interval as λ_U, where

$$\lambda_U = \text{observed number} + 1.96\sqrt{\lambda_U} \qquad (8\text{-}7)$$

Only 2.5 percent of all possible samples can be expected to result in an observed number smaller than $1.96\sqrt{\text{parameter}}$ below the parameter value. Thus, unless we happen to have a sample among this 2.5 percent, we can estimate the parameter value to be no greater than the observed number plus $1.96\sqrt{\text{parameter}}$, as in Equation 8-7.

Similarly, we can define a lower limit to our 95 percent confidence interval as λ_L, where

$$\lambda_L = \text{observed number} - 1.96\sqrt{\lambda_L} \qquad (8\text{-}8)$$

These equations are easy to solve if we recognize that Equation 8-7, for example, is a quadratic equation in $\sqrt{\lambda_U}$. In relation to the standard quadratic form $ax^2 + bx + c = 0$, $x = \sqrt{\lambda_U}$ and $x^2 = \lambda_U$. Putting Equation 8-7 into standard form and substituting 36, the observed number of cases from the cataract example, for c we have

$$\lambda_U - 1.96\sqrt{\lambda_U} - 36 = 0$$

with $a = 1$, $b = -1.96$, and $c = -36$ the solution to the quadratic equation is then

$$\sqrt{\lambda_U} = \frac{-b \pm \sqrt{b^2 - 4ac}}{2a} = \frac{1.96 \pm \sqrt{3.84 - 4(1)(-36)}}{2(1)}$$

$$= 7.06 \text{ and } -5.10$$

Therefore $\lambda_U = 49.84$ or 26.01. Clearly our choice for λ_U is 49.84.

Following the same procedure for $\sqrt{\lambda_L}$, the equation to be solved is

$$\lambda_L + 1.96\sqrt{\lambda_L} - 36 = 0$$

and the solutions for $\sqrt{\lambda_L}$ turn out to be 5.10 and -7.06 with $\lambda_L = 26.01$ or 49.84. We now choose 26.01 for λ_L. (Because of the symmetry of the equations for $\sqrt{\lambda_U}$ and $\sqrt{\lambda_L}$, it was not necessary to solve both.)

By using the Poisson assumption, we have obtained 95 percent confidence limits of 26.01 and 49.84. Recalling that these are confidence limits on the numerator of the rate, i.e., the number of cataract cases occurring, we divide each of these by 1300 (considered not a sampling variable but a constant) to get 95 percent confidence limits on the person-year rate (via the Poisson approximation). These turn out to be .020 and .038, almost identical to the limits of .019 and .037 obtained with Equation 8-6. In both calculations, the presumption that ±1.96 standard errors would yield 95 percent confidence limits depends on the distribution of all possible sample values being approximately normal. If the number of events is 20 or more (in our example it is 36), the normality assumption is probably satisfactory. To obtain more exact confidence limits for Poisson variables, see *Documenta Geigy* [1970] and Bailar and Ederer [1964] for methods and tables of values.

RELATIVE RISK FROM PERSON-YEAR DATA

We now describe how to estimate a summary relative risk, based on person-year data, after adjustment for confounding variables. The methods to be used are similar to those previously described for the Mantel–Haenszel procedure. First arrange the person-year data for the *i*th stratum as follows:

	Events	Person-years
Risk factor +	a_i	y_{1i}
Risk factor −	b_i	y_{2i}
Total	n_i	t_i

As noted in Chapter 5, the existence of a common relative risk is impossible unless the risks in individual strata are low. A common relative risk of 2.00 could apply to strata with risks of .01, .10, or .30 for those negative for the risk factor. But if the risk for those negative for the risk factor is .55, it is impossible to double it. Assuming that individual risks are sufficiently low (e.g., a risk of .40 can not be tripled), the common relative risk is estimated as in Equation 8-9 [Rothman and Boice 1979].

$$RR = [\sum (a_i y_{2i}/t_i)]/[\sum (b_i y_{1i}/t_i)] \tag{8-9}$$

A significance test for this adjusted relative risk can be based on a one degree of freedom χ^2 [Oleinick and Mantel 1970]. The formula for this summary χ^2 is given in Equation 8-10.

$$\chi^2 = \frac{\left\{\sum a_i - \sum [n_i(y_{1i}/t_i)]\right\}^2}{\sum [n_i(y_{1i}/t_i)(y_{2i}/t_i)]} \tag{8-10}$$

Table 8-4. Person-Year Data for the Framingham Heart Study Comparing Age 55–62 to 45–49 Adjusted for Blood Pressure and Sex: Rate of Developing Coronary Heart Disease

SBP	Sex	Observation period	Cases (d_x) (a)	Person-years (y_1)	Cases (d_x) (b)	Person-years (y_2)	Total person-years (t)
			Age 55+		**Age 45–49**		
<165	M	0–9	26	1408.5	12	1471.5	2880.0
		9–18	23	877.5	24	1093.5	1971.0
	F	0–9	12	1368.0	1	1611.0	2979.0
		9–18	13	954.0	12	1278.0	2332.0
≥165	M	0–9	17	265.5	3	202.5	468.0
		9–18	4	94.5	6	103.5	198.0
	F	0–9	17	666.0	2	333.0	999.0
		9–18	11	423.0	5	225.0	648.0
Total			123		65		

Confidence limits for the adjusted relative risk can be obtained using Miettinen's significance test based limits as described in Chapter 5. To illustrate these methods we examine the relative risk of CHD comparing those aged 55 or over to those aged 45–49. The basic data consist of eight 2×2 tables, each comparing cases and person-years exposure at risk for the two age groups, and specific for blood pressure level, sex, and whether the observation is within the time interval 0–9 or 9–18. To save space we arrange each 2×2 table on a single line in Table 8-4.

Using Equation 8-9 the adjusted relative risk is

$$RR = \frac{(26)(1471.5)/2880 + (23)(1093.5)1971 + \cdots}{(12)(1408.5)/2880 + (24)(877.5)1971 + \cdots} = \frac{58.91}{31.30} = 1.88$$

A significance test for this adjusted relative risk is described in Equation 8-10. Applying it to Table 8-4 data we have

$$\chi^2 = \frac{\{(26 + 23 + \cdots) - [38(1408.5)/2880.0 + 47(877.5)/1971.0 + \cdots]\}^2}{38(1408.5/2880)(1471.5/2880) + 47(877.5/1971)(1093.5/1971) + \cdots} = 16.67$$

This value of 16.67 for a χ^2 with one degree of freedom is extremely rare as a chance occurrence if the true RR were 1.00. The χ^2 value can be used to calculate confidence limits on the estimated summary relative risk according to Miettinen's test-based procedure as explained and illustrated in Chapter 5.

REVIEW OF ASSUMPTIONS

In Table 8-5, we recapitulate the assumptions underlying the calculation of person-year rates and compare them with the assumptions required for life table calculations. As can be noted from Table 8-5, if there are withdrawals, there are no differences of any practical importance. Since the methods for summarizing longitudinal observations by life table analysis or person-year analysis rest on the same assumptions, and since probability of risk is often numerically identical to rate of risk, does it make any difference which method is used? In our opinion there is no important distinction between the two methods and the choice between them need rest on nothing more than personal preference. Our own preference is to use life table analysis when the cases observed have a common point for initiating observation (such as date of diagnosis or date of surgery) and where the dominant factor controlling risk is likely to be the time since that original date. For observation lacking this common initial date and where a major factor of risk tends to be age at observation, we prefer person-year methods.

APPLICATION TO FRAMINGHAM HEART STUDY DATA

In looking at person-year data for an 18-year observation period, we recognize that the interval of analysis has to meet the requirement that risk is approximately constant within intervals. To demonstrate the use of

Table 8-5. Assumptions Required for Summarizing Longitudinal Observations

Assumption	Life table method	Person-year method
1. Experience of persons after withdrawal (for any reason) is same as that of persons remaining under observation	x	x
2. Pooling relates to individuals with similar risk experience within interval of analysis	x	x
3. Withdrawals occur uniformly within interval of analysis	x	x
4. Constant risk within interval of analysis	x (only if there are any withdrawals)	x[a]

[a] Risk must be sufficiently low within intervals of analysis to permit *k* years of observation to reflect *k* times the risk of one year of observation.

person-year rates in comparing various groups as to the risk of developing coronary disease, we are using nine-year intervals. Five-year intervals would be better but nine-year intervals are not unreasonable and they help to simplify the data presentation. Data on blood pressure groups specific for eight age–sex strata are in Table 8-6.

Using the data in Table 8-6 it is easy to compare the two blood pressure groups after indirect adjustment for age–sex differences. Person-year rates for the lower blood pressure group are the standard rates. The expected number of CHD cases in the high blood pressure group is calculated by multiplying the person-year rate for the low blood pressure group by the person-years of observation in the high blood pressure group, as follows:

$$\text{Expected cases (SBP} \geq 165) = \sum_i \left[\frac{d_{xi}/L_{xi}}{\text{for SBP} < 165}\right]\left[\frac{L_{xi}}{\text{for SBP} \geq 165}\right]$$

where i = the ith age–sex class. For Table 8-6 data the expected number of cases equals 35.19. Since 95 cases were observed in the SBP $\geq$ 165 group the standardized morbidity ratio (SMR) = 95/35.19 = 2.70. The SMR is comparable to an (indirectly) adjusted relative risk, which was calculated to be 2.02 when computed without regard to the time of the event.

Table 8-6. Person-Year Data for Framingham Heart Study Comparing SBP $\geq$ 165 with SBP < 165: Rate of Developing Coronary Heart Disease

Sex	Age	Period	d_x	L_x	d_x/L_x	d_x	L_x	d_x/L_x
	Stratum		SBP < 165			SBP $\geq$ 165		
Men	45–49	0–9	12	1471.5	.00815	3	202.5	.01481
		9–18	24	1093.5	.02195	6	103.5	.05797
	50–54	0–9	12	1354.5	.00886	5	265.5	.01883
		9–18	23	967.5	.02377	9	139.5	.06452
	55–59	0–9	18	1084.5	.01660	13	211.5	.06147
		9–18	18	729.0	.02469	3	81.0	.03704
	60–62	0–9	8	324.0	.02469	4	54.0	.07407
		9–18	5	148.5	.03367	1	13.5	.07407
Women	45–49	0–9	1	1611.0	.00062	2	333.0	.00601
		9–18	12	1278.0	.00939	5	225.0	.02222
	50–54	0–9	2	1395.0	.00143	6	477.0	.01258
		9–18	13	1089.0	.01194	10	319.5	.03130
	55–59	0–9	9	1089.0	.00826	15	531.0	.02825
		9–18	9	765.0	.01176	10	351.0	.02849
	60–62	0–9	3	279.0	.01075	2	135.0	.01481
		9–18	4	189.0	.02116	1	72.0	.01389
Total			173			95		

The substantial increase, from 2.02 to 2.70, flows from the distribution of event times in the two blood pressure groups. The high blood pressure group not only has proportionately more cases but also proportionately more of them occurred in the first nine-year interval (53 versus 38 percent).

Rothman and Boice [1979] have proposed another method for estimating an adjusted summary relative risk based on person-year data. It is similar to the Mantel–Haenszel procedure for estimating a summary odds ratio. The summary relative risk comparing SBP $\geq$ 165 to SBP < 165 can easily be calculated from Table 8-6 and we emphasize its relation to Mantel–Haenszel by first converting each line of Table 8-6 into a 2 × 2 table, thus:

		Cases (d_x)	Person-years (L_x)
(From line 1	SBP $\geq$ 165	3	202.5
of Table 8-6)	SBP < 165	12	1471.5
	Total		1674.0
(From line 2	SBP $\geq$ 165	6	103.5
of Table 8-6)	SBP < 165	24	1093.5
	Total		1197.0
(From line 3	SBP $\geq$ 165	5	265.5
of Table 8-6)	SBP < 165	12	1354.5
	Total		1620.0 etc.

The adjusted summary relative risk using Equation 8-9 is then estimated as

$$\hat{RR} = \frac{(3)(1471.5)/1674 + (6)(1093.5)/1197 + (5)(1354.5)/1620 + \cdots}{(12)(202.5)/1674 + (24)(103.5)/1197 + (12)(265.5)/1620 + \cdots}$$

Using all 16 2 × 2 tables obtainable from Table 8-6

$$\hat{RR} = \frac{75.21}{27.98} = 2.69$$

This is almost the same result as we obtained from these person-year data using indirect adjustment and the low pressure group as the standard (2.70).

To illustrate the calculation of standard errors for person-year rates, we choose a rate per person-year of developing coronary heart disease taken from Table 8-6. It is for women aged 55–59 with high blood pressure and relates to the first nine years of observation with a numerical value of .0282. Using Equation 8-6 the standard error of this rate is

$$SE(_9m_0) = \left\{\frac{_9m_0[2 - n_9m_0]}{_9L_0[2 + n_9m_0]}\right\}^{1/2} = \left\{\frac{.0282[2 - 9(.0282)]}{531[2 + 9(.0282)]}\right\}^{1/2} = .00641$$

and $1.96\ SE(_9m_0) = .0126$ with .95 confidence limits of $.0282 \pm .0126$ or .016 and .041.

Alternatively, using Equations 8-7 and 8-8 applied to the above rate, which is based on 15 events, we begin with the following:

$$\lambda_U - 1.96\sqrt{\lambda_U} - 15 = 0$$

$$\lambda_L + 1.96\sqrt{\lambda_L} - 15 = 0$$

These are quadratic equations in standard form with $\sqrt{\lambda_L}$ and $\sqrt{\lambda_U}$ as equivalent to x. Solving them we get

$$\sqrt{\lambda_U} = \frac{1.96 \pm \sqrt{(-1.96)^2 - (4)(1)(-15)}}{2(1)}$$

$$\sqrt{\lambda_U} = 4.98 \quad \text{or} \quad -3.02$$

$$\lambda_U = 24.80 \quad \text{or} \quad 9.12$$

As discussed earlier, we choose the larger value for λ_U and due to symmetry in the equations, the smaller value is our estimate of λ_L. Since these are .95 confidence limits on the numerator of the person-year rate, dividing by the number of person-years (531), which is not a sampling variable, results in

$$9.12/531 \quad \text{and} \quad 24.80/531 = .017 \quad \text{and} \quad .047$$

Based on only 15 cases these limits are reasonably close to the limits of .016 and .041 obtained with the use of Equation 8-6.

EXERCISES

Ex. 8-1. The denominator for a single year's mortality rates is the estimated midyear population. What is the relationship between the midyear population and person-years of observation?

Ex. 8-2. Use the Appendix data for men aged 45–49 to count the number of CHD incidence cases and person-years at risk of developing CHD for each two-year period through examination 6 (year 10). Then assuming events and withdrawals are at interval midpoints

a. Compute $_2d_x$, $_2L_x$, and $_2m_x$ for each two-year period.
b. Compute $_{10}d_0$, $_{10}L_0$, and $_{10}m_0$ for the ten-year period.

Ex. 8-3. Repeat Exercise 8-2 but now assume that all events and withdrawals occur at the beginning of the interval. Compare results for the different assumptions.

Ex. 8-4. Repeat the calculations specified in Exercise 8-2 for men aged 55-59. Compare the results for the two age groups.

Ex. 8-5. Using Table 8-3 as a model, compute the person-years of observation by *attained age* for ages 45–54, 55–64, 65–74, and 75 or over for the following 10 individuals.

Number	Age at exam 1	CHD at exam no.	YRS_CHD
1	45	0	14
2	48	0	6
3	47	3	3
4	52	0	18
5	51	7	11
6	56	0	8
7	59	10	17
8	57	5	8
9	61	0	18
10	62	7	11

NOTE

* To clarify the relationship between probability and rate, we consider identical populations at the start of an interval with no additions during the interval. The possibility of additions during the interval is not a serious problem for the person-year method, which uses average number at risk. For the life table method, however, additions during the interval are conceptually confusing at best. For this reason, one basis for choosing person-year analysis or life table analysis can be whether or not the data include additions to observation after the start of periods used for analysis. For more precise definitions of rate and risk see [Kleinbaum et al 1982].

9
Comparison of Numerical Results for Various Methods of Adjustment

Throughout the preceding chapters we have applied the methods discussed to estimating the association of systolic blood pressure, adjusted for age and sex, to 18-year risk of coronary heart disease using Framingham Heart Study data. Up to this point we have observed how methods differed among those considered within any chapter. Now we undertake a global comparison of methods from the entire book.

Table 9-1 summarizes the extent to which various methods of adjustment for confounding produce similar results when applied to the Framingham Heart Study data listed herein. Odds ratios and relative risks are used to quantify the relationship of three risk factors to the incidence of coronary heart disease. Each of the three risk factors—age, sex, and systolic blood pressure—is adjusted for potential confounding by the other two. Some methods lead to estimated odds ratios and others to estimated relative risks. Methods that lead to estimated risks for specific categories (e.g., the risk for men after direct adjustment) can provide both relative risks (p_1/p_2) and odds ratios $[p_1/(1 - p_1)]/[p_2/(1 - p_2)]$. Crude rates are included for comparison.

Details regarding Table 9-1 are as follows:

1. It relates to the 1363 individuals in the listing that are at risk of developing coronary heart disease.
2. As potential confounders, age and blood pressure were sometimes categorical variables with classes for age of 45–49, 50–54, 55–59, 60–62, and classes for systolic blood pressure of <165 and ≥165.
3. When age and blood pressure were treated as continuous variables in some multivariate models, odds ratios or relative risks were computed

Table 9-1. Relationship of Systolic Blood Pressure (≥165/<165), Age (≥55/<55), and Sex (M/F) to Coronary Heart Disease, Each of the Three Risk Factors Adjusted for the Other Two: Numerical Results for Various Methods of Adjustment, Eighteen-Year Framingham Heart Study Data

Method of Adjustment	Odds ratios			Relative risks		
	SBP ≥165 / SBP ≥165	Age ≥55 / Age <55	Male / Female	SBP ≥165 / SBP <165	Age ≥55 / Age <55	Male / Female
Without regard for the time of event occurrence						
Direct adjustment (combined weights)	2.54	1.54	2.27	2.04	1.41	1.93
Direct adjustment (wts inversely ∝ variance)	2.61	1.53	2.28	2.09	1.40	1.95
Indirect adjustment (combined rates[a])	2.51	1.52	2.23	2.02	1.40	1.90
Woolf	2.71	1.56	2.36	—	—	—
Mantel–Haenszel	2.69	1.56	2.37	—	—	—
Multiple regression (categorical)	2.56	1.53	2.27	2.05	1.40	1.93
Multiple regression (multivariate strata)	2.66	1.49	2.42	—	—	—
Multiple logistic (all categorical)	2.72	1.57	2.37	—	—	—
Multiple logistic (only sex categorical)	2.45	1.54	2.50	—	—	—
With regard for the time of event occurrence						
Person-years (indirect adjustment)	—	—	—	2.70	1.71	2.37
Person-years (Rothman–Boice)	—	—	—	2.69	1.69	2.34
Life table stratification	2.80	1.68	2.54	—	—	—
Cox regression (all categorical)	—	—	—	2.72	1.66	2.42
Cox regression (only sex categorical)	—	—	—	2.19	1.65	2.54
Crude (unadjusted for potential confounding)						
Unadjusted	2.45	1.66	2.03	1.98	1.50	1.77

[a] Technically incorrect to compare a risk factor category to anything other than the standard population, which in this case is the total population.

using the difference in average value for the classes being compared. Thus, the mean systolic blood for those with SBP ≥ 165 is 188.4 and the mean SBP for those with SBP < 165 is 136.5. The difference of 51.9 was used to estimate *OR* and *RR* comparing the two blood pressure classes. Similarly for age. The average age for those 55 or more is 57.7 and for those under age 55 it is 49.4. The difference of 8.3 was used as a multiplier of the fitted coefficient to estimate *OR* and *RR*.

4. Strata based on a multivariate function were computed using multiple regression coefficients with age and systolic blood pressure as continuous variables.
5. Person-years were accumulated separately for the first and second nine-year periods of observation.
6. Life tables were computed using four-year time intervals.
7. Indirect adjustment for *person-year data* used rates for SBP < 165, for age <55, or for females as the standard.

Several points regarding the relationships among methods are illustrated by Table 9-1. Based on our experience with moderate to large data sets these findings are about what we expected.

The differences between crude and adjusted estimates range from slight to moderate. Great differences are not seen. All crude relationships of risk factor to disease occurrence are positive and remain so after adjustment.

All of the methods that omitted consideration of the time an event occurred produced similar results *when applied to categorical variables.* All of the methods that used the time of the event as part of the analysis produced similar results *when applied to categorical variables.*

The results derived from multivariate models may or may not differ to an appreciable degree depending on whether continuous variables are treated in the model as categorical or continuous. Whenever the difference is of consequence, we recommend the use of categories.

Inclusion in the analysis of the time when the event occurred makes an important difference in these data. It will do so whenever the group with the highest risk also has events occurring, on the average, appreciably earlier (or later) in the observation period than is true for the low risk group. In other data sets this may not be the case [Kahn et al 1984] and analytical results will be similar whether or not the time of the event is part of the analysis.

Odds ratios are larger than the comparable relative risks for methods that do not take account of the time events occurred. This is understandable and expected since the overall 18-year risk of CHD is about 20 percent in these data. All but one of the methods that do take account of the time of event produce only relative risk. The one method that leads to an odds ratio, after including time of event in the analysis, demonstrates numerical equality with the comparable relative risks. This seeming anomaly is due to the fact that the analyses using time of event are making comparisons *at specific times*. The risk at any specific time is much less than 20 percent and, as previously stated, odds ratios and relative risks are approximately equal for rare diseases.

10
The Primacy of Data Collection

INTRODUCTION

Upon completing this book, you should have a fair understanding of the principal analytical techniques used in epidemiologic studies of chronic disease. While the additional information obtainable as a result of proper analysis is always to be sought, the additional information resulting from careful and thorough data collection is potentially much greater. Because we are anxious not to be misunderstood, we repeat that appropriate analytical methods should be used and it is important to understand them. Up to now this book has dealt only with such topics. Nevertheless we agree with the following quotation from Sir Austin Bradford Hill [1953]: "One must go seek more facts, paying less attention to techniques of handling the data and far more to the . . . methods of obtaining them."

To do justice to the topic of data collection could well require another book, but we limit ourselves to this modest addendum in order to encourage a suitable perspective. Important topics in data collection are listed below, followed by a brief discussion of each.

Important Components of Data Collection

1. Clearly defined objectives
2. Study population
3. Sample size
4. Written protocol
5. Training of the study staff
6. Pilot study

7. Completeness of response
8. Adherence to protocol
9. Data review and clean-up

CLEARLY DEFINED OBJECTIVES

This element and many others in this chapter are so obvious that they are infrequently stated. Obvious or not, they are too often ignored with disastrous results. Nothing can be more fundamental than maximum practical clarification of the objective the study is attempting to reach. Be careful not to attempt too much. The studies with the greatest probability of contributing to knowledge are those with limited specific aims that are well planned and carried out with strict attention to all details. Alternatively, studies that aim to accomplish many objectives are necessarily unable to be as careful and complete for all aspects of data collection as the more limited studies. Thus, the "grandiose" studies tend to result in confusion and/or uncertainty rather than progress. Our advice is to do less but to do it at the highest quality level that you can. Nobel prize winner Arthur Kornberg has said this very well [Kornberg 1976]: "ask a small and modest question, focus on it in laser beam fashion, and then maintain the focus until the beam burns through."

Never lose sight of your objective even though it may not be completely attainable. For example, your study objective may be to relate diet to disease but your data do not describe what study subjects have eaten. Instead they describe what study subjects *say* they have eaten. Recognize the difference and to the maximum practical extent try to determine how valid the data collection process is to the underlying objective.

Errors of measurement, in terms of your real objective, can lead to classifying individuals in the wrong category. For example, a study subject might be incorrectly classified as an above average consumer of saturated fat because he reported an exaggerated frequency of hamburger consumption. His classification is correct from the perspective of reported diet but not in terms of actual diet, which is the variable related to the objective. Misclassification error can obscure the discovery of the association between disease and the risk factor of interest. If the misclassification results from a random process, estimates of relative risk or odds ratio will be biased toward unity, i.e., toward a finding of no association. However, nonrandom classification errors can lead to bias in any direction [Fleiss 1981, Liu et al 1978]. Unfortunately we usually do not know whether the measurements actually made are adequate stand-ins for the variables of real interest, e.g., reported diet versus actual diet, reported physical activity versus kilocalories of energy expenditure, reported cause of death versus actual cause of death, etc.

STUDY POPULATION

This choice needs to be made dependent on the study objectives. For example, suppose you wish to verify the claim that Seventh Day Adventists (SDAs) have lower mortality rates than the nonSeventh Day Adventist population after suitable adjustment for age, sex, race, smoking, and geographic area. For logistic reasons you have decided to conduct the study in ABC county, California where approximately 10 percent of the population are Seventh Day Adventists. Should all SDAs in the county be eligible to participate in the study? What about recent converts to the SDA church? What about children and young adults or persons recently migrating to ABC county from elsewhere? Since the claim as to lower mortality risk derives from the SDA lifestyle, which includes prohibition of tobacco and alcohol and encouragement of vegetarianism, it seems appropriate to exclude recent converts to the SDA church. Recent immigrants would be difficult to standardize as to background risk associated with geographic area. If the claims as to lower mortality risk relate to cancer and heart disease and follow-up is planned for only fifteen years, it would be sensible to exclude young people from the population to be studied. A decision is also needed with respect to persons who have left the church and no longer consider themselves to be Seventh Day Adventists. For this illustrative study, the population could be defined as all residents of ABC county for ten years or more but excluding:

SDA members who were converts to the church within the past five
     years.
Those who have left the church and no longer consider themselves to be
     SDAs.
All persons under age 50.

The time and age references are in relation to the beginning date of the study.

   Alternative choices for these time and age references are certainly possible and could be considered from the viewpoint of effect on study objectives. However, it is from the specified population that study subjects are selected and it is to this same restricted population that study findings should be referred. Whatever the study findings they have no necessary relation to recent SDA converts, persons under age 50, etc. The basic principles are:

The population should be specifically defined.
It should be specified so as to aid study objectives.
All findings relate back to the specified population.

Whether or not the study findings have wider application than to the defined population is, strictly speaking, unknown, but logic can provide some guidance. In the above example it is reasonable to presume that the study findings might not apply to recent converts. It is much less reasonable to presume that the findings do not apply to counties adjacent to ABC.

SAMPLE SIZE

The sample size that is appropriate to the study objective has been discussed in Chapter 2. Since sample size is so closely connected with both analytical and data collection aspects of a study, we list it again here. Although it is usually impossible or at least impractical to have a sample size that is adequate for all questions of interest, be certain that you have a sample size that is adequate for at least the major question.

WRITTEN PROTOCOL

The protocol needs to specify study objective; population to be sampled; when applicable, the method of random allocation and how it is guarded; method of approaching individuals to invite cooperation; procedure for maximizing participation of invited individuals; forms and procedures for obtaining informed consent, conducting examinations, interviewing, or abstracting records; laboratory methods; plans for coding, data processing, and analysis; methods for staff training; methods for evaluating adherence to protocol specifications, and plans for a pilot study. Epidemiologic studies of chronic disease are almost always too complex to be carried out by a single individual. Typically several disciplines need to be involved and *all* study personnel should review the complete protocol so as to minimize misunderstanding with regard to the relationship among various study elements. Although it is important for the study protocol to be specific, it should not be so detailed that the fundamental points are obscured and overlooked by the staff. By circulating a copy of the draft protocol to colleagues with experience in the area of the proposed study, it is possible to obtain valuable advice and avoid much unnecessary grief.

As an illustration of the specificity needed for the study protocol, consider the matter of measuring visual acuity by reading letters on a wall chart. This is something most of us have experienced in a clinical rather than an epidemiologic setting. In addition to the obvious points about the specific chart to be used, the lighting on the chart and in the room, and the distance the subject is from the chart the protocol must specify items such as:

What constitutes successful reading of a line? Must every letter be read correctly?
If mistakes are made should the subject be asked to try again?

If subject says he cannot see, should the examiner coax him to try? Should guessing be encouraged?

The difference in results following from alternative decisions with regard to these choices is substantial. For those without experience in protocol drafting, the protocol for the Framingham Eye Study has been published and could be useful as a guide without regard to its particular application to ophthalmic measurements [Leibowitz et al 1980].

TRAINING OF THE STUDY STAFF

With possible rare exceptions, conducting a medical examination on, or obtaining questionnaire information from an epidemiologic study subject is not analogous to the procedure used in clinical practice. For the epidemiologic study, which often includes multiple examiners, standardization is essential. All examiners (or interviewers, technicians, etc.) should be following the same procedures so that results can be combined and other investigators can replicate the study on other populations. This is impossible without *training*. After the protocol has been tentatively established (changes may be desirable following experience gained in training sessions, pilot study etc.), the appropriate study staff should be exposed to formal training sessions that should include demonstrations by the principal investigator or his designated expert, replicate examinations, discussion of unclear details, and trial operations. It should not be taken for granted that ophthalmologists can diagnose eye disease, or that cardiologists can read electrocardiograms. Of course they can do these things *but usually not to the standard of an epidemiologic study,* unless specifically trained to do so. Clinicians even tend to be biased against standardized procedures because they "know" that in certain unusual cases mistakes will be made by following the rules. They are right, but this occasional mistake has to be weighed against the values of a well-defined procedure (clinical practice often includes undefined elements) that can be clearly reported and also replicated elsewhere. It is probably not an exaggeration to say that there will never be a single definitive epidemiologic study of chronic disease. The conclusion that tobacco is a general poison associated with increased risk of several diseases does not rest on any one study. Replication of studies and confirmation of findings are essential components of the scientific method as applied to chronic disease epidemiology. Without staff training we cannot know that the protocol is being followed nor whether replicate study results are actually comparable.

PILOT STUDY

It is nothing short of remarkable how often it is presumed that complex plans can be carried out as intended. Experience teaches us that

Murphy's Law (anything that can go wrong will go wrong) is unrelenting. Until a protocol has been tried out under conditions as close to realistic as practical, the study is not ready to start. Be prepared to revise record forms, procedures, the sequence of activities, or anything else in the light of pilot study results. The sample size for a pilot study is difficult to state in the abstract, but a one- or two-week trial will be more than repaid in subsequent improvements. In the planning schedule, time is needed after the pilot to make suitable changes and arrange for final printing of forms before beginning full operations. In extreme cases the pilot will indicate that the study is not feasible and it will be necessary to decide whether to attempt major revisions (requiring a new pilot study) or to abandon the project. For example, The National Diet Heart Study, which was a feasibility or pilot study, found that the costs and logistic problems would make it impossible to conduct a full-scale double-blind substantive study of the effect of diet on coronary heart disease incidence and mortality [National Diet-Heart Study 1968].

COMPLETENESS OF RESPONSE

If you plan a study of sample size 300 and the study requires that a questionnaire be answered, will all 300 reply? If it requires an examination, will all 300 submit to it? If the study requires merely abstracting information from existing records, is the specific information recorded for all 300? Perhaps the information is in the record but the record is missing from the file or otherwise unavailable. What is the importance of incomplete response and what can the investigator do about it?

Nonresponse is important because of the unknown differences between responders and nonresponders. The term nonresponse is used here in a general sense, without regard to the specific reasons for nonresponse. One sample individual may refuse an examination. Another may be impossible to locate. In either case we should be concerned that those actually examined may differ in some important aspect from those not examined.

The problem of nonresponse is a general one. It applies to studies of total populations and of samples, to individuals lost from observation in longitudinal studies, and to those not cooperative in cross-sectional studies. Writing specifically about incomplete follow-up, Lilienfeld and Lilienfeld state that differences between responders and nonresponders vary "in different studies and perhaps with different types of disease entities so that a general rule cannot be established" [Lilienfeld and Lilienfeld 1980].

The use of data derived from studies with moderate to large nonresponse rates usually presumes that the nonresponders are similar to those included, which may or may not be true. The investigator reporting sample data involving appreciable nonresponse has the burden of defending them and should supply supportive evidence with respect to the presumption of similarity. Dorn's comment on loss to follow-up can be generalized as, "The only correct way to deal with nonresponse is not to have any" [Dorn 1950]. There exists no certain method "not to have any," but the following guidelines may be useful.

a. Before embarking on any extensive study, conduct a pilot investigation, which among other benefits will provide some indication of the response rate. If it seems to be seriously low and cannot be improved, perhaps the study plan should be abandoned. If the study is to include long-term follow-up, a pilot investigation to test how many will stay under observation for ten years is clearly impractical. However, careful planning with respect to factors that may impair long-term follow-up can be helpful in defining the study population. A proposal to conduct a five-year study on the incidence of coronary disease among the Bedouin nomads of Israel was abandoned as soon as serious thought was given to the near impossibility of locating these wanderers some years after their initial examination.

b. Exert all practical effort toward obtaining cooperation from sampled individuals. A smaller sample intensively contacted with respect to cooperation may be preferable to a larger sample with a high nonresponse rate resulting from lack of resources to motivate cooperation.

c. If unable to obtain the cooperation of a sample individual with respect to the item under investigation, collect, where possible, the reason for responding and such other information as may be helpful in judging whether or not the nonrespondent group differs substantially from the respondents. A seroepidemiologic study of hepatitis B prevalence among recruits for military service in Italy included the collection of data on education, residence, etc., from all recruits, although 20 percent were rejected withot being blood-tested. Comparison of those whose sera were tested with those whose sera were not tested with respect to the variables measured for both groups was helpful in calculating weighted estimates of the overall prevalence [Pasquini et al 1983]. At times, information on variables such as age, sex, race, or census tract may exist for the study population, even before data collection is started. Such data also provide an opportunity to compare respondents and nonrespondents. Extensive use of supplementary variables to compare respondents and nonrespondents has been reported in publications of the National Health and Nutrition Surveys [Forthofer 1983, Hadden and Harris 1987].

d. Intensive effort directed toward a subsample of the nonrespondent population is sometimes recommended and may help in estimating the extent of bias among nonrespondents. However, suppose n was the sample size considered appropriate for the study in order to measure a variable with adequate precision. Suppose that $n/3$ are nonrespondents and 25 percent of these ($n/12$) are intensively approached to obtain cooperation, with 100 percent success in the effort. The intensive effort will be costly, but since it applies to only one-twelfth of the sample, it may be practical to carry out. This will result in $n/12$ individuals upon which to base estimates of the nonrespondents to see if they differ from the respondents. This, however, is 1/12 the sample size believed necessary for adequate precision in measuring the variables of interest, as stated above. A further complication is that the intensive follow-up is unlikely to achieve 100 percent response. Intensive efforts are most often useful as a method for reducing the size of the nonresponse group.

The preceding discussion relates to moderate or large nonresponse rates. In this imperfect world, small nonresponse rates are necessarily accepable. What then constitutes a response rate that is unacceptable or a cause for serious concern? There is no specific answer to that question in this book, or in any source that we are familiar with, and it is the investigators responsibility to make a judgment as to the value of data based on a particular response rate.

Bias Potential in Prevalence or Incidence Studies

The potential for bias is quite large in surveys of disease prevalence with high nonresponse rates. It is understandable that those with known disease may be uninterested, unable to reach the examination site, or unwilling to respond. However, it is equally easy to appreciate that the sick may be specially interested in a study related to their condition and will therefore participate more readily than those who are well. Thus, good explanations exist for potential biases in opposite directions in the estimation of population prevalence of disease.

When the study objective is related to the association of two conditions, such as the development of myocardial infarction among those with and without high blood pressure, the likelihood of bias due to nonresponse seems less. Consider the population described by the simple cross-classification in Table 10-1. Using the number in a group as a convenient label for that group, we have two groups of persons who currently have high blood pressure:

1. The A group is those persons who will develop myocardial infarction in the next five years.
2. The B group is those persons who will not.

At present, these two groups cannot be distinguished, and there is only the single group with high blood pressure, $A + B$. Estimates of the current prevalence of high blood pressure will be affected if the $A + B$

Table 10-1. Blood Pressure and Incidence of Myocardial Infarction in a *Population*

Present blood pressure	Will develop MI in next 5 years		
	Yes	No	Total
High	A	B	A + B
Normal	C	D	C + D

Odds ratio relating MI and blood pressure level in population = AD/BC

group responds to the sample invitation to a greater or lesser extent than the group without high blood pressure labeled C + D in Table 10-1. For the reasons previously cited, this is quite probable.

As shown in Table 10-2, however, even if the sample includes 10 percent of those with high blood pressure (A + B) and as many as 90 percent of those without high blood pressure (C + D), estimates of the degree of association of blood pressure with myocardial infarction incidence will be almost unbiased. If, on the other hand, the 10 percent response for the A + B group is much greater than 10 percent for either the A or the B component of the group and much less than 10 percent for the other, bias will exist. Similarly, if the 90 percent response in the C + D group differs substantially between C and D, bias will be introduced. Although such variation cannot be ruled out, it is less likely than the differential participation of those currently sick relative to those

Table 10-2. Blood Pressure and Incidence of Myocardial Infarction in a *Sample*

Present blood pressure	Will develop MI in next 5 years		
	Yes	No	Total
High	$\dfrac{A^a}{10}$	$\dfrac{B}{10}$	$\dfrac{A + B}{10}$
Normal	$\dfrac{9C}{10}$	$\dfrac{9D}{10}$	$\dfrac{9(C + D)}{10}$

Odds ratio relating MI and blood pressure level in sample = $(A/10)(9D/10) \div (B/10)(9C/10)$
$= [AD(9)/100][100/BC(9)] = AD/BC$, as in Table 10-1 for the population

[a] Ten percent of high blood pressure population and 90 percent of normal blood pressure population are in the sample.

currently well, as previously stated. For additional discussion see Kelsey et al [1986].

ADHERENCE TO PROTOCOL

No matter how great the effort expended in training study staff, this does not ensure that the protocol is being followed. Without training the probability that study examiners or interviewers are all doing the same thing, in conformity with the written protocol, is quite low. With training the probability is much higher but still uncertain. Because training may be unsuccessful for specific examiners or specific elements of data, methods are needed for discovering such failures. One possible approach makes use of replicate measurements and another the variance among examiners.

Replicate Measurements and Technical Error

Periodically perform independent replicate examinations (or interviews) on the same patient. These replications are to compare the staff examiner (or interviewer) with an acknowledged expert who is familiar with and instructed to follow the protocol. This expert might be the principal investigator but not necessarily. Disagreement between the two replicate results presumably shows the extent to which the staff person is departing from protocol. There are several drawbacks to this approach. It is difficult enough to get subjects to accept the basic study procedures and even more difficult to get them to accept replicate examinations or interviews. Getting around this difficulty by using study staff, their family, or friends (of similar age and sex to the study subjects as the patients to be replicated) introduces serious problems of representativeness. Furthermore it is not always correct to presume the subject has not changed between replications even though they may be less than one hour apart. For example, changes in systolic blood pressure can occur in a minute. With regard to interview data, the second interview response is not an independent piece of information since the subject may remember all or part of his previous response. Usually, the method of replicate measurements is difficult and expensive and unlikely to result in a sufficient number for adequate analysis.

One specific type of replicate measurement that does have wide practical application is laboratory testing on aliquots of the same specimen. For example, if a laboratory test requires 5 ml of blood, draw 10 ml and divide it into two specimens of 5 ml each. Assign randomly chosen identification numbers to each specimen or in some other way prevent the laboratory from knowing that the two specimens are related.* Properly performed laboratory tests should produce similar results for the two replicates. A common method for evaluating the

extent to which the replicates differ from each other requires calculation
of the technical error of the test as given in Equation 10-1.

$$\text{Technical error} = \sqrt{\frac{\sum\limits_{i=1}^{n} d_i^2}{2n}} \tag{10-1}$$

where

d_i = difference in test results between the two specimens for the ith
individual
n = the number of individuals
$i = 1, 2, 3 \cdots n$

The technical error calculated as in Equation 10-1 is the standard
deviation of the two replicates pooled over all individuals. Since the test
is on the identical blood specimen (divided into two portions), any
variation between the two test results can be considered as variation due
to the test procedure. The technical error formula is easily derived from
elementary definitions.
Let

x_{i1} = first replicate test result for the ith individual
x_{i2} = second replicate test result for the ith individual
$\bar{x}_i$ = average of the two results for the ith individual

The estimated variance between replicate tests, in accordance with
Equation 1-5 is

$$\frac{(x_{i1} - \bar{x}_i)^2 + (x_{i2} - \bar{x}_i)^2}{2 - 1} \tag{10-2}$$

If we assume, as seems reasonable, that laboratory variability is the
same for all study subjects, we can pool the estimate of variance stated in
Equation 10-2 over all individuals. This is done by summing the squared
deviations in the numerator over all persons in the study and also
summing the one degree of freedom in the denominator over all persons
in the study. This pooled variance within individuals (i.e., variation due
to the test procedure) is

$$\begin{matrix}\text{Pooled within} \\ \text{specimen} \\ \text{variance}\end{matrix} = \frac{\sum\limits_{i=1}^{n} [(x_{i1} - \bar{x}_i)^2 + (x_{i2} - \bar{x}_i)^2]}{n} \tag{10-3}$$

Recognizing that $(x_{i1} - \bar{x}_i)^2$ is exactly equal to $(x_{i2} - \bar{x}_i)^2$

Pooled within specimen variance $= \dfrac{2 \sum\limits_{i=1}^{n} (x_{i1} - \bar{x}_i)^2}{n} = \dfrac{2 \sum\limits_{i=1}^{n} [x_{i1} - (x_{i1} + x_{i2})/2]^2}{n}$

$$= \dfrac{2 \sum\limits_{i=1}^{n} [x_{i1} - (x_{i1}/2) - (x_{i2}/2)]^2}{n} = \dfrac{2 \sum\limits_{i=1}^{n} [(x_{i1}/2) - (x_{i2}/2)]^2}{n}$$

$$= \dfrac{\frac{2}{4} \sum\limits_{i=1}^{n} (x_{i1} - x_{i2})^2}{n} = \dfrac{\sum\limits_{i=1}^{n} (d_i)^2}{2n}$$

The square root of the pooled within specimen variance is the technical error of the test, as given in Equation 10-1.

If the repeated measures are in triplicate or quadruplicate the above simplification applicable to duplicates does not apply but Equation 10-3 is generalizable as follows:

$$\text{Pooled within specimen variance} = \dfrac{\sum\limits_{i=1}^{n} \sum\limits_{j=1}^{m} (x_{ij} - \bar{x}_i)^2}{n(m-1)} \qquad (10\text{-}4)$$

where

$x_{ij} = j$th replicate value for the ith subject
$\bar{x}_i = $ average value for the ith subject
$m = $ the number of replicates
$n = $ the number of subjects

The technical error of the test equals the square root of Equation 10-4.

After the technical error has been calculated, how is it to be evaluated? Although it is often expressed as a ratio relative to the mean value, we prefer relating it to the total standard deviation among individuals. If a large fraction of the total variation among individuals is due to variability in the test rather than to variability among persons, the test is a poor one and consideration should be given to abandoning it. To calculate the standard deviation among persons, it is not correct to use all the data as if they were independent measurements. However all the data can be used if the replicate values are kept separate. We illustrate this with duplicate tests. Designate one of each replicate pair as belonging to "set one" and the other as belonging to "set two." Calculate the variance of each set using Equation 1-5 and designate the results as var(1) and var(2). The ratio of technical error to

$$\sqrt{\dfrac{\text{var}(1) + \text{var}(2)}{2}}^{\dagger}$$

can then be evaluated in the light of subject matter knowledge, to judge whether the technical error is acceptable.

The technical error of laboratory tests should be evaluated (along with everything else) in the pilot phase of the study. During the course of the study, replication of 10 percent of the specimens is often sufficient to detect whether laboratory quality control is being maintained. The caution stated previously with respect to replicate measurements certainly applies as well to replicate laboratory tests. If replication is poor, that constitutes evidence that adherence to the protocol may not be complete. However, even if replication is perfect, that does *not* prove complete adherence to the protocol. Perhaps the wrong procedures are being carried out in a meticulous fashion. A low ratio of technical error to total individual variation indicates high reliability of the measurement procedure. Whether or not the protocol is being adhered to is more difficult to determine and is not always capable of objective measurement. See Lilienfeld and Lilienfeld [1980] or Kelsey et al [1986] for further discussion.

Variance among Examiners

If study subjects are allocated to examiners at random or by any procedure unrelated to their study status (e.g., order of arrival at examination center, odd or even day of birth), all examiners should obtain similar average results if they are all following the same procedure. During the first three months of the Framingham Eye Study, five examiners reported 0, 2, 3, 7, and 53 percent, respectively, as the proportion of their patients showing myopic cupping of the optic disk. In spite of substantial training activity, the examiner reporting 53 percent had completely misunderstood this particular aspect of the protocol. Discussion of the above results led to curing the problem [Kahn et al 1975]. This example shows the importance of monitoring for data quality throughout the study. Investigators should not wait until the end of the study before "cleaning up" the data. It is also important to retest, and when necessary reeducate examiners as a continuous process throughout the study. For example, although in the Hypertension Detection and Follow-up Program, blood pressure examiners had to pass a training course before being employed, they had to be certified again every six months [Hypertension Detection 1976].

The basic difficulty with excessive variation among examiners is that we often do not know who, if anyone, is correct. If all examiner averages are in approximate agreement, they may be all following the protocol *or* all departing from it in the same way. This method does not really detect failure to follow protocol but only differences among examiners. Further investigation and discussion with the examiners will probably identify the correction required but it would be wise to maintain an open mind about who is wrong. In addition to using either of the above methods or some combination of them, the principal investigator should personally observe all operations periodically in an effort to detect departures from protocol.

Patient Compliance

The investigator's concern for adherence to the protocol is not limited to staff activities. In studies that require the subjects to take a medication or limit their diet or behave in any particular proscribed way, it is necessary to verify that they are acting as required. This may be attempted through periodic interview, but objective evaluations are preferable whenever practical. For example, if pills are being taken, participants should be encouraged to bring all pill bottles and their contents back to the study center at each appointment. This allows the investigator to do a pill count and identify at least some of the individuals who are taking too few or too many pills. It may also be possible to test for the presence, in the subject's blood or urine, and the absence, in the control's blood or urine, of the substance being investigated.

DATA REVIEW AND CLEAN-UP

It is essential to have complete verification, conducted as independently as possible, of all coding, data entry into the computer, or any other form of data handling. Having gone to the labor and expense of collecting the data, it would be unfortunate to process it incorrectly. Editing programs can list all cases that have suspect values for one or more variables. After investigation and possible correction, it is necessary to put everything through the editing process again to minimize the possibility that the corrections made have inadvertently caused an error to be introduced elsewhere. In any event the guiding principle should be to build quality into the framework of the study, rather than to simply edit out wild values. Procedures such as reviewing a study form for completeness and appropriateness of entries *while the patient is still present* are very important. The forms on which study information is to be entered should be arranged so that accidental overlooking of required entries will be at a minimum. Always remember how much effort and expense went into collecting the data, so be sure to *handle with care*!

A FINAL WORD AS TO DATA COLLECTION

There seem to be an unlimited number of possible ways for data collection procedures to go wrong. During the course of an investigation, you should maintain a high degree of suspicion that all is not progressing satisfactorily because it often is not. Some sage has remarked that if all appears to be going well in an epidemiologic study, you have forgotten something. According to Cornfield [1959], the principle underlying research operations can be expressed in two words, "Be careful." It is excellent advice.

NOTES

* In a large prospective study, masked replicate blood samples were sent to the laboratory. In addition the laboratory also ran duplicate tests on every specimen received. The technical error for serum cholesterol measurement was then calculated separately for masked replicates and for known replicates. Not surprisingly the technical error was 7.1 mg/100 ml for known replicate pairs and 13.3 mg/100 ml for masked replicate pairs [Kahn et al 1969].

† This ratio is approximately equal to $(1 - r')^{1/2}$ where r' is the intraclass correlation coefficient [Snedecor and Cochran 1980].

Appendix

DESCRIPTION OF VARIABLES IN THE FRAMINGHAM HEART STUDY DATA SET

The listing and summary tabulations included herein contain data for 13 variables including 18-year follow-up for CHD incidence and total mortality. A brief description of the definition, coding, and range of values for each variable is presented below. Where abbreviations are used to describe variables, they are shown preceding the variable name. The listing is in sequence by age–sex group, within each age–sex group by CHD code, and within each CHD code by systolic blood pressure on examination 1. For further description and discussion of these data, see Gordon and Shurtleff [1973] and Shurtleff [1974].

SEX   1   Men

              2   Women (in most tabulations we have set $2 = 0$)

CHD   Coronary heart disease diagnosis

              0   No evidence of CHD through examination 10

              1   Preexisting CHD at examination 1 (prevalence cases)

              2–10   Examination at which definite CHD is first diagnosed (incidence cases). A participant was diagnosed as an incidence case if, after review of all available information, a panel of investigators agreed upon a definite diagnosis of myocardial infarction, coronary insufficiency, angina pectoris, or CHD death.

AGE   Age at examination 1

              45–62   Age in years

SBP   Systolic blood pressure, first examiner, examination 1

              90–300 mm Hg

SBP10   Systolic blood pressure, first examiner, examination 10

              ·   Missing data (635 persons)

              94–264 mm Hg

DBP   Diastolic blood pressure, first examiner, examination 1
             50–160 mm Hg
CHOL   Serum cholesterol, examination 1
             96–430 mg/100 ml
FRW   Framingham relative weight, examination 1, expressed as a
             percentage
             · Missing data (11 persons)
             52–222   FRW was calculated from the ratio of the subjects' body
                      weight to the median weight for their sex–height group.
CIG   Number of cigarettes smoked per day, examination 1
             · Missing data (1 person)
             0   No cigarettes smoked
             1–60
YRS_CHD   Person years observation until withdrawal or first CHD event
             · Preexisting CHD at examination 1 (43 persons not at risk)
             0–18   Years (See Chapter 7 for an explanation of how YRS_CHD
                    was calculated.)
YRS_DTH   Person–years observation for mortality
             1–18   Years (See Chapter 7 for an explanation of how YRS_DTH
                    was calculated.)
DEATH
             0   Alive at examination 10
             2–10   First examination that had been scheduled following the
                    date of death.
CAUSE   Cause of death
             · Missing data (19 persons)
             0   Alive at examination 10
             1   CHD (sudden)
             2   CHD (not sudden)
             3   Stroke
             4   Other cardiovascular disease
             5   Cancer
             6   Other

Framingham Data Subset for Exams 1 through 10 (n=1406)
Includes All Persons Age 45 and Above with a Valid
Serum Cholesterol Value at Exam 1.

------------------ GROUP=Men 45-49 ------------------------

OBS	CHD	AGE	SBP	SBP10	DBP	CHOL	FRW	CIG	YRS CHD	YRS DTH	DEATH	CAUSE
1	0	45	90	112	50	216	76	5	18	18	0	0
2	0	49	100	108	64	237	97	0	18	18	0	0
3	0	47	100	112	70	215	86	50	18	18	0	0
4	0	48	108	120	70	340	93	0	18	18	0	0
5	0	49	108	118	75	149	95	0	18	18	0	0
6	0	47	108	110	68	165	88	0	18	18	0	0
7	0	48	108	140	70	196	79	20	18	18	0	0
8	0	48	110	130	70	229	85	25	18	18	0	0
9	0	46	110	125	80	204	112	0	18	18	0	0
10	0	45	110	136	72	183	93	20	18	18	0	0
11	0	45	110	134	88	183	90	0	18	18	0	0
12	0	47	110	.	68	182	83	30	2	18	0	0
13	0	49	110	130	80	218	114	20	18	18	0	0
14	0	45	112	152	78	162	109	20	18	18	0	0
15	0	46	112	130	80	195	128	0	18	18	0	0
16	0	45	112	126	80	194	108	0	18	18	0	0
17	0	45	114	112	78	256	97	20	18	18	0	0
18	0	46	114	134	76	192	90	20	18	18	0	0
19	0	48	114	115	78	173	96	0	18	18	0	0
20	0	46	114	.	80	205	88	0	14	18	0	0
21	0	45	114	115	74	217	112	0	18	18	0	0
22	0	48	115	138	80	232	93	20	18	18	0	0
23	0	45	116	.	76	140	83	35	0	18	0	0
24	0	46	116	.	74	270	83	20	12	18	0	0
25	0	45	116	124	84	237	79	0	18	18	0	0
26	0	48	118	110	88	243	109	0	18	18	0	0
27	0	48	118	130	90	223	116	0	18	18	0	0
28	0	46	118	.	70	246	86	60	0	18	0	0
29	0	48	118	.	90	242	96	0	0	9	6	.
30	0	46	118	.	84	195	105	15	12	18	0	0
31	0	47	120	150	72	185	93	20	18	18	0	0
32	0	48	120	130	80	200	90	15	18	18	0	0
33	0	47	120	.	80	224	91	20	4	5	4	5
34	0	45	120	144	80	200	96	0	18	18	0	0
35	0	49	120	150	85	184	80	15	18	18	0	0
36	0	45	120	120	70	200	82	30	18	18	0	0
37	0	48	120	120	80	180	104	20	18	18	0	0
38	0	47	120	140	90	284	99	50	18	18	0	0
39	0	45	120	.	85	199	91	20	16	18	0	0
40	0	49	120	118	84	201	100	20	18	18	0	0
41	0	48	120	124	76	258	.	20	18	18	0	0
42	0	48	120	128	80	240	99	0	18	18	0	0
43	0	48	122	140	80	200	117	0	18	18	0	0
44	0	45	122	124	80	302	100	20	18	18	0	0
45	0	45	122	.	74	225	92	30	10	11	7	4
46	0	46	122	130	84	210	84	20	18	18	0	0
47	0	46	124	.	90	194	97	40	4	18	0	0
48	0	46	124	138	78	250	85	5	18	18	0	0
49	0	46	124	.	86	192	109	20	16	18	0	0
50	0	46	124	120	80	230	80	15	18	18	0	0
51	0	47	124	134	84	243	90	30	18	18	0	0
52	0	46	125	120	85	280	110	10	18	18	0	0

Framingham Data Subset for Exams 1 through 10 (n=1406)
Includes All Persons Age 45 and Above with a Valid
Serum Cholesterol Value at Exam 1.

------------------ GROUP=Men 45-49 -----------------------

OBS	CHD	AGE	SBP	SBP10	DBP	CHOL	FRW	CIG	YRS CHD	YRS DTH	DEATH	CAUSE
53	0	46	125	.	80	258	97	40	2	3	3	5
54	0	45	126	.	92	250	102	50	2	3	3	3
55	0	48	126	.	80	212	101	20	10	18	0	0
56	0	45	126	120	90	225	107	0	18	18	0	0
57	0	48	126	.	90	248	95	40	12	18	0	0
58	0	49	126	.	90	221	99	0	16	18	0	0
59	0	47	126	156	84	225	108	15	18	18	0	0
60	0	45	128	110	90	216	119	25	18	18	0	0
61	0	46	128	106	84	275	107	20	18	18	0	0
62	0	45	128	136	88	280	109	25	18	18	0	0
63	0	49	128	130	82	172	118	0	18	18	0	0
64	0	49	128	145	96	209	103	0	18	18	0	0
65	0	48	130	146	84	195	95	20	18	18	0	0
66	0	49	130	145	80	142	94	0	18	18	0	0
67	0	45	130	118	80	227	100	25	18	18	0	0
68	0	47	130	120	88	243	131	0	18	18	0	0
69	0	46	130	.	70	227	128	40	0	18	0	0
70	0	46	130	132	86	227	105	30	18	18	0	0
71	0	48	130	.	75	198	79	20	8	9	6	6
72	0	47	132	.	82	183	101	30	4	18	0	0
73	0	46	134	160	84	247	105	0	18	18	0	0
74	0	46	134	175	74	255	96	30	18	18	0	0
75	0	49	134	148	86	230	105	0	18	18	0	0
76	0	46	135	124	95	270	82	20	18	18	0	0
77	0	45	136	160	84	256	98	0	18	18	0	0
78	0	47	136	.	84	255	88	0	8	18	0	0
79	0	46	136	144	74	231	80	20	18	18	0	0
80	0	49	136	144	80	276	93	0	18	18	0	0
81	0	46	136	.	98	225	105	25	10	13	8	3
82	0	45	136	164	80	204	111	20	18	18	0	0
83	0	47	138	126	94	215	106	10	18	18	0	0
84	0	48	138	120	82	149	96	20	18	18	0	0
85	0	49	138	148	86	232	93	20	18	18	0	0
86	0	48	138	116	94	232	109	0	18	18	0	0
87	0	47	138	.	90	288	113	20	16	18	0	0
88	0	47	138	.	72	240	83	20	12	13	8	5
89	0	49	140	136	90	183	107	0	18	18	0	0
90	0	45	140	150	76	198	100	20	18	18	0	0
91	0	48	140	130	80	250	133	15	18	18	0	0
92	0	45	140	150	94	198	98	0	18	18	0	0
93	0	48	140	158	110	220	123	0	18	18	0	0
94	0	47	140	150	98	243	93	0	18	18	0	0
95	0	47	140	.	92	250	119	5	4	5	4	5
96	0	49	140	160	80	237	106	0	18	18	0	0
97	0	46	140	120	90	174	103	0	18	18	0	0
98	0	46	140	.	96	180	87	10	0	18	0	0
99	0	47	142	.	94	224	90	40	14	18	0	0
100	0	45	142	122	100	237	97	0	18	18	0	0
101	0	45	142	.	85	263	87	10	8	18	0	0
102	0	47	142	106	100	225	98	0	18	18	0	0
103	0	46	142	130	98	238	115	40	18	18	0	0
104	0	46	142	.	90	278	107	20	2	18	0	0

Framingham Data Subset for Exams 1 through 10 (n=1406)
Includes All Persons Age 45 and Above with a Valid
Serum Cholesterol Value at Exam 1.

------------------- GROUP=Men 45-49 -----------------------

OBS	CHD	AGE	SBP	SBP10	DBP	CHOL	FRW	CIG	YRS CHD	YRS DTH	DEATH	CAUSE
105	0	45	144	140	104	249	120	30	18	18	0	0
106	0	47	144	150	82	198	99	0	18	18	0	0
107	0	46	144	120	110	187	90	30	18	18	0	0
108	0	46	144	160	90	198	91	30	18	18	0	0
109	0	48	144	.	94	213	131	30	6	7	5	5
110	0	47	144	135	86	238	115	35	18	18	0	0
111	0	46	144	.	70	165	96	25	0	18	0	0
112	0	47	144	.	92	255	.	20	2	3	3	.
113	0	49	144	160	84	188	128	0	18	18	0	0
114	0	48	145	136	85	194	92	30	18	18	0	0
115	0	46	145	130	90	276	106	0	18	18	0	0
116	0	45	145	.	95	248	120	10	0	18	0	0
117	0	48	146	150	84	232	106	20	18	18	0	0
118	0	47	146	.	94	244	99	30	2	3	3	6
119	0	49	148	.	88	263	108	15	2	13	8	5
120	0	45	150	142	104	220	127	0	18	18	0	0
121	0	47	150	146	80	216	103	0	18	18	0	0
122	0	46	150	134	86	191	110	0	18	18	0	0
123	0	47	150	166	90	170	109	0	18	18	0	0
124	0	46	150	.	102	284	123	50	16	18	0	0
125	0	45	150	.	88	301	90	20	16	18	0	0
126	0	47	150	120	88	207	112	20	18	18	0	0
127	0	45	150	110	98	255	89	20	18	18	0	0
128	0	47	152	.	90	155	88	20	0	1	2	6
129	0	47	152	125	100	265	109	5	10	18	0	0
130	0	46	152	164	78	221	75	20	18	18	0	0
131	0	46	154	100	100	145	107	0	18	18	0	0
132	0	49	154	.	92	174	104	40	2	18	0	0
133	0	49	154	.	94	265	103	10	12	18	0	0
134	0	45	154	144	100	232	79	20	18	18	0	0
135	0	48	154	160	102	259	113	0	18	18	0	0
136	0	47	155	142	90	256	92	20	18	18	0	0
137	0	45	155	.	95	250	87	20	2	18	0	0
138	0	48	156	150	108	302	98	0	18	18	0	0
139	0	45	156	.	90	255	83	15	6	7	5	3
140	0	48	160	146	100	225	92	1	18	18	0	0
141	0	49	160	.	94	209	71	20	16	18	0	0
142	0	49	160	120	106	213	90	30	18	18	0	0
143	0	45	160	.	98	208	104	20	16	17	10	.
144	0	48	160	.	98	217	89	40	10	11	7	6
145	0	45	160	.	110	221	95	20	0	7	5	6
146	0	47	162	.	88	259	125	50	16	18	0	0
147	0	49	164	.	90	256	108	0	16	18	0	0
148	0	47	170	.	100	232	102	50	12	15	9	4
149	0	49	170	.	110	292	143	10	0	17	10	6
150	0	46	170	146	115	326	102	35	18	18	0	0
151	0	45	170	.	96	196	125	0	12	13	8	3
152	0	49	172	.	100	174	106	5	2	18	0	0
153	0	48	172	166	108	294	111	0	18	18	0	0
154	0	45	172	.	110	221	99	20	6	9	6	.
155	0	47	174	.	120	292	113	20	16	18	0	0
156	0	46	174	150	90	238	98	30	18	18	0	0

Framingham Data Subset for Exams 1 through 10 (n=1406)
Includes All Persons Age 45 and Above with a Valid
Serum Cholesterol Value at Exam 1.

------------------ GROUP=Men 45-49 ------------------------

OBS	CHD	AGE	SBP	SBP10	DBP	CHOL	FRW	CIG	YRS CHD	YRS DTH	DEATH	CAUSE
157	0	47	175	.	95	227	92	20	14	18	0	0
158	0	46	175	.	115	263	116	0	10	18	0	0
159	0	45	184	.	108	216	119	25	14	15	9	5
160	0	45	185	.	105	296	103	0	16	18	0	0
161	0	46	185	.	118	232	96	20	14	15	9	4
162	0	48	194	.	100	217	109	5	14	18	0	0
163	0	48	200	170	130	305	119	0	18	18	0	0
164	0	46	200	.	100	212	130	50	0	1	2	6
165	1	49	124	.	84	232	91	5	.	18	0	0
166	1	48	142	.	100	216	129	50	.	3	3	2
167	1	48	154	130	100	271	106	25	.	18	0	0
168	2	47	170	156	108	166	106	20	1	18	0	0
169	2	46	195	.	124	189	95	0	1	1	2	2
170	4	45	130	136	82	161	107	0	5	18	0	0
171	4	48	142	.	100	183	100	30	5	13	8	5
172	4	45	142	.	90	207	112	0	5	13	8	1
173	4	45	150	.	100	287	103	40	5	15	9	2
174	4	47	158	202	92	386	94	15	5	18	0	0
175	5	47	115	130	78	276	103	25	7	18	0	0
176	5	48	122	130	64	196	85	20	7	18	0	0
177	5	45	132	.	84	249	98	5	7	7	5	1
178	5	48	146	126	92	192	113	20	7	18	0	0
179	5	48	152	156	94	270	107	30	7	18	0	0
180	5	47	155	.	105	175	113	5	7	7	5	1
181	5	46	160	156	112	260	125	5	7	18	0	0
182	5	47	195	.	130	194	134	10	7	18	0	0
183	6	46	124	140	90	326	97	0	9	18	0	0
184	6	47	125	.	90	227	113	10	9	17	10	6
185	6	46	128	.	84	292	112	20	9	13	8	1
186	6	48	128	.	80	200	106	40	9	11	7	2
187	6	46	134	.	94	160	104	5	9	9	6	1
188	6	49	138	.	84	211	86	40	9	9	6	1
189	6	47	140	100	78	170	83	20	9	18	0	0
190	6	45	140	170	85	267	106	20	9	18	0	0
191	6	46	142	.	80	178	82	30	9	18	0	0
192	6	46	142	140	94	246	105	30	9	18	0	0
193	6	48	155	150	85	192	93	20	9	18	0	0
194	6	47	156	190	96	234	109	30	9	18	0	0
195	6	49	226	.	102	305	128	0	9	9	6	1
196	7	47	122	.	78	198	95	20	11	18	0	0
197	7	49	208	.	114	234	118	20	11	11	7	1
198	8	46	144	.	94	243	84	5	13	18	0	0
199	8	46	146	160	90	260	104	35	13	18	0	0
200	8	46	160	.	90	183	126	20	13	18	0	0
201	8	46	166	.	108	213	112	5	13	13	8	1
202	8	46	180	156	110	211	110	0	13	18	0	0
203	9	45	118	146	74	196	99	20	15	18	0	0
204	9	49	125	115	80	255	95	20	15	18	0	0
205	9	45	132	160	84	226	98	15	15	18	0	0
206	9	45	152	.	98	200	120	5	15	15	9	1
207	9	45	180	200	110	234	84	20	15	18	0	0
208	9	48	215	.	120	225	96	0	15	17	10	1

Framingham Data Subset for Exams 1 through 10 (n=1406)
Includes All Persons Age 45 and Above with a Valid
Serum Cholesterol Value at Exam 1.

------------------ GROUP=Men 45-49 ------------------------

| | | | | | | | | YRS | YRS | | |
OBS	CHD	AGE	SBP	SBP10	DBP	CHOL	FRW	CIG	CHD	DTH	DEATH	CAUSE
209	10	49	128	.	76	212	101	20	17	17	10	1
210	10	49	134	.	96	200	97	0	17	17	10	1
211	10	47	145	.	90	228	77	20	17	18	0	0
212	10	48	156	146	84	200	88	40	17	18	0	0

------------------ GROUP=Men 50-54 ------------------------

| | | | | | | | | YRS | YRS | | |
OBS	CHD	AGE	SBP	SBP10	DBP	CHOL	FRW	CIG	CHD	DTH	DEATH	CAUSE
213	0	51	96	114	68	265	76	20	18	18	0	0
214	0	53	105	134	65	234	108	1	18	18	0	0
215	0	51	108	126	80	292	85	5	18	18	0	0
216	0	51	108	116	64	148	119	0	18	18	0	0
217	0	50	110	130	70	224	110	0	18	18	0	0
218	0	51	110	100	70	249	99	5	18	18	0	0
219	0	52	110	120	68	196	88	15	18	18	0	0
220	0	54	110	.	76	271	102	20	14	18	0	0
221	0	52	110	128	80	175	105	20	18	18	0	0
222	0	52	110	126	60	209	87	10	18	18	0	0
223	0	52	110	.	70	200	100	0	6	7	5	6
224	0	53	114	120	80	149	108	25	18	18	0	0
225	0	50	114	180	80	178	78	0	18	18	0	0
226	0	51	115	160	90	285	101	0	18	18	0	0
227	0	53	116	.	76	270	94	20	14	17	10	4
228	0	50	118	110	70	227	114	20	18	18	0	0
229	0	52	118	130	78	183	92	0	18	18	0	0
230	0	52	118	.	82	249	94	0	0	18	0	0
231	0	53	118	.	82	212	95	20	12	13	8	5
232	0	52	118	.	72	260	103	0	16	17	10	6
233	0	53	120	120	70	137	89	30	18	18	0	0
234	0	53	120	152	80	220	114	20	18	18	0	0
235	0	52	120	142	80	243	96	20	18	18	0	0
236	0	50	120	105	86	265	112	0	18	18	0	0
237	0	51	120	.	80	174	97	5	10	18	0	0
238	0	54	120	124	82	165	78	10	18	18	0	0
239	0	50	120	.	76	196	82	20	10	18	0	0
240	0	52	120	.	70	271	85	0	10	13	8	5
241	0	53	120	120	70	184	91	35	18	18	0	0
242	0	52	124	170	84	187	117	0	18	18	0	0
243	0	51	124	.	76	235	86	15	6	18	0	0
244	0	53	124	.	72	142	116	30	8	18	0	0
245	0	54	124	128	84	225	98	0	18	18	0	0
246	0	50	124	130	84	315	90	20	18	18	0	0
247	0	51	124	116	78	242	118	0	18	18	0	0
248	0	50	124	.	80	280	100	0	8	18	0	0
249	0	50	125	.	85	187	92	0	2	18	0	0
250	0	54	125	114	85	213	92	5	18	18	0	0
251	0	53	125	130	75	213	106	20	18	18	0	0
252	0	51	126	150	92	141	93	20	18	18	0	0
253	0	50	126	.	84	237	111	0	12	13	8	4
254	0	50	126	156	90	166	106	0	18	18	0	0

Framingham Data Subset for Exams 1 through 10 (n=1406)
Includes All Persons Age 45 and Above with a Valid
Serum Cholesterol Value at Exam 1.

------------------ GROUP=Men 50-54 ------------------------

OBS	CHD	AGE	SBP	SBP10	DBP	CHOL	FRW	CIG	YRS CHD	YRS DTH	DEATH	CAUSE
255	0	53	126	132	90	211	108	0	18	18	0	0
256	0	52	128	118	90	178	96	0	18	18	0	0
257	0	53	128	138	80	230	137	0	18	18	0	0
258	0	53	128	.	70	209	91	20	14	18	0	0
259	0	51	130	164	82	256	102	20	18	18	0	0
260	0	52	130	146	80	216	90	35	18	18	0	0
261	0	52	130	130	85	302	118	0	18	18	0	0
262	0	51	130	136	80	285	111	0	18	18	0	0
263	0	54	130	120	80	237	91	0	18	18	0	0
264	0	54	130	.	70	172	93	20	12	13	8	6
265	0	54	130	124	88	170	105	0	18	18	0	0
266	0	52	130	.	80	172	88	20	12	18	0	0
267	0	50	130	150	98	334	108	15	18	18	0	0
268	0	50	130	.	80	225	97	30	4	18	0	0
269	0	53	130	.	80	196	82	20	12	13	8	5
270	0	51	130	134	88	213	105	0	18	18	0	0
271	0	50	132	.	86	266	107	0	14	18	0	0
272	0	52	134	100	82	172	110	0	18	18	0	0
273	0	51	134	166	82	198	90	20	18	18	0	0
274	0	54	134	140	80	183	109	10	18	18	0	0
275	0	51	134	.	84	194	90	20	16	18	0	0
276	0	54	134	.	82	250	102	0	6	7	5	5
277	0	51	134	.	94	234	109	40	10	18	0	0
278	0	52	135	136	85	296	95	20	18	18	0	0
279	0	53	135	125	80	259	109	0	18	18	0	0
280	0	52	135	139	95	221	113	0	18	18	0	0
281	0	50	136	170	80	250	97	10	18	18	0	0
282	0	51	136	142	80	220	109	15	18	18	0	0
283	0	50	136	.	86	309	111	0	16	18	0	0
284	0	54	136	138	80	234	104	20	18	18	0	0
285	0	52	138	180	76	248	110	5	18	18	0	0
286	0	53	138	118	90	159	138	0	18	18	0	0
287	0	50	140	.	86	244	108	0	0	18	0	0
288	0	50	140	166	84	186	114	0	18	18	0	0
289	0	51	140	170	96	191	96	5	18	18	0	0
290	0	54	140	.	86	200	105	20	2	5	4	6
291	0	53	140	150	90	170	116	0	18	18	0	0
292	0	54	140	120	100	212	119	0	18	18	0	0
293	0	53	140	.	75	178	94	1	16	18	0	0
294	0	50	140	131	90	285	91	0	18	18	0	0
295	0	52	140	.	98	155	143	20	0	1	2	6
296	0	51	140	.	80	211	89	40	12	13	8	6
297	0	51	140	140	90	175	103	20	18	18	0	0
298	0	52	140	.	84	182	102	20	8	18	0	0
299	0	51	140	110	98	301	101	35	18	18	0	0
300	0	54	140	.	82	238	99	5	12	13	8	4
301	0	52	140	135	84	221	111	0	18	18	0	0
302	0	50	142	170	80	270	93	40	18	18	0	0
303	0	51	142	.	88	149	111	20	10	11	7	6
304	0	53	142	150	72	157	103	10	18	18	0	0
305	0	53	144	131	90	229	97	0	18	18	0	0
306	0	52	144	.	94	265	93	20	10	13	8	4

Framingham Data Subset for Exams 1 through 10 (n=1406)
Includes All Persons Age 45 and Above with a Valid
Serum Cholesterol Value at Exam 1.

------------------ GROUP=Men 50-54 ------------------------

OBS	CHD	AGE	SBP	SBP10	DBP	CHOL	FRW	CIG	YRS CHD	YRS DTH	DEATH	CAUSE
307	0	51	144	120	90	259	101	1	18	18	0	0
308	0	50	145	152	120	243	103	0	18	18	0	0
309	0	52	145	.	100	213	99	20	14	18	0	0
310	0	51	145	.	105	250	99	20	10	11	7	6
311	0	51	145	144	105	167	89	20	18	18	0	0
312	0	51	146	128	90	263	113	20	18	18	0	0
313	0	54	146	130	100	194	112	20	18	18	0	0
314	0	50	148	148	92	204	98	0	18	18	0	0
315	0	50	150	170	90	250	100	0	18	18	0	0
316	0	52	150	.	100	249	94	40	0	18	0	0
317	0	50	150	.	108	249	126	0	12	13	8	6
318	0	51	150	150	100	315	110	30	18	18	0	0
319	0	51	150	200	90	187	99	0	18	18	0	0
320	0	51	150	160	100	296	93	60	18	18	0	0
321	0	51	150	.	98	284	104	20	14	18	0	0
322	0	53	150	.	90	238	102	10	14	15	9	4
323	0	54	152	.	88	217	99	0	2	3	3	5
324	0	53	155	156	88	170	94	30	18	18	0	0
325	0	52	155	.	80	265	122	20	2	3	3	4
326	0	50	156	.	100	224	148	5	6	18	0	0
327	0	54	156	.	110	200	103	20	14	18	0	0
328	0	52	156	.	78	121	88	20	2	3	3	4
329	0	52	158	166	90	237	84	5	18	18	0	0
330	0	53	158	140	102	200	115	0	18	18	0	0
331	0	51	158	148	106	259	114	20	18	18	0	0
332	0	54	158	.	88	276	114	20	0	5	4	5
333	0	54	160	.	100	292	77	20	16	17	10	4
334	0	52	160	.	94	249	105	20	10	13	8	6
335	0	51	160	.	98	216	100	30	10	11	7	3
336	0	53	160	.	90	292	106	20	14	15	9	5
337	0	50	160	170	108	238	111	15	18	18	0	0
338	0	53	160	154	96	164	95	0	18	18	0	0
339	0	51	160	140	105	255	106	20	18	18	0	0
340	0	54	160	.	110	205	112	0	6	7	5	3
341	0	54	160	138	102	167	118	0	18	18	0	0
342	0	54	160	.	105	243	106	10	16	18	0	0
343	0	51	164	180	96	334	118	20	18	18	0	0
344	0	52	165	150	94	178	76	5	18	18	0	0
345	0	50	165	.	95	187	89	20	0	1	2	5
346	0	53	165	.	110	148	116	0	12	18	0	0
347	0	50	166	.	104	232	132	10	10	18	0	0
348	0	51	166	.	104	200	104	25	6	7	5	5
349	0	50	170	172	104	198	128	0	18	18	0	0
350	0	51	172	160	92	232	107	0	18	18	0	0
351	0	51	172	.	108	217	94	30	4	18	0	0
352	0	50	174	.	106	192	95	5	8	13	8	3
353	0	52	175	.	120	284	103	0	14	18	0	0
354	0	54	180	.	120	235	102	20	14	17	10	3
355	0	54	180	.	96	284	101	0	6	7	5	4
356	0	54	184	.	100	213	115	0	12	18	0	0
357	0	54	184	.	110	217	90	0	10	18	0	0
358	0	54	184	170	86	304	85	0	18	18	0	0

Framingham Data Subset for Exams 1 through 10 (n=1406)
Includes All Persons Age 45 and Above with a Valid
Serum Cholesterol Value at Exam 1.

------------------ GROUP=Men 50-54 ------------------------

OBS	CHD	AGE	SBP	SBP10	DBP	CHOL	FRW	CIG	YRS CHD	YRS DTH	DEATH	CAUSE
359	0	50	190	208	104	221	119	0	18	18	0	0
360	0	53	200	.	125	284	122	0	14	18	0	0
361	0	54	204	.	102	242	104	5	8	11	7	4
362	0	50	220	160	120	243	124	0	18	18	0	0
363	0	54	220	236	130	232	113	0	18	18	0	0
364	0	52	220	.	160	259	115	1	16	18	0	0
365	1	52	118	.	66	330	86	20	.	11	7	1
366	1	53	122	100	78	292	94	25	.	18	0	0
367	1	54	128	.	75	275	102	0	.	11	7	2
368	1	53	130	120	90	227	124	0	.	18	0	0
369	1	52	136	.	90	256	101	25	.	11	7	5
370	1	50	140	.	88	220	88	20	.	9	6	4
371	1	54	165	.	105	243	105	0	.	3	3	4
372	1	54	165	.	90	240	90	15	.	15	9	2
373	1	53	190	.	120	149	135	10	.	7	5	1
374	1	51	228	.	122	246	139	40	.	7	5	1
375	2	52	120	150	80	224	96	20	1	18	0	0
376	2	54	140	.	88	267	.	40	1	1	2	1
377	2	52	146	.	94	243	105	35	1	3	3	2
378	2	54	160	.	95	174	82	20	1	15	9	2
379	2	52	175	.	114	233	88	0	1.	3	3	2
380	2	54	180	.	100	220	101	0	1	3	3	1
381	3	53	114	112	74	292	95	0	3	18	0	0
382	3	50	130	.	90	191	108	20	3	7	5	3
383	3	53	130	.	84	288	107	20	3	15	9	5
384	3	54	182	.	100	271	152	45	3	3	3	1
385	4	54	122	139	68	203	86	20	5	18	0	0
386	4	53	124	110	94	299	109	0	5	18	0	0
387	4	52	152	.	100	155	119	0	5	18	0	0
388	4	54	180	190	100	263	104	30	4	18	0	0
389	5	50	135	.	98	232	109	20	7	18	0	0
390	5	52	145	.	103	200	111	20	7	18	0	0
391	5	52	190	.	104	280	135	25	7	7	5	2
392	6	50	120	.	74	217	89	30	9	9	6	1
393	6	52	130	170	82	280	98	40	9	18	0	0
394	6	51	132	.	86	265	107	15	9	18	0	0
395	6	51	142	.	90	217	125	5	9	9	6	1
396	6	50	148	.	95	280	102	30	9	9	6	1
397	6	50	164	150	104	220	105	0	9	18	0	0
398	6	53	168	168	90	195	115	15	9	18	0	0
399	6	54	174	.	86	194	127	0	9	9	6	1
400	6	50	175	.	110	187	113	0	9	9	6	1
401	7	51	110	110	76	302	92	0	11	18	0	0
402	7	52	130	.	90	351	108	0	11	11	7	2
403	7	51	140	.	82	209	92	30	11	11	7	1
404	7	54	140	.	84	217	88	5	11	11	7	2
405	7	52	142	120	100	237	95	0	11	18	0	0
406	7	52	156	.	104	333	128	0	11	17	10	2
407	7	54	170	144	100	222	107	20	11	18	0	0
408	7	52	175	.	105	216	106	15	11	18	0	0
409	8	50	108	118	82	243	103	20	13	18	0	0
410	8	50	134	136	88	225	112	0	13	18	0	0

Framingham Data Subset for Exams 1 through 10 (n=1406)
Includes All Persons Age 45 and Above with a Valid
Serum Cholesterol Value at Exam 1.

```
----------------- GROUP=Men 50-54 ----------------------
```

									YRS	YRS		
OBS	CHD	AGE	SBP	SBP10	DBP	CHOL	FRW	CIG	CHD	DTH	DEATH	CAUSE
411	8	53	138	.	86	199	93	0	13	13	8	2
412	8	53	155	.	90	263	99	0	13	13	8	2
413	8	50	174	.	115	213	97	0	13	17	10	2
414	9	52	122	140	92	200	105	20	15	18	0	0
415	9	53	125	.	90	225	111	0	15	17	10	2
416	9	53	130	160	80	195	103	30	15	18	0	0
417	9	54	166	.	104	196	113	40	15	15	9	2
418	9	53	174	.	98	228	107	5	15	15	9	1
419	10	54	110	168	68	275	91	0	17	18	0	0
420	10	51	124	156	84	198	93	30	17	18	0	0
421	10	52	150	.	95	209	99	30	17	17	10	2
422	10	52	156	160	80	217	102	15	17	18	0	0
423	10	52	176	.	100	230	90	0	17	17	10	1

```
-------         ---- GROUP-Men 55-59 ---------------------
```

									YRS	YRS		
OBS	CHD	AGE	SBP	SBP10	DBP	CHOL	FRW	CIG	CHD	DTH	DEATH	CAUSE
424	0	58	108	120	76	217	91	20	18	18	0	0
425	0	56	108	.	72	165	112	0	8	11	7	5
426	0	57	110	148	82	183	99	0	18	18	0	0
427	0	57	110	134	75	166	86	0	18	18	0	0
428	0	55	110	170	80	217	101	20	18	18	0	0
429	0	56	112	146	70	149	90	40	18	18	0	0
430	0	56	112	116	66	296	78	15	18	18	0	0
431	0	58	114	125	64	238	97	20	18	18	0	0
432	0	58	115	100	80	209	101	0	18	18	0	0
433	0	56	116	124	74	205	72	5	18	18	0	0
434	0	58	116	120	80	217	.	20	18	18	0	0
435	0	57	118	148	76	163	98	0	18	18	0	0
436	0	55	118	144	86	194	113	0	18	18	0	0
437	0	56	120	134	68	237	91	0	18	18	0	0
438	0	57	120	.	70	243	96	50	8	9	6	5
439	0	57	120	150	66	191	102	0	18	18	0	0
440	0	57	120	150	78	224	97	0	18	18	0	0
441	0	58	120	.	65	266	111	0	12	18	0	0
442	0	56	120	130	80	255	100	15	18	18	0	0
443	0	57	120	.	80	288	96	20	2	3	3	5
444	0	56	120	135	72	234	92	35	18	18	0	0
445	0	55	124	160	88	236	101	30	18	18	0	0
446	0	59	124	118	80	200	164	0	18	18	0	0
447	0	58	124	.	75	178	111	0	16	17	10	5
448	0	57	124	120	74	227	99	0	18	18	0	0
449	0	56	125	120	80	224	92	20	18	18	0	0
450	0	59	125	130	80	196	92	5	18	18	0	0
451	0	57	125	110	85	213	91	0	18	18	0	0
452	0	58	125	135	65	199	94	20	18	18	0	0
453	0	58	126	.	80	225	95	40	6	7	5	5
454	0	57	126	.	78	161	113	5	16	18	0	0
455	0	56	128	144	78	232	88	0	18	18	0	0
456	0	56	128	.	82	232	83	40	8	17	10	5

Framingham Data Subset for Exams 1 through 10 (n=1406)
Includes All Persons Age 45 and Above with a Valid
Serum Cholesterol Value at Exam 1.

------------------ GROUP=Men 55-59 ------------------------

OBS	CHD	AGE	SBP	SBP10	DBP	CHOL	FRW	CIG	YRS CHD	YRS DTH	DEATH	CAUSE
457	0	55	128	.	78	167	110	20	12	18	0	0
458	0	58	128	.	82	134	72	5	0	1	2	5
459	0	57	130	146	90	254	82	0	18	18	0	0
460	0	57	130	156	78	295	91	5	18	18	0	0
461	0	56	130	.	72	240	85	15	14	17	10	6
462	0	56	130	142	80	227	92	20	18	18	0	0
463	0	56	130	158	90	212	81	20	18	18	0	0
464	0	57	130	.	75	96	101	20	4	5	4	5
465	0	58	130	186	80	175	82	20	18	18	0	0
466	0	56	130	.	75	271	84	0	14	15	9	6
467	0	59	130	140	82	264	101	0	18	18	0	0
468	0	58	130	.	88	260	139	40	10	18	0	0
469	0	55	132	140	88	231	98	10	18	18	0	0
470	0	58	132	120	88	180	114	0	18	18	0	0
471	0	56	132	.	90	326	93	20	12	18	0	0
472	0	55	134	200	84	224	101	0	18	18	0	0
473	0	57	134	170	84	233	119	0	18	18	0	0
474	0	58	134	160	84	209	104	0	18	18	0	0
475	0	55	136	140	96	250	102	0	18	18	0	0
476	0	58	136	130	80	183	103	0	18	18	0	0
477	0	57	136	137	88	242	96	20	18	18	0	0
478	0	55	136	150	80	247	95	0	18	18	0	0
479	0	55	138	.	82	195	88	10	0	1	2	5
480	0	59	138	104	90	270	88	0	18	18	0	0
481	0	56	138	.	100	175	95	20	2	9	6	5
482	0	59	138	.	86	175	84	20	10	18	0	0
483	0	57	138	.	78	182	91	50	0	9	6	6
484	0	55	138	180	80	126	94	0	18	18	0	0
485	0	58	138	.	80	279	122	10	14	15	9	5
486	0	56	140	.	80	166	95	20	16	17	10	5
487	0	55	140	120	92	300	108	0	18	18	0	0
488	0	55	140	.	80	256	112	30	8	15	9	.
489	0	59	140	110	70	170	86	5	18	18	0	0
490	0	58	140	130	85	237	80	1	18	18	0	0
491	0	57	140	.	84	250	102	0	16	18	0	0
492	0	59	140	162	80	163	95	0	18	18	0	0
493	0	56	140	.	84	200	113	0	14	18	0	0
494	0	55	140	145	90	213	93	0	18	18	0	0
495	0	56	140	120	90	276	112	5	18	18	0	0
496	0	59	140	.	80	228	123	10	12	18	0	0
497	0	55	142	186	88	217	99	20	18	18	0	0
498	0	55	142	170	92	221	98	20	18	18	0	0
499	0	58	144	.	102	126	120	0	14	15	9	6
500	0	57	144	.	96	184	88	20	2	3	3	3
501	0	59	145	.	90	200	104	25	6	9	6	3
502	0	59	146	.	80	250	117	0	4	7	5	3
503	0	59	146	.	84	226	89	20	16	18	0	0
504	0	57	147	.	68	188	104	20	6	7	5	4
505	0	55	148	.	92	268	105	20	8	9	6	6
506	0	55	148	150	100	187	109	0	18	18	0	0
507	0	58	148	.	84	217	97	20	0	18	0	0
508	0	59	150	.	88	200	81	5	14	18	0	0

Framingham Data Subset for Exams 1 through 10 (n=1406)
Includes All Persons Age 45 and Above with a Valid
Serum Cholesterol Value at Exam 1.

------------------ GROUP=Men 55-59 ------------------------

OBS	CHD	AGE	SBP	SBP10	DBP	CHOL	FRW	CIG	YRS CHD	YRS DTH	DEATH	CAUSE
509	0	59	150	170	90	200	116	0	18	18	0	0
510	0	55	150	210	90	232	108	0	18	18	0	0
511	0	59	150	136	80	200	88	0	18	18	0	0
512	0	58	150	150	94	292	83	20	18	18	0	0
513	0	58	152	.	74	196	77	0	0	18	0	0
514	0	58	152	.	90	192	98	20	10	18	0	0
515	0	56	154	154	88	271	111	10	18	18	0	0
516	0	57	154	152	100	232	114	15	18	18	0	0
517	0	55	156	.	94	243	105	25	8	18	0	0
518	0	57	156	194	78	265	87	5	18	18	0	0
519	0	58	157	165	80	213	108	0	18	18	0	0
520	0	58	158	.	96	142	107	5	16	18	0	0
521	0	56	158	.	100	292	111	0	0	18	0	0
522	0	55	158	159	98	267	121	0	18	18	0	0
523	0	59	160	180	96	237	88	20	18	18	0	0
524	0	57	160	.	94	216	102	0	10	17	10	6
525	0	55	160	160	110	212	136	0	18	18	0	0
526	0	57	160	.	80	230	98	40	6	11	7	5
527	0	59	160	.	110	209	95	25	0	3	3	6
528	0	56	160	.	90	290	80	5	6	11	7	.
529	0	58	166	.	115	216	109	0	2	3	3	6
530	0	57	168	.	86	221	137	20	8	9	6	.
531	0	55	170	.	88	183	84	20	8	18	0	0
532	0	56	170	200	86	196	111	1	18	18	0	0
533	0	56	172	.	114	213	125	0	8	9	6	.
534	0	55	172	164	104	230	109	0	18	18	0	0
535	0	58	174	.	92	193	128	0	2	18	0	0
536	0	55	174	182	90	173	78	0	18	18	0	0
537	0	58	176	.	104	234	118	15	8	9	6	3
538	0	56	180	150	100	178	124	0	18	18	0	0
539	0	59	180	.	104	194	85	20	10	11	7	5
540	0	59	180	148	110	205	112	0	18	18	0	0
541	0	57	184	.	100	162	109	0	4	7	5	4
542	0	59	184	.	120	207	100	0	16	17	10	4
543	0	56	190	.	70	217	97	30	8	9	6	4
544	0	58	200	.	112	166	106	0	0	11	7	4
545	0	56	200	220	100	202	93	10	18	18	0	0
546	0	57	234	.	134	260	110	0	10	15	9	5
547	0	55	246	.	110	246	109	25	2	3	3	3
548	1	59	108	.	68	209	98	20	.	3	3	1
549	1	56	124	.	86	284	121	35	.	15	9	2
550	1	59	128	120	72	340	82	0	.	18	0	0
551	1	55	135	.	80	237	101	0	.	5	4	2
552	1	59	136	.	72	167	98	20	.	7	5	2
553	1	59	150	.	94	189	75	20	.	5	4	.
554	1	58	156	156	110	237	123	0	.	18	0	0
555	1	59	170	.	90	229	76	0	.	7	5	2
556	2	57	120	.	74	219	94	15	1	1	2	1
557	2	59	124	130	84	227	98	20	1	18	0	0
558	2	59	146	.	94	300	106	25	1	9	6	.
559	2	56	160	.	94	267	108	20	1	5	4	2
560	2	56	176	.	90	182	79	15	1	9	6	1

Framingham Data Subset for Exams 1 through 10 (n=1406)
Includes All Persons Age 45 and Above with a Valid
Serum Cholesterol Value at Exam 1.

------------------ GROUP=Men 55-59 ------------------------

OBS	CHD	AGE	SBP	SBP10	DBP	CHOL	FRW	CIG	YRS CHD	YRS DTH	DEATH	CAUSE
561	2	57	185	.	105	272	113	0	1	15	9	6
562	2	55	186	.	124	263	120	20	1	1	2	1
563	2	58	200	.	130	213	125	5	1	13	8	1
564	2	59	260	.	130	246	111	20	1	13	8	6
565	3	58	124	.	80	195	97	0	3	7	5	6
566	3	58	126	.	70	280	119	20	3	9	6	2
567	3	55	140	.	85	288	91	30	3	3	3	2
568	3	59	155	130	90	223	94	50	3	18	0	0
569	3	59	158	.	89	326	116	0	3	9	6	2
570	3	56	172	.	104	221	113	0	3	18	0	0
571	3	57	182	.	112	184	102	0	3	3	3	6
572	3	56	216	.	126	309	130	15	3	7	5	6
573	4	57	130	120	90	187	109	0	5	18	0	0
574	4	59	130	.	80	324	102	0	5	15	9	5
575	4	56	135	.	104	217	119	15	5	5	4	1
576	4	55	140	.	82	280	85	30	5	9	6	2
577	4	57	140	120	76	188	93	5	5	18	0	0
578	4	58	148	144	98	232	109	0	5	18	0	0
579	4	59	148	186	86	226	83	40	5	18	0	0
580	4	58	150	198	95	296	100	15	5	18	0	0
581	4	59	172	.	108	319	122	0	5	17	10	2
582	4	56	178	.	100	172	97	15	5	9	6	2
583	4	57	220	162	118	194	119	0	5	18	0	0
584	4	57	230	.	138	221	96	20	5	17	10	2
585	5	56	140	.	92	191	97	20	7	17	10	1
586	5	57	180	.	100	301	115	15	7	18	0	0
587	6	59	135	170	75	249	122	5	9	18	0	0
588	6	55	142	148	88	221	97	40	9	18	0	0
589	6	55	148	.	84	232	95	20	9	9	6	2
590	7	58	105	115	75	225	84	20	11	18	0	0
591	7	58	132	130	84	227	97	40	11	18	0	0
592	7	56	132	150	78	204	121	0	11	18	0	0
593	7	57	138	142	85	198	71	5	11	18	0	0
594	7	56	190	.	110	292	87	20	10	15	9	4
595	7	59	200	.	130	250	109	0	10	15	9	1
596	8	58	110	.	72	282	91	0	13	15	9	4
597	8	58	124	128	82	178	98	0	13	18	0	0
598	8	56	150	.	90	187	130	0	13	15	9	1
599	8	57	150	.	90	174	99	5	13	13	8	2
600	8	57	154	.	66	192	82	20	13	13	8	5
601	9	55	138	130	70	221	105	0	15	18	0	0
602	9	56	158	116	100	246	112	0	15	18	0	0
603	9	57	164	.	94	246	98	15	15	17	10	2
604	9	58	170	120	116	194	126	30	15	18	0	0
605	10	59	120	152	86	229	105	0	17	18	0	0
606	10	56	125	130	75	305	88	0	17	18	0	0
607	10	57	158	178	100	267	128	20	17	18	0	0

Framingham Data Subset for Exams 1 through 10 (n=1406)
Includes All Persons Age 45 and Above with a Valid
Serum Cholesterol Value at Exam 1.

------------------ GROUP=Men 60-62 ------------------------

OBS	CHD	AGE	SBP	SBP10	DBP	CHOL	FRW	CIG	YRS CHD	YRS DTH	DEATH	CAUSE
608	0	62	110	.	70	198	100	15	10	11	7	4
609	0	60	120	.	80	200	73	50	6	13	8	4
610	0	60	120	132	70	198	110	0	18	18	0	0
611	0	60	122	.	78	209	115	0	0	17	10	6
612	0	61	124	.	74	263	104	0	4	18	0	0
613	0	60	125	.	85	199	76	20	2	3	3	5
614	0	60	126	.	74	188	74	5	14	15	9	4
615	0	60	126	.	82	163	78	20	16	18	0	0
616	0	60	130	.	98	237	105	25	10	11	7	4
617	0	60	130	.	85	264	98	20	16	18	0	0
618	0	61	134	.	88	276	92	0	4	18	0	0
619	0	60	134	.	78	326	111	10	12	13	8	5
620	0	60	136	130	80	234	100	20	18	18	0	0
621	0	60	136	.	82	230	112	0	14	18	0	0
622	0	60	138	94	98	187	136	30	18	18	0	0
623	0	60	138	.	92	238	121	0	2	15	9	6
624	0	60	140	.	78	249	85	0	16	18	0	0
625	0	61	140	.	80	191	95	0	12	18	0	0
626	0	60	140	200	80	175	108	20	18	18	0	0
627	0	60	142	150	94	237	124	0	18	18	0	0
628	0	60	142	.	66	209	103	0	8	9	6	4
629	0	60	148	.	86	159	77	5	8	9	6	.
630	0	60	150	.	90	237	102	30	6	18	0	0
631	0	60	150	.	86	188	118	0	14	15	9	5
632	0	60	150	.	100	180	122	0	16	17	10	3
633	0	61	150	180	52	246	91	0	18	18	0	0
634	0	60	152	.	88	142	98	0	2	18	0	0
635	0	60	154	.	90	183	100	0	8	9	6	5
636	0	60	154	184	82	159	112	5	18	18	0	0
637	0	61	154	138	100	313	101	20	18	18	0	0
638	0	61	155	.	75	230	103	5	4	18	0	0
639	0	62	156	.	90	255	87	0	6	7	5	3
640	0	60	156	.	96	248	115	20	4	5	4	5
641	0	60	160	.	75	242	91	0	12	17	10	5
642	0	60	172	.	100	276	106	0	8	9	6	5
643	0	61	175	.	95	243	91	0	2	9	6	.
644	0	60	180	.	120	275	118	20	6	18	0	0
645	0	60	190	170	105	198	146	0	18	18	0	0
646	0	60	200	.	85	255	101	0	2	18	0	0
647	1	61	140	.	68	248	104	20	.	1	2	2
648	1	60	160	.	80	263	107	0	.	11	7	1
649	1	60	160	.	90	244	109	20	.	3	3	1
650	1	60	190	.	100	246	102	15	.	1	2	4
651	1	60	208	.	130	213	124	10	.	11	7	6
652	2	60	140	.	72	216	113	15	1	18	0	0
653	2	60	150	.	90	194	130	0	1	18	0	0
654	2	60	175	.	70	224	101	0	1	5	4	1
655	3	61	98	.	78	179	90	20	3	13	8	6
656	3	61	116	138	76	228	96	0	3	18	0	0
657	3	60	176	.	94	255	87	0	3	3	3	1
658	4	61	148	.	80	284	.	0	5	13	8	2
659	4	61	150	.	95	207	97	0	5	5	4	2

Framingham Data Subset for Exams 1 through 10 (n=1406)
Includes All Persons Age 45 and Above with a Valid
Serum Cholesterol Value at Exam 1.

------------------ GROUP=Men 60-62 ------------------------

OBS	CHD	AGE	SBP	SBP10	DBP	CHOL	FRW	CIG	YRS CHD	YRS DTH	DEATH	CAUSE
660	4	60	164	.	96	257	.	5	5	9	6	2
661	4	60	166	.	110	216	80	30	3	11	7	2
662	5	61	145	.	85	299	119	10	7	11	7	4
663	5	61	276	.	112	232	116	0	7	7	5	2
664	6	60	144	150	92	232	121	20	9	18	0	0
665	7	61	135	.	75	224	111	20	11	13	8	1
666	9	60	140	.	92	217	126	0	15	15	9	2
667	10	60	158	.	76	200	81	0	17	17	10	1
668	10	60	160	.	100	200	117	0	17	17	10	1
669	10	60	202	.	108	255	121	0	17	17	10	4

------------------ GROUP=Women 45-49 ------------------------

OBS	CHD	AGE	SBP	SBP10	DBP	CHOL	FRW	CIG	YRS CHD	YRS DTH	DEATH	CAUSE
670	0	48	90	.	60	271	110	10	0	13	8	5
671	0	45	100	110	62	220	93	0	18	18	0	0
672	0	45	100	124	70	149	102	0	18	18	0	0
673	0	48	105	112	75	172	96	0	18	18	0	0
674	0	49	105	.	80	170	85	30	0	18	0	0
675	0	48	106	.	70	167	90	0	14	15	9	5
676	0	45	110	130	75	205	90	0	18	18	0	0
677	0	45	112	.	80	309	133	0	2	18	0	0
678	0	46	112	112	72	230	88	0	18	18	0	0
679	0	46	114	110	80	200	113	0	18	18	0	0
680	0	48	114	139	84	221	96	15	18	18	0	0
681	0	46	114	150	76	150	97	20	18	18	0	0
682	0	46	115	122	75	217	87	10	18	18	0	0
683	0	45	115	110	80	188	94	1	18	18	0	0
684	0	45	116	.	80	158	99	0	16	18	0	0
685	0	46	116	132	70	237	93	0	18	18	0	0
686	0	45	116	124	70	260	92	0	18	18	0	0
687	0	46	118	156	80	141	107	15	18	18	0	0
688	0	46	118	130	76	183	79	0	18	18	0	0
689	0	49	118	120	76	155	98	20	18	18	0	0
690	0	47	118	114	70	226	118	0	18	18	0	0
691	0	49	120	133	76	220	98	5	18	18	0	0
692	0	45	120	220	90	214	117	0	18	18	0	0
693	0	47	120	.	85	167	101	0	8	9	6	5
694	0	49	120	134	88	227	122	20	18	18	0	0
695	0	45	120	160	82	149	94	0	18	18	0	0
696	0	45	120	.	80	224	101	0	12	18	0	0
697	0	47	120	100	80	324	107	10	18	18	0	0
698	0	46	120	170	80	232	97	20	18	18	0	0
699	0	46	120	.	68	234	95	0	12	18	0	0
700	0	47	120	.	90	267	125	0	16	18	0	0
701	0	46	120	.	74	232	95	20	16	18	0	0
702	0	49	120	.	80	207	94	10	16	18	0	0
703	0	47	122	.	80	199	107	20	6	18	0	0
704	0	46	122	142	70	214	95	0	18	18	0	0
705	0	45	122	130	88	220	79	0	18	18	0	0

Framingham Data Subset for Exams 1 through 10 (n=1406)
Includes All Persons Age 45 and Above with a Valid
Serum Cholesterol Value at Exam 1.

---------------- GROUP=Women 45-49 ---------------------

OBS	CHD	AGE	SBP	SBP10	DBP	CHOL	FRW	CIG	YRS CHD	YRS DTH	DEATH	CAUSE
706	0	45	122	138	76	220	85	10	18	18	0	0
707	0	45	122	146	70	166	90	0	18	18	0	0
708	0	45	122	.	74	178	88	5	14	18	0	0
709	0	45	122	.	78	217	76	15	16	18	0	0
710	0	46	124	.	66	232	94	20	14	18	0	0
711	0	46	124	.	84	198	91	10	14	15	9	5
712	0	45	124	120	82	200	89	0	18	18	0	0
713	0	47	124	142	76	196	91	0	18	18	0	0
714	0	47	124	.	74	216	88	0	14	18	0	0
715	0	46	124	.	80	234	52	0	0	9	6	6
716	0	48	125	188	85	200	99	0	18	18	0	0
717	0	45	125	110	75	167	102	0	18	18	0	0
718	0	45	125	104	80	221	104	1	18	18	0	0
719	0	49	126	200	80	183	93	20	18	18	0	0
720	0	49	126	160	84	232	134	0	18	18	0	0
721	0	46	126	180	92	187	120	20	18	18	0	0
722	0	47	126	.	80	309	97	5	14	18	0	0
723	0	48	126	.	88	215	111	0	14	15	9	5
724	0	45	126	144	80	242	111	0	18	18	0	0
725	0	45	128	125	90	224	69	0	18	18	0	0
726	0	48	128	150	82	351	85	20	18	18	0	0
727	0	46	128	.	80	263	102	5	0	18	0	0
728	0	49	128	112	80	217	85	10	18	18	0	0
729	0	47	130	.	80	257	84	10	6	7	5	6
730	0	45	130	156	78	216	109	0	18	18	0	0
731	0	48	130	140	86	299	94	25	18	18	0	0
732	0	46	130	150	80	250	92	0	18	18	0	0
733	0	48	130	116	85	243	119	0	18	18	0	0
734	0	45	130	140	85	200	83	20	18	18	0	0
735	0	48	130	.	86	224	85	20	6	18	0	0
736	0	47	130	120	70	232	81	0	18	18	0	0
737	0	45	130	142	90	212	86	0	18	18	0	0
738	0	45	130	.	70	183	94	5	16	18	0	0
739	0	45	130	.	85	194	73	0	16	18	0	0
740	0	45	130	152	86	232	100	0	18	18	0	0
741	0	47	130	155	80	232	84	0	18	18	0	0
742	0	46	130	.	90	183	118	0	0	18	0	0
743	0	46	130	160	90	288	116	0	18	18	0	0
744	0	46	130	138	78	173	91	0	18	18	0	0
745	0	47	132	150	86	301	104	0	18	18	0	0
746	0	48	132	134	92	217	110	0	18	18	0	0
747	0	49	132	176	90	250	104	0	18	18	0	0
748	0	46	132	.	82	262	133	5	12	18	0	0
749	0	49	132	.	84	243	77	0	8	18	0	0
750	0	45	132	.	66	285	90	0	16	18	0	0
751	0	48	134	140	84	259	99	1	18	18	0	0
752	0	45	134	220	76	183	117	20	18	18	0	0
753	0	45	134	114	86	315	99	10	18	18	0	0
754	0	45	134	144	88	194	112	0	18	18	0	0
755	0	45	134	180	86	211	104	20	18	18	0	0
756	0	45	135	134	80	155	76	1	18	18	0	0
757	0	47	135	.	82	249	111	0	2	18	0	0

Framingham Data Subset for Exams 1 through 10 (n=1406)
Includes All Persons Age 45 and Above with a Valid
Serum Cholesterol Value at Exam 1.

---------------- GROUP=Women 45-49 -----------------------

OBS	CHD	AGE	SBP	SBP10	DBP	CHOL	FRW	CIG	YRS CHD	YRS DTH	DEATH	CAUSE
758	0	48	135	.	90	265	113	20	16	18	0	0
759	0	45	135	.	85	315	127	0	14	18	0	0
760	0	48	135	.	100	198	111	0	16	17	10	5
761	0	48	135	174	90	146	.	0	18	18	0	0
762	0	49	135	152	90	305	114	10	18	18	0	0
763	0	48	135	134	90	244	109	10	18	18	0	0
764	0	46	135	139	80	180	122	0	18	18	0	0
765	0	47	136	150	80	257	91	1	18	18	0	0
766	0	47	136	140	86	227	90	0	18	18	0	0
767	0	47	136	130	70	140	87	5	18	18	0	0
768	0	45	136	.	86	198	99	20	14	18	0	0
769	0	45	136	126	86	246	108	0	18	18	0	0
770	0	48	136	148	84	217	131	0	18	18	0	0
771	0	46	136	156	86	244	101	0	18	18	0	0
772	0	46	136	130	74	192	102	0	18	18	0	0
773	0	49	136	.	80	212	125	0	4	13	8	6
774	0	49	136	154	94	161	89	0	18	18	0	0
775	0	48	136	.	90	238	106	0	12	13	8	5
776	0	45	138	160	88	260	110	0	18	18	0	0
777	0	49	138	136	90	232	95	0	18	18	0	0
778	0	47	138	146	96	220	91	20	18	18	0	0
779	0	49	138	164	95	280	107	30	18	18	0	0
780	0	49	138	148	94	223	99	0	18	18	0	0
781	0	46	138	.	82	269	106	0	16	18	0	0
782	0	47	140	95	80	157	101	0	18	18	0	0
783	0	45	140	148	80	257	113	5	18	18	0	0
784	0	49	140	.	88	249	112	0	6	18	0	0
785	0	47	140	140	90	170	116	0	18	18	0	0
786	0	48	140	144	98	302	129	0	18	18	0	0
787	0	47	140	136	90	237	103	0	18	18	0	0
788	0	45	140	.	104	211	122	0	14	18	0	0
789	0	45	140	170	95	196	93	0	18	18	0	0
790	0	48	140	.	90	184	97	0	14	18	0	0
791	0	46	140	.	82	221	102	0	16	18	0	0
792	0	49	140	.	82	246	102	0	16	18	0	0
793	0	45	140	126	86	275	100	30	18	18	0	0
794	0	48	140	.	70	271	94	5	16	17	10	4
795	0	49	142	134	90	154	97	0	18	18	0	0
796	0	47	142	144	90	217	96	5	18	18	0	0
797	0	45	142	150	72	223	80	20	18	18	0	0
798	0	47	144	190	94	220	114	20	18	18	0	0
799	0	47	144	.	88	276	99	0	16	18	0	0
800	0	49	144	146	96	238	94	0	18	18	0	0
801	0	49	144	150	84	213	92	0	18	18	0	0
802	0	45	144	144	92	213	95	0	18	18	0	0
803	0	49	145	134	105	243	95	5	18	18	0	0
804	0	47	145	160	85	238	100	0	18	18	0	0
805	0	49	145	.	90	263	97	5	12	18	0	0
806	0	48	146	160	90	187	109	0	18	18	0	0
807	0	47	146	160	106	275	111	5	18	18	0	0
808	0	48	146	130	84	280	81	20	18	18	0	0
809	0	47	148	.	82	194	87	0	6	18	0	0

Framingham Data Subset for Exams 1 through 10 (n=1406)
Includes All Persons Age 45 and Above with a Valid
Serum Cholesterol Value at Exam 1.

---------------- GROUP=Women 45-49 ----------------------

OBS	CHD	AGE	SBP	SBP10	DBP	CHOL	FRW	CIG	YRS CHD	YRS DTH	DEATH	CAUSE
810	0	45	148	160	90	319	104	0	18	18	0	0
811	0	45	148	130	90	220	121	0	18	18	0	0
812	0	47	148	164	86	292	99	0	18	18	0	0
813	0	49	150	144	100	200	116	20	18	18	0	0
814	0	49	150	.	105	243	121	0	16	18	0	0
815	0	48	150	120	96	178	116	0	18	18	0	0
816	0	45	150	150	90	212	99	15	18	18	0	0
817	0	49	150	.	86	249	191	0	2	18	0	0
818	0	47	150	.	90	200	117	0	0	18	0	0
819	0	48	150	.	115	237	128	0	12	18	0	0
820	0	49	150	142	90	217	97	0	18	18	0	0
821	0	49	150	150	90	330	84	0	18	18	0	0
822	0	48	150	.	90	242	76	10	14	18	0	0
823	0	48	150	.	90	163	97	5	10	15	9	5
824	0	45	150	.	90	284	111	20	12	18	0	0
825	0	46	152	166	100	185	118	0	18	18	0	0
826	0	47	154	150	100	265	96	0	18	18	0	0
827	0	46	154	171	86	163	134	0	18	18	0	0
828	0	48	154	130	90	194	104	20	18	18	0	0
829	0	45	155	130	96	187	105	0	18	18	0	0
830	0	47	155	144	95	265	120	0	18	18	0	0
831	0	48	155	138	90	194	100	0	18	18	0	0
832	0	45	156	168	94	174	103	0	18	18	0	0
833	0	47	156	160	82	140	99	0	18	18	0	0
834	0	47	158	.	98	256	125	0	14	18	0	0
835	0	48	158	180	92	230	86	5	18	18	0	0
836	0	45	158	.	88	217	94	0	14	18	0	0
837	0	45	160	.	100	171	91	0	14	15	9	4
838	0	46	160	.	90	216	122	5	14	18	0	0
839	0	48	160	.	116	225	151	1	2	18	0	0
840	0	49	160	.	100	238	102	0	16	18	0	0
841	0	45	160	146	100	198	155	0	18	18	0	0
842	0	46	160	.	110	225	103	0	4	18	0	0
843	0	45	160	150	90	242	121	0	18	18	0	0
844	0	48	162	.	100	330	102	0	10	18	0	0
845	0	49	164	170	96	230	131	0	18	18	0	0
846	0	49	165	.	105	178	109	5	2	18	0	0
847	0	48	165	.	84	196	130	20	4	17	10	6
848	0	45	165	124	95	192	93	0	18	18	0	0
849	0	45	165	177	95	209	93	0	18	18	0	0
850	0	45	165	.	95	265	100	1	16	18	0	0
851	0	48	168	160	90	249	100	0	18	18	0	0
852	0	47	168	182	100	166	136	5	18	18	0	0
853	0	48	170	174	100	207	92	0	18	18	0	0
854	0	49	170	162	100	220	124	0	18	18	0	0
855	0	48	170	.	84	187	125	0	14	15	9	4
856	0	46	170	140	114	200	150	0	18	18	0	0
857	0	49	170	150	100	225	126	0	18	18	0	0
858	0	49	170	.	98	250	100	0	16	18	0	0
859	0	49	170	170	110	317	99	0	18	18	0	0
860	0	46	172	.	110	232	107	10	6	18	0	0
861	0	46	172	140	120	264	170	0	18	18	0	0

Framingham Data Subset for Exams 1 through 10 (n=1406)
Includes All Persons Age 45 and Above with a Valid
Serum Cholesterol Value at Exam 1.

----------------- GROUP=Women 45-49 -----------------------

OBS	CHD	AGE	SBP	SBP10	DBP	CHOL	FRW	CIG	YRS CHD	YRS DTH	DEATH	CAUSE
862	0	48	174	.	108	234	124	10	10	11	7	5
863	0	47	175	190	115	174	112	10	18	18	0	0
864	0	46	176	.	96	213	102	0	12	18	0	0
865	0	49	178	140	100	329	105	0	18	18	0	0
866	0	49	178	164	94	363	94	0	18	18	0	0
867	0	45	180	.	104	198	72	20	16	18	0	0
868	0	46	180	.	106	271	97	25	14	18	0	0
869	0	49	180	.	80	231	99	0	8	11	7	4
870	0	49	182	.	106	249	130	0	12	18	0	0
871	0	48	182	.	104	296	150	1	0	18	0	0
872	0	49	184	180	100	280	107	5	18	18	0	0
873	0	49	184	180	114	317	119	5	18	18	0	0
874	0	45	185	.	105	326	99	20	8	17	10	.
875	0	48	185	.	115	238	98	0	12	18	0	0
876	0	47	190	.	110	211	119	0	6	7	5	6
877	0	49	192	.	92	271	79	10	0	18	0	0
878	0	49	210	180	110	319	104	0	18	18	0	0
879	0	45	250	170	115	200	86	0	18	18	0	0
880	0	49	300	170	150	326	166	0	18	18	0	0
881	1	46	120	112	90	285	128	0	.	18	0	0
882	1	48	150	185	92	220	82	0	.	18	0	0
883	1	47	160	164	90	255	139	0	.	18	0	0
884	3	47	160	142	95	265	104	0	3	18	0	0
885	4	49	165	140	95	225	108	0	5	18	0	0
886	4	47	184	.	96	259	100	0	5	18	0	0
887	6	45	114	.	72	227	95	10	9	18	0	0
888	6	46	114	132	82	225	102	0	9	18	0	0
889	6	48	130	160	70	179	115	0	9	18	0	0
890	6	49	164	222	90	182	105	0	9	18	0	0
891	7	47	150	170	100	333	133	5	11	18	0	0
892	7	47	172	180	84	243	99	0	11	18	0	0
893	7	49	175	.	100	405	104	0	11	11	7	2
894	8	49	136	130	84	225	109	0	13	18	0	0
895	8	49	172	.	104	211	103	0	13	18	0	0
896	9	47	146	162	88	291	91	15	15	18	0	0
897	9	45	160	190	90	292	97	0	15	18	0	0
898	9	47	208	199	120	170	222	0	15	18	0	0
899	10	49	134	130	74	173	110	0	17	18	0	0
900	10	49	135	140	90	302	91	0	17	18	0	0
901	10	49	145	144	85	211	109	20	17	18	0	0
902	10	45	150	134	90	200	101	0	17	18	0	0
903	10	47	175	140	105	305	135	0	17	18	0	0

Framingham Data Subset for Exams 1 through 10 (n=1406)
Includes All Persons Age 45 and Above with a Valid
Serum Cholesterol Value at Exam 1.

---------------- GROUP=Women 50-54 ----------------------

OBS	CHD	AGE	SBP	SBP10	DBP	CHOL	FRW	CIG	YRS CHD	YRS DTH	DEATH	CAUSE
904	0	52	96	114	68	225	85	0	18	18	0	0
905	0	50	102	.	80	232	88	0	12	13	8	6
906	0	51	104	120	66	280	138	0	18	18	0	0
907	0	51	108	.	70	175	83	0	12	18	0	0
908	0	52	110	160	80	232	82	10	18	18	0	0
909	0	54	110	.	68	155	75	35	2	9	6	6
910	0	51	110	114	80	250	99	0	18	18	0	0
911	0	53	110	134	80	196	83	0	18	18	0	0
912	0	50	110	100	75	276	94	20	18	18	0	0
913	0	51	110	.	78	213	102	0	0	18	0	0
914	0	52	110	112	70	219	115	5	18	18	0	0
915	0	50	110	116	70	184	81	30	18	18	0	0
916	0	54	114	138	72	309	114	0	18	18	0	0
917	0	53	116	140	70	232	90	0	18	18	0	0
918	0	54	116	132	82	209	99	0	18	18	0	0
919	0	50	118	124	80	227	136	0	18	18	0	0
920	0	52	120	146	78	318	102	0	18	18	0	0
921	0	51	120	128	70	170	109	0	18	18	0	0
922	0	54	120	110	80	270	96	0	18	18	0	0
923	0	51	120	136	76	226	84	5	18	18	0	0
924	0	50	120	140	82	263	89	5	18	18	0	0
925	0	51	120	154	84	271	104	0	18	18	0	0
926	0	52	120	140	82	217	119	0	18	18	0	0
927	0	54	120	155	76	288	128	0	18	18	0	0
928	0	50	120	.	75	178	72	0	16	18	0	0
929	0	53	122	.	68	270	79	0	16	18	0	0
930	0	52	122	160	70	270	76	0	18	18	0	0
931	0	52	122	138	78	233	90	15	18	18	0	0
932	0	54	122	140	75	194	109	0	18	18	0	0
933	0	54	124	130	80	237	116	0	18	18	0	0
934	0	53	124	120	78	192	149	15	18	18	0	0
935	0	53	125	.	75	133	87	0	10	18	0	0
936	0	52	125	.	85	309	85	30	8	9	6	4
937	0	53	125	.	85	255	74	0	16	18	0	0
938	0	52	125	154	90	292	125	5	18	18	0	0
939	0	51	126	120	92	212	.	1	18	18	0	0
940	0	53	126	.	80	299	99	0	10	18	0	0
941	0	51	126	.	98	194	94	10	2	18	0	0
942	0	50	126	.	80	280	113	0	10	18	0	0
943	0	54	126	140	86	263	103	5	18	18	0	0
944	0	52	126	.	80	301	112	0	0	1	2	4
945	0	54	126	130	76	309	94	5	18	18	0	0
946	0	51	126	170	86	279	140	0	18	18	0	0
947	0	50	128	146	90	260	124	0	10	18	0	0
948	0	54	128	140	82	221	122	20	18	18	0	0
949	0	50	128	135	100	223	110	0	18	18	0	0
950	0	54	130	130	70	308	99	0	18	18	0	0
951	0	52	130	.	76	224	95	0	8	11	7	5
952	0	52	130	130	90	198	131	0	18	18	0	0
953	0	54	130	.	70	216	100	0	6	18	0	0
954	0	51	130	148	80	212	99	5	18	18	0	0
955	0	54	130	180	76	198	98	5	18	18	0	0

Framingham Data Subset for Exams 1 through 10 (n=1406)
Includes All Persons Age 45 and Above with a Valid
Serum Cholesterol Value at Exam 1.

---------------- GROUP=Women 50-54 ----------------------

OBS	CHD	AGE	SBP	SBP10	DBP	CHOL	FRW	CIG	YRS CHD	YRS DTH	DEATH	CAUSE
956	0	50	130	134	94	212	96	0	18	18	0	0
957	0	52	130	.	90	227	126	0	14	18	0	0
958	0	52	130	130	74	319	102	25	18	18	0	0
959	0	52	130	176	80	243	85	10	18	18	0	0
960	0	50	130	140	78	271	82	0	18	18	0	0
961	0	52	130	.	70	232	98	0	16	18	0	0
962	0	54	130	.	70	267	95	15	16	18	0	0
963	0	53	130	.	90	271	91	20	16	18	0	0
964	0	53	130	.	80	246	97	20	16	18	0	0
965	0	54	130	112	70	221	93	0	18	18	0	0
966	0	52	130	.	92	208	121	0	12	18	0	0
967	0	51	132	.	70	242	80	5	6	7	5	4
968	0	52	132	.	90	284	85	15	10	13	8	5
969	0	50	134	158	86	220	120	15	18	18	0	0
970	0	51	134	.	86	267	114	1	8	9	6	5
971	0	53	134	154	82	330	112	0	18	18	0	0
972	0	50	134	.	80	267	96	5	2	3	3	6
973	0	51	134	178	94	167	93	0	18	18	0	0
974	0	51	134	.	84	159	98	0	16	18	0	0
975	0	50	135	140	85	198	125	5	18	18	0	0
976	0	52	135	124	95	260	117	0	18	18	0	0
977	0	50	135	.	85	227	88	20	16	18	0	0
978	0	50	135	144	95	357	96	0	18	18	0	0
979	0	52	136	138	84	220	120	20	18	18	0	0
980	0	54	138	126	82	430	98	0	18	18	0	0
981	0	54	138	154	88	224	122	0	18	18	0	0
982	0	51	138	146	78	233	112	0	18	18	0	0
983	0	50	140	.	95	248	88	0	0	3	3	5
984	0	50	140	166	94	215	102	0	18	18	0	0
985	0	52	140	124	88	270	107	0	18	18	0	0
986	0	52	140	120	90	270	105	5	18	18	0	0
987	0	54	140	160	86	232	104	0	18	18	0	0
988	0	52	140	.	100	237	99	1	6	18	0	0
989	0	51	140	150	94	223	113	0	18	18	0	0
990	0	51	140	160	88	180	93	0	18	18	0	0
991	0	50	140	160	84	255	120	0	18	18	0	0
992	0	51	140	120	90	217	113	0	18	18	0	0
993	0	52	140	.	85	321	97	5	16	18	0	0
994	0	54	140	.	90	213	115	5	8	13	8	.
995	0	50	142	120	94	170	96	0	18	18	0	0
996	0	53	142	140	95	285	106	1	18	18	0	0
997	0	51	142	144	98	288	95	0	18	18	0	0
998	0	50	142	146	90	224	115	0	18	18	0	0
999	0	51	142	.	90	234	93	35	4	13	8	.
1000	0	52	144	.	94	362	105	15	16	18	0	0
1001	0	51	144	179	82	280	102	0	18	18	0	0
1002	0	50	144	.	85	205	104	0	8	18	0	0
1003	0	50	144	173	90	210	104	0	18	18	0	0
1004	0	54	145	.	95	191	87	0	4	7	5	5
1005	0	51	145	140	75	237	124	0	18	18	0	0
1006	0	54	145	.	80	276	107	1	16	18	0	0
1007	0	54	146	160	90	220	100	0	18	18	0	0

Framingham Data Subset for Exams 1 through 10 (n=1406)
Includes All Persons Age 45 and Above with a Valid
Serum Cholesterol Value at Exam 1.

---------------- GROUP=Women 50-54 -----------------------

| | | | | | | | | | YRS | YRS | | |
OBS	CHD	AGE	SBP	SBP10	DBP	CHOL	FRW	CIG	CHD	DTH	DEATH	CAUSE
1008	0	51	146	152	86	265	105	15	18	18	0	0
1009	0	51	146	138	76	265	101	0	18	18	0	0
1010	0	53	146	132	80	301	113	0	18	18	0	0
1011	0	50	146	154	80	318	107	0	18	18	0	0
1012	0	54	146	150	98	326	86	0	18	18	0	0
1013	0	50	148	142	90	172	95	0	18	18	0	0
1014	0	52	148	154	86	227	79	0	18	18	0	0
1015	0	53	148	170	92	242	135	0	18	18	0	0
1016	0	52	148	.	78	270	96	0	0	18	0	0
1017	0	52	148	144	78	209	121	5	18	18	0	0
1018	0	50	150	170	96	160	141	0	18	18	0	0
1019	0	54	150	124	90	167	112	0	18	18	0	0
1020	0	51	150	142	96	260	116	0	18	18	0	0
1021	0	51	150	208	90	299	145	0	18	18	0	0
1022	0	53	150	180	100	223	114	1	18	18	0	0
1023	0	50	150	132	106	291	121	5	18	18	0	0
1024	0	53	152	130	86	285	112	0	18	18	0	0
1025	0	52	152	142	90	207	108	0	18	18	0	0
1026	0	53	152	.	100	242	120	0	10	18	0	0
1027	0	51	152	.	90	199	95	1	8	18	0	0
1028	0	50	154	.	96	227	98	0	14	17	10	5
1029	0	52	154	.	84	183	114	5	4	13	8	6
1030	0	50	154	132	94	302	110	0	18	18	0	0
1031	0	52	154	.	102	234	126	20	16	18	0	0
1032	0	54	154	.	96	248	132	0	4	18	0	0
1033	0	51	155	144	102	232	123	0	18	18	0	0
1034	0	51	156	156	88	200	101	0	18	18	0	0
1035	0	50	156	180	82	194	118	0	18	18	0	0
1036	0	51	156	.	96	305	90	30	0	1	2	3
1037	0	52	156	.	84	260	79	0	4	18	0	0
1038	0	53	156	.	94	221	146	0	12	18	0	0
1039	0	52	156	.	80	199	97	20	16	18	0	0
1040	0	52	158	.	92	260	82	0	16	17	10	3
1041	0	52	160	180	100	294	100	0	18	18	0	0
1042	0	52	160	166	100	330	101	0	18	18	0	0
1043	0	52	160	.	100	224	112	0	14	15	9	5
1044	0	50	160	.	90	216	88	5	4	18	0	0
1045	0	52	160	160	94	250	100	0	18	18	0	0
1046	0	50	160	.	90	409	96	5	0	18	0	0
1047	0	51	160	140	98	370	71	15	18	18	0	0
1048	0	50	160	.	100	334	118	20	14	18	0	0
1049	0	51	160	120	95	205	104	0	18	18	0	0
1050	0	50	160	125	90	284	135	0	18	18	0	0
1051	0	51	160	160	104	221	150	0	18	18	0	0
1052	0	53	162	138	90	255	108	15	18	18	0	0
1053	0	51	162	142	98	190	156	0	18	18	0	0
1054	0	53	164	.	96	149	128	0	16	17	10	3
1055	0	52	164	128	96	198	135	0	18	18	0	0
1056	0	53	164	204	102	258	139	5	18	18	0	0
1057	0	54	165	126	100	178	78	20	18	18	0	0
1058	0	54	165	130	104	260	89	0	18	18	0	0
1059	0	53	165	164	80	299	100	0	18	18	0	0

Framingham Data Subset for Exams 1 through 10 (n=1406)
Includes All Persons Age 45 and Above with a Valid
Serum Cholesterol Value at Exam 1.

---------------- GROUP=Women 50-54 ----------------------

OBS	CHD	AGE	SBP	SBP10	DBP	CHOL	FRW	CIG	YRS CHD	YRS DTH	DEATH	CAUSE
1060	0	53	165	188	80	174	101	0	18	18	0	0
1061	0	53	166	180	78	276	108	0	18	18	0	0
1062	0	54	168	170	96	305	138	20	18	18	0	0
1063	0	52	168	150	110	326	86	0	18	18	0	0
1064	0	50	168	180	96	179	121	0	18	18	0	0
1065	0	53	170	134	98	214	83	0	18	18	0	0
1066	0	50	170	154	90	280	107	0	18	18	0	0
1067	0	50	170	174	100	270	108	0	18	18	0	0
1068	0	54	170	180	90	232	99	0	18	18	0	0
1069	0	52	170	.	104	280	102	15	10	11	7	.
1070	0	50	172	.	110	300	91	5	8	9	6	4
1071	0	50	174	.	106	280	142	0	6	7	5	5
1072	0	54	174	.	108	334	108	0	10	18	0	0
1073	0	50	175	158	88	265	119	0	18	18	0	0
1074	0	53	175	.	75	216	117	0	4	5	4	4
1075	0	52	178	154	98	242	82	0	18	18	0	0
1076	0	51	178	.	98	221	81	0	8	9	6	6
1077	0	54	180	150	96	224	119	5	18	18	0	0
1078	0	53	180	130	95	217	98	0	18	18	0	0
1079	0	50	180	.	105	276	135	0	12	18	0	0
1080	0	50	180	.	100	211	127	0	4	18	0	0
1081	0	54	182	160	100	207	132	0	18	18	0	0
1082	0	54	186	.	102	263	120	10	16	18	0	0
1083	0	52	188	160	138	149	101	15	18	18	0	0
1084	0	52	188	.	96	263	108	0	8	18	0	0
1085	0	51	190	210	110	290	135	15	18	18	0	0
1086	0	50	190	196	110	191	115	0	18	18	0	0
1087	0	51	190	.	104	310	145	5	14	15	9	4
1088	0	53	190	148	104	246	108	0	18	18	0	0
1089	0	50	198	130	120	242	121	0	18	18	0	0
1090	0	54	200	.	116	265	139	.	0	18	0	0
1091	0	51	208	.	110	209	74	15	10	11	7	3
1092	0	52	210	180	120	250	97	5	18	18	0	0
1093	0	54	210	.	110	221	102	0	0	3	3	4
1094	0	54	215	.	110	292	100	0	2	5	4	5
1095	0	50	220	158	110	260	129	0	18	18	0	0
1096	0	51	220	.	130	250	150	1	4	18	0	0
1097	0	53	225	220	125	315	106	0	18	18	0	0
1098	0	50	236	242	140	284	91	5	18	18	0	0
1099	0	53	246	.	130	166	204	0	14	18	0	0
1100	0	52	286	.	104	263	153	0	14	18	0	0
1101	0	50	290	.	124	221	107	15	14	15	9	4
1102	1	50	140	140	84	200	109	0	.	18	0	0
1103	1	53	164	.	98	221	150	0	.	15	9	2
1104	1	51	186	250	108	249	113	20	.	18	0	0
1105	1	51	200	.	110	183	.	0	.	17	10	5
1106	1	51	250	240	130	265	111	0	.	18	0	0
1107	2	50	188	.	128	184	116	0	1	18	0	0
1108	2	53	270	.	135	292	152	20	1	5	4	4
1109	4	52	160	185	100	213	132	0	5	18	0	0
1110	4	54	170	.	75	328	115	5	5	11	7	6
1111	4	54	170	168	60	165	116	0	5	18	0	0

Framingham Data Subset for Exams 1 through 10 (n=1406)
Includes All Persons Age 45 and Above with a Valid
Serum Cholesterol Value at Exam 1.

---------------- GROUP=Women 50-54 ----------------------

OBS	CHD	AGE	SBP	SBP10	DBP	CHOL	FRW	CIG	YRS CHD	YRS DTH	DEATH	CAUSE
1112	4	54	192	180	78	234	138	0	4	18	0	0
1113	5	53	164	184	104	317	142	0	7	18	0	0
1114	5	54	194	140	116	237	115	0	7	18	0	0
1115	6	52	130	.	70	300	99	0	9	18	0	0
1116	6	51	140	160	88	220	90	5	9	18	0	0
1117	7	51	140	120	90	313	102	20	11	18	0	0
1118	7	50	148	135	95	220	140	1	11	18	0	0
1119	7	53	155	180	100	198	91	10	11	18	0	0
1120	7	52	160	.	104	150	99	10	11	18	0	0
1121	7	51	214	170	114	288	113	0	11	18	0	0
1122	7	52	240	190	112	237	131	0	11	18	0	0
1123	8	54	150	.	94	220	115	0	13	13	8	1
1124	8	52	170	178	110	166	84	0	13	18	0	0
1125	8	51	190	186	124	270	139	40	13	18	0	0
1126	8	54	240	.	130	275	154	0	13	17	10	2
1127	9	54	132	.	88	346	100	0	15	15	9	2
1128	9	51	138	120	82	255	100	0	15	18	0	0
1129	9	52	160	.	106	271	103	0	15	15	9	1
1130	9	50	166	.	110	321	113	5	15	15	9	2
1131	9	50	195	150	125	248	132	0	15	18	0	0
1132	10	50	132	130	84	267	101	0	17	18	0	0
1133	10	54	142	.	76	305	88	20	17	17	10	2
1134	10	52	160	.	102	187	113	20	17	17	10	1
1135	10	51	168	208	100	177	91	0	17	18	0	0
1136	10	54	220	176	116	292	131	0	16	18	0	0
1137	10	54	220	.	112	219	100	0	17	17	10	2

---------------- GROUP=Women 55-59 ----------------------

OBS	CHD	AGE	SBP	SBP10	DBP	CHOL	FRW	CIG	YRS CHD	YRS DTH	DEATH	CAUSE
1138	0	56	90	110	50	292	91	5	18	18	0	0
1139	0	59	100	.	55	292	93	5	16	17	10	5
1140	0	56	104	112	70	298	104	0	18	18	0	0
1141	0	56	106	.	54	226	118	5	8	17	10	4
1142	0	58	108	136	70	313	110	20	18	18	0	0
1143	0	55	108	.	74	231	111	0	0	18	0	0
1144	0	59	110	.	70	240	124	5	16	18	0	0
1145	0	55	110	130	82	430	101	0	18	18	0	0
1146	0	57	110	140	78	243	93	0	18	18	0	0
1147	0	57	110	.	62	200	91	0	16	18	0	0
1148	0	58	112	.	94	250	75	0	10	11	7	5
1149	0	57	112	.	88	207	97	0	14	18	0	0
1150	0	59	114	130	78	304	112	0	18	18	0	0
1151	0	56	118	.	76	267	90	0	0	18	0	0
1152	0	55	118	.	80	274	115	30	16	18	0	0
1153	0	58	120	126	86	216	112	0	18	18	0	0
1154	0	55	120	112	68	292	101	0	18	18	0	0
1155	0	55	120	158	72	200	84	0	18	18	0	0
1156	0	58	120	.	80	211	117	5	2	18	0	0
1157	0	57	120	160	74	190	76	0	18	18	0	0

Framingham Data Subset for Exams 1 through 10 (n=1406)
Includes All Persons Age 45 and Above with a Valid
Serum Cholesterol Value at Exam 1.

---------------- GROUP=Women 55-59 ----------------------

OBS	CHD	AGE	SBP	SBP10	DBP	CHOL	FRW	CIG	YRS CHD	YRS DTH	DEATH	CAUSE
1158	0	56	122	160	80	280	113	0	18	18	0	0
1159	0	55	122	144	62	317	101	20	18	18	0	0
1160	0	59	124	120	78	192	117	0	18	18	0	0
1161	0	57	124	179	80	317	116	0	18	18	0	0
1162	0	59	126	.	74	227	82	20	16	18	0	0
1163	0	58	126	170	86	227	119	0	18	18	0	0
1164	0	59	126	170	86	265	99	0	18	18	0	0
1165	0	56	126	120	82	296	102	0	18	18	0	0
1166	0	57	130	150	80	265	94	0	18	18	0	0
1167	0	55	130	150	86	285	102	0	18	18	0	0
1168	0	56	130	.	95	309	98	1	16	18	0	0
1169	0	56	130	.	80	209	120	0	8	9	6	5
1170	0	55	130	150	75	217	95	0	18	18	0	0
1171	0	58	130	.	106	296	117	0	8	18	0	0
1172	0	55	130	.	70	217	102	15	12	18	0	0
1173	0	55	132	143	82	250	107	0	18	18	0	0
1174	0	59	132	.	72	270	96	0	8	9	6	5
1175	0	55	132	160	85	275	95	0	18	18	0	0
1176	0	55	132	130	80	220	99	5	18	18	0	0
1177	0	59	132	124	94	220	101	0	18	18	0	0
1178	0	56	132	180	84	263	116	0	18	18	0	0
1179	0	59	132	139	72	192	113	0	18	18	0	0
1180	0	58	134	.	98	250	102	0	16	18	0	0
1181	0	55	135	.	85	292	93	5	4	7	5	.
1182	0	59	136	170	84	250	100	0	18	18	0	0
1183	0	56	136	138	80	235	102	0	18	18	0	0
1184	0	56	136	154	84	166	114	0	18	18	0	0
1185	0	55	136	164	76	232	92	10	18	18	0	0
1186	0	55	138	164	76	244	101	0	18	18	0	0
1187	0	58	138	100	92	237	123	0	18	18	0	0
1188	0	57	138	.	80	310	105	5	6	18	0	0
1189	0	57	138	158	90	259	101	1	18	18	0	0
1190	0	56	138	.	70	227	111	5	16	18	0	0
1191	0	55	140	168	90	365	95	0	18	18	0	0
1192	0	56	140	.	100	208	101	0	16	18	0	0
1193	0	55	140	.	78	227	99	0	12	13	8	5
1194	0	55	140	200	90	250	136	5	18	18	0	0
1195	0	58	140	.	84	260	129	0	16	18	0	0
1196	0	57	140	.	80	191	80	20	6	18	0	0
1197	0	56	140	.	90	249	82	0	14	18	0	0
1198	0	55	140	160	85	302	130	0	18	18	0	0
1199	0	56	140	120	86	209	122	0	18	18	0	0
1200	0	58	140	.	90	246	86	0	0	18	0	0
1201	0	58	140	.	90	211	134	0	14	18	0	0
1202	0	59	140	156	80	148	139	0	18	18	0	0
1203	0	57	142	150	84	296	115	0	18	18	0	0
1204	0	58	142	122	92	181	115	0	18	18	0	0
1205	0	57	142	.	84	203	129	0	2	18	0	0
1206	0	59	144	170	84	250	122	5	18	18	0	0
1207	0	55	144	164	96	224	113	0	18	18	0	0
1208	0	56	144	.	84	376	96	0	0	18	0	0
1209	0	59	144	.	86	326	102	0	10	11	7	5

Framingham Data Subset for Exams 1 through 10 (n=1406)
Includes All Persons Age 45 and Above with a Valid
Serum Cholesterol Value at Exam 1.

------------------ GROUP=Women 55-59 ----------------------

OBS	CHD	AGE	SBP	SBP10	DBP	CHOL	FRW	CIG	YRS CHD	YRS DTH	DEATH	CAUSE
1210	0	56	144	160	86	284	105	0	18	18	0	0
1211	0	59	145	128	95	263	102	0	18	18	0	0
1212	0	56	145	162	95	259	83	0	18	18	0	0
1213	0	57	145	.	85	296	107	0	16	18	0	0
1214	0	57	146	.	80	265	126	0	8	9	6	6
1215	0	58	146	170	94	227	98	5	18	18	0	0
1216	0	58	146	.	90	221	112	0	16	18	0	0
1217	0	57	148	130	68	267	89	5	18	18	0	0
1218	0	55	148	148	98	228	106	0	18	18	0	0
1219	0	58	148	132	86	284	104	0	18	18	0	0
1220	0	56	150	.	90	220	120	0	8	18	0	0
1221	0	58	150	.	90	340	112	0	4	18	0	0
1222	0	55	150	130	80	220	106	0	18	18	0	0
1223	0	56	150	160	88	292	117	0	18	18	0	0
1224	0	57	150	150	115	319	99	0	18	18	0	0
1225	0	55	150	.	95	266	105	30	2	18	0	0
1226	0	56	150	190	110	276	96	0	18	18	0	0
1227	0	59	150	156	95	192	102	0	18	18	0	0
1228	0	57	150	.	83	317	.	0	8	11	7	5
1229	0	56	150	180	82	263	104	5	18	18	0	0
1230	0	55	152	160	96	242	116	0	18	18	0	0
1231	0	58	152	.	74	221	111	0	10	15	9	4
1232	0	59	152	.	100	167	205	0	6	7	5	4
1233	0	57	154	210	96	242	101	0	18	18	0	0
1234	0	56	154	.	104	226	99	10	0	18	0	0
1235	0	55	154	.	90	196	146	0	16	18	0	0
1236	0	55	155	.	110	310	124	0	6	18	0	0
1237	0	57	155	142	95	227	88	0	18	18	0	0
1238	0	57	155	178	100	249	117	0	18	18	0	0
1239	0	55	155	176	95	301	109	0	18	18	0	0
1240	0	59	155	.	95	250	101	0	16	18	0	0
1241	0	58	155	.	85	280	95	0	16	17	10	6
1242	0	55	156	.	100	242	111	0	14	18	0	0
1243	0	55	156	.	86	271	115	0	0	18	0	0
1244	0	59	158	.	88	244	111	0	0	15	9	3
1245	0	56	160	.	100	227	112	5	14	15	9	6
1246	0	56	160	170	100	187	120	0	18	18	0	0
1247	0	55	160	160	100	220	117	5	18	18	0	0
1248	0	56	160	.	90	237	91	0	16	18	0	0
1249	0	55	160	154	102	236	137	0	18	18	0	0
1250	0	56	160	.	92	227	91	0	4	5	4	4
1251	0	56	160	.	85	280	75	20	16	18	0	0
1252	0	57	160	165	92	353	88	0	18	18	0	0
1253	0	58	160	230	90	242	99	0	10	18	0	0
1254	0	56	162	.	80	216	113	0	16	17	10	4
1255	0	58	162	.	84	211	133	0	0	1	2	5
1256	0	56	162	.	94	325	125	0	12	15	9	5
1257	0	55	164	160	92	309	160	0	18	18	0	0
1258	0	59	165	170	98	266	89	0	18	18	0	0
1259	0	59	165	.	100	225	86	0	10	13	8	6
1260	0	57	168	168	96	335	88	0	18	18	0	0
1261	0	56	168	196	85	249	124	0	18	18	0	0

Framingham Data Subset for Exams 1 through 10 (n=1406)
Includes All Persons Age 45 and Above with a Valid
Serum Cholesterol Value at Exam 1.

---------------- GROUP=Women 55-59 ----------------------

OBS	CHD	AGE	SBP	SBP10	DBP	CHOL	FRW	CIG	YRS CHD	YRS DTH	DEATH	CAUSE
1262	0	57	168	.	104	259	106	0	14	17	10	5
1263	0	59	168	.	100	217	134	0	8	9	6	4
1264	0	58	170	160	112	270	95	0	18	18	0	0
1265	0	57	170	150	108	237	194	0	18	18	0	0
1266	0	58	170	.	86	238	99	0	14	15	9	3
1267	0	56	170	186	100	330	116	0	18	18	0	0
1268	0	55	170	190	90	225	111	0	18	18	0	0
1269	0	55	170	.	97	196	109	0	12	13	8	5
1270	0	55	174	144	88	259	113	0	18	18	0	0
1271	0	57	174	194	94	200	126	0	18	18	0	0
1272	0	55	175	200	95	220	124	0	18	18	0	0
1273	0	56	175	136	105	250	127	0	18	18	0	0
1274	0	56	176	174	106	250	145	5	18	18	0	0
1275	0	58	176	.	100	263	94	5	4	7	5	5
1276	0	55	176	140	100	288	131	0	18	18	0	0
1277	0	58	180	140	110	220	121	0	18	18	0	0
1278	0	58	180	150	120	198	143	0	18	18	0	0
1279	0	57	182	204	92	250	119	0	18	18	0	0
1280	0	55	182	146	100	302	160	0	18	18	0	0
1281	0	57	186	120	80	270	102	0	18	18	0	0
1282	0	55	190	146	110	220	118	20	18	18	0	0
1283	0	56	190	.	130	305	116	0	8	18	0	0
1284	0	56	190	150	100	234	94	5	18	18	0	0
1285	0	59	195	155	115	267	105	5	18	18	0	0
1286	0	58	195	.	105	405	76	0	14	15	9	4
1287	0	59	200	170	104	221	153	0	18	18	0	0
1288	0	59	200	.	100	167	160	0	16	17	10	4
1289	0	56	205	.	115	265	124	5	16	18	0	0
1290	0	56	205	170	140	267	98	0	18	18	0	0
1291	0	56	206	200	94	270	109	0	18	18	0	0
1292	0	56	210	144	110	183	92	10	18	18	0	0
1293	0	56	210	.	120	150	202	20	10	18	0	0
1294	0	57	210	.	94	205	88	0	0	18	0	0
1295	0	56	214	.	120	255	106	0	16	18	0	0
1296	0	58	220	170	125	270	120	0	18	18	0	0
1297	0	59	220	190	114	285	91	1	18	18	0	0
1298	0	55	230	.	155	215	128	0	4	15	9	4
1299	0	58	236	150	114	284	106	0	18	18	0	0
1300	0	55	280	.	145	305	144	0	16	17	10	4
1301	0	57	294	264	144	220	112	45	18	18	0	0
1302	1	59	128	.	74	150	129	0	.	15	9	3
1303	1	55	154	.	84	278	99	0	.	1	2	5
1304	1	55	170	.	95	255	128	0	.	18	0	0
1305	1	55	176	230	104	200	81	0	.	18	0	0
1306	1	57	186	.	120	150	135	0	.	11	7	.
1307	1	56	194	.	120	182	154	0	.	11	7	4
1308	1	57	230	.	110	232	134	0	.	18	0	0
1309	2	55	158	150	90	347	104	0	1	18	0	0
1310	2	59	216	.	150	285	138	0	1	9	6	4
1311	2	55	250	160	140	260	118	0	1	18	0	0
1312	3	55	124	.	90	400	113	0	3	3	3	2
1313	3	58	148	250	80	259	90	0	3	18	0	0

Framingham Data Subset for Exams 1 through 10 (n=1406)
Includes All Persons Age 45 and Above with a Valid
Serum Cholesterol Value at Exam 1.

---------------- GROUP=Women 55-59 ----------------------

OBS	CHD	AGE	SBP	SBP10	DBP	CHOL	FRW	CIG	YRS CHD	YRS DTH	DEATH	CAUSE
1314	3	55	155	.	100	249	87	5	3	11	7	3
1315	3	59	170	.	100	192	148	0	3	17	10	6
1316	3	57	230	.	124	217	97	20	3	9	6	6
1317	4	57	165	.	95	305	103	0	5	7	5	2
1318	4	57	170	.	90	292	117	0	5	13	8	1
1319	4	56	178	.	94	274	92	0	5	18	0	0
1320	4	56	190	184	94	249	121	15	5	18	0	0
1321	4	57	210	138	100	221	107	20	5	18	0	0
1322	4	59	216	.	106	212	91	20	5	15	9	2
1323	5	58	126	.	70	279	106	0	7	13	8	1
1324	5	56	130	110	86	232	93	0	7	18	0	0
1325	5	57	146	.	86	224	112	0	6	18	0	0
1326	5	55	158	.	104	184	79	15	7	7	5	2
1327	5	59	160	.	95	321	104	0	7	18	0	0
1328	5	59	170	.	100	140	92	0	7	18	0	0
1329	5	55	170	.	100	351	127	35	7	17	10	3
1330	5	55	172	158	100	309	130	0	7	18	0	0
1331	5	58	185	.	90	334	88	0	7	7	5	2
1332	5	57	204	.	104	237	111	0	7	9	6	1
1333	6	59	164	150	104	292	102	0	9	18	0	0
1334	6	56	165	166	80	309	113	1	9	18	0	0
1335	6	57	174	.	90	266	105	0	9	18	0	0
1336	6	58	260	.	145	250	148	0	9	13	8	2
1337	7	58	126	115	82	334	100	0	11	18	0	0
1338	7	58	138	.	82	192	119	0	11	18	0	0
1339	7	57	152	190	88	234	118	0	11	18	0	0
1340	7	58	190	.	110	250	106	0	11	15	9	4
1341	8	59	154	.	94	285	114	0	13	13	8	1
1342	8	57	160	165	92	227	114	1	13	18	0	0
1343	8	58	165	170	105	194	142	0	13	18	0	0
1344	8	58	180	.	120	346	98	0	13	18	0	0
1345	8	59	212	.	108	263	127	0	13	17	10	2
1346	9	59	138	160	86	238	77	0	15	18	0	0
1347	9	57	156	146	86	232	114	0	15	18	0	0
1348	9	59	240	210	120	200	145	0	15	18	0	0
1349	10	59	158	148	98	267	94	0	17	18	0	0
1350	10	56	196	184	118	342	96	10	17	18	0	0
1351	10	56	200	144	100	250	163	0	17	18	0	0

---------------- GROUP=Women 60-62 ----------------------

OBS	CHD	AGE	SBP	SBP10	DBP	CHOL	FRW	CIG	YRS CHD	YRS DTH	DEATH	CAUSE
1352	0	61	120	.	80	211	116	0	8	15	9	5
1353	0	62	128	.	72	288	81	15	16	17	10	4
1354	0	60	130	.	85	324	142	0	14	15	9	5
1355	0	60	130	124	80	264	94	20	18	18	0	0
1356	0	61	130	.	76	243	92	5	6	17	10	6
1357	0	62	130	160	78	238	115	0	18	18	0	0
1358	0	61	132	170	84	246	134	0	18	18	0	0
1359	0	60	134	.	72	221	142	0	16	18	0	0

Framingham Data Subset for Exams 1 through 10 (n=1406)
Includes All Persons Age 45 and Above with a Valid
Serum Cholesterol Value at Exam 1.

------------------ GROUP=Women 60-62 ------------------------

OBS	CHD	AGE	SBP	SBP10	DBP	CHOL	FRW	CIG	YRS CHD	YRS DTH	DEATH	CAUSE
1360	0	61	134	172	72	255	123	0	18	18	0	0
1361	0	61	135	.	85	200	130	0	12	18	0	0
1362	0	60	138	.	88	267	106	0	14	18	0	0
1363	0	61	140	128	82	256	78	0	18	18	0	0
1364	0	60	140	140	90	220	112	5	18	18	0	0
1365	0	60	140	.	90	230	117	0	8	18	0	0
1366	0	61	140	.	85	165	66	0	12	18	0	0
1367	0	62	146	.	94	221	104	0	4	18	0	0
1368	0	60	148	180	90	249	104	0	18	18	0	0
1369	0	60	148	.	90	209	139	0	6	7	5	6
1370	0	60	150	120	84	260	87	20	18	18	0	0
1371	0	60	150	152	80	276	115	0	18	18	0	0
1372	0	61	154	162	94	333	110	0	18	18	0	0
1373	0	61	154	.	80	284	105	0	14	18	0	0
1374	0	60	156	136	94	265	122	0	18	18	0	0
1375	0	60	158	.	90	265	96	0	16	18	0	0
1376	0	60	160	138	90	192	122	0	18	18	0	0
1377	0	61	160	134	85	246	77	0	18	18	0	0
1378	0	61	160	195	100	213	110	0	18	18	0	0
1379	0	62	160	198	92	228	100	0	18	18	0	0
1380	0	60	165	.	100	167	123	25	16	17	10	.
1381	0	61	168	196	96	234	135	0	18	18	0	0
1382	0	61	170	.	95	213	132	0	0	17	10	6
1383	0	62	170	.	100	256	101	0	0	18	0	0
1384	0	62	176	230	104	255	121	0	18	18	0	0
1385	0	60	180	154	100	234	102	10	18	18	0	0
1386	0	61	180	.	120	182	73	0	16	18	0	0
1387	0	60	182	.	94	250	106	0	10	18	0	0
1388	0	60	185	.	110	309	104	0	16	18	0	0
1389	0	60	190	.	100	234	.	0	12	13	8	6
1390	0	62	194	.	140	199	72	0	16	17	10	.
1391	0	60	196	.	110	221	137	0	4	7	5	5
1392	0	60	208	.	108	205	144	0	12	17	10	6
1393	0	60	225	139	120	238	148	0	18	18	0	0
1394	0	62	230	.	120	261	117	0	4	5	4	3
1395	1	60	170	.	92	328	129	0	.	5	4	2
1396	1	61	182	.	104	263	93	0	.	17	10	5
1397	3	60	150	.	85	256	113	0	3	3	3	1
1398	4	61	152	.	88	218	88	5	5	9	6	3
1399	4	61	170	.	100	305	86	15	5	5	4	2
1400	5	60	155	.	90	255	111	0	7	7	5	2
1401	5	61	195	185	95	223	121	0	7	18	0	0
1402	6	60	140	130	84	260	119	0	9	18	0	0
1403	7	62	140	116	90	267	108	0	11	18	0	0
1404	8	61	185	.	115	233	140	0	13	13	8	2
1405	9	61	152	.	95	263	139	0	15	15	9	2
1406	10	61	130	138	80	296	158	0	16	18	0	0

Table A-1. Number, Mean, and Standard Deviation for Specified Variables: Eighteen-Year Framingham Heart Study Data

	AGE	SPB	SPB10	DBP	CHOL	FRW	CIG	YRS_CHD	YRS_DTH
				Total prevalence population					
N	1406	1406	771	1406	1406	1395	1405	1363	1406
μ	52.4	148.1	148.0	90.2	234.7	105.4	8.0	13.3	16.2
σ	4.8	28.0	25.7	14.2	46.3	17.8	11.6	5.9	4.0
				Prevalence population men 45–49					
N	212	212	125	212	212	210	212	209	212
μ	46.8	140.2	137.4	89.1	226.0	101.4	16.3	13.3	16.3
σ	1.4	22.4	19.3	12.6	39.6	13.5	14.3	6.0	3.9
				Prevalence population men 50–54					
N	211	211	107	211	211	210	211	201	211
μ	52.0	143.3	142.4	89.9	227.9	103.5	12.2	13.1	15.6
σ	1.4	23.7	24.1	13.8	44.4	13.3	12.7	5.7	4.5
				Prevalence population men 55–59					
N	184	184	91	184	184	183	184	176	184
μ	57.0	146.4	146.7	88.3	223.4	101.3	11.3	11.6	14.8
σ	1.4	26.7	25.2	14.5	43.4	14.8	12.8	6.5	5.0
				Prevalence population men 60–62					
N	62	62	11	62	62	60	62	57	62
μ	60.3	151.0	151.5	87.0	226.0	104.2	8.5	9.4	13.5
σ	0.5	27.3	30.1	13.6	37.7	15.8	11.2	6.1	5.3
				Prevalence population woman 45–49					
N	234	234	152	234	234	233	234	231	234
μ	46.9	143.2	148.1	88.5	229.3	104.7	4.4	14.9	17.6
σ	1.5	24.3	23.7	12.1	46.9	19.4	7.6	5.0	1.7
				Prevalence population women 50–54					
N	234	234	147	234	234	232	233	229	234
μ	51.9	153.4	151.6	91.8	245.7	108.4	4.1	14.3	16.8
σ	1.4	32.4	26.8	14.9	49.3	19.7	7.8	5.5	3.3
				Prevalence population women 55–59					
N	214	214	115	214	214	213	214	207	214
μ	56.8	158.1	158.8	93.2	253.5	110.9	2.5	13.3	16.6
σ	1.4	32.8	28.2	16.8	48.9	20.7	6.6	5.9	3.4
				Prevalence population women 60–62					
N	55	55	23	55	55	54	55	53	55
μ	60.7	159.0	156.4	93.0	245.3	112.2	2.2	12.9	15.8
σ	0.7	24.9	30.0	13.4	37.0	21.4	5.8	5.6	4.3

Table A-1 (continued)

	AGE	SPB	SPB10	DBP	CHOL	FRW	CIG	YRS_CHD	YRS_DTH
				Total incidence population					
N	1363	1363	759	1363	1363	1353	1363	1363	1363
μ	52.4	147.8	147.7	90.0	234.6	105.2	8.0	13.3	16.3
σ	4.8	27.8	25.1	14.1	46.4	17.7	11.5	5.9	3.8
				Incidence population men 45–49					
M	209	209	124	209	209	207	209	209	209
μ	46.8	140.2	137.4	89.0	225.8	101.3	16.2	13.3	16.4
σ	1.4	22.5	19.4	12.6	39.8	13.4	14.2	6.0	3.9
				Incidence population men 50–54					
N	201	201	105	201	201	200	201	201	201
μ	52.0	142.8	143.1	89.8	226.9	103.4	12.0	13.1	15.8
σ	1.4	23.0	23.9	13.6	44.1	13.0	12.7	5.7	4.3
				Incidence population men 55–59					
N	176	176	89	176	176	175	176	176	176
μ	57.0	146.8	146.9	88.5	222.8	101.5	11.3	11.6	15.0
σ	1.4	27.0	25.3	14.5	43.0	14.6	12.7	6.5	4.9
				Incidence population men 60–62					
N	57	57	11	57	57	55	57	57	57
μ	60.3	149.2	151.5	86.5	224.9	103.7	8.1	9.4	14.2
σ	0.5	26.8	30.1	12.6	39.0	16.3	11.4	6.1	4.7
				Incidence population women 45–49					
N	231	231	149	231	231	230	231	231	231
μ	46.9	143.2	147.9	88.4	228.9	104.5	4.5	14.9	17.6
σ	1.5	24.4	23.5	12.2	47.1	19.2	7.6	5.0	1.7
				Incidence population women 50–54					
N	229	229	144	229	229	228	228	229	229
μ	51.9	152.7	150.4	91.5	246.2	108.1	4.1	14.3	16.8
σ	1.4	31.9	24.7	14.7	49.5	19.7	7.8	5.5	3.4
				Incidence population women 55–59					
N	207	207	114	207	207	206	207	207	207
μ	56.8	157.5	158.2	92.9	255.1	110.4	2.6	13.3	16.7
σ	1.4	32.7	27.5	16.7	48.2	20.5	6.7	5.9	3.2
				Incidence population women 60–62					
N	53	53	23	53	53	52	53	53	53
μ	60.7	158.4	156.4	92.8	243.5	112.2	2.3	12.9	16.0
σ	0.7	25.1	30.0	13.6	35.8	21.6	5.8	5.6	4.1

Table A-2. Number of Individuals in Specified Categories: Eighteen-Year Framingham Heart Study Data

Category	Total	Men				Women			
		45–49	50–54	55–59	60–62	45–49	50–54	55–59	60–62
Total population including prevalence cases (N = 1406)									
CHD exam 1	43	3	10	8	5	3	5	7	2
CHD exam 2–10	268	45	49	52	18	20	31	43	10
SBP ≥ 140	825	107	112	100	43	115	151	154	43
SBP ≥ 165	313	26	39	36	12	42	64	74	20
DBP ≥ 90	717	104	106	76	27	113	132	125	34
DBP ≥ 115	82	8	10	11	2	8	17	21	5
CHOL ≥ 220	875	117	119	96	35	133	164	168	43
CHOL ≥ 260	397	37	51	39	9	55	97	90	19
FRW ≥ 120	244	21	18	22	10	40	59	54	20
Smoker	633	150	128	106	29	83	80	48	9
Died	351	44	67	72	37	20	41	50	20
Total	1406	212	211	184	62	234	234	214	55
Incidence population excluding prevalence cases (N = 1363)									
CHD exams 2–10	268	45	49	52	18	20	31	43	10
SBP ≥ 140	795	105	107	97	38	113	146	148	41
SBP ≥ 165	296	26	35	35	10	42	61	69	18
DBP ≥ 90	689	102	100	73	24	110	128	120	32
DBP ≥ 115	76	8	8	11	1	8	16	19	5
CHOL ≥ 220	844	115	110	91	31	130	161	165	41
CHOL ≥ 260	386	36	48	37	9	54	96	89	17
FRW ≥ 120	228	20	15	20	9	38	58	49	19
Smoker	614	147	121	102	25	83	79	48	9
Died	323	43	59	66	32	20	39	46	18
Total	1363	209	201	176	87	231	229	207	53

Table A-3. U.S. Resident Population by Age and Sex (in Thousands)

Age	April 1, 1940[a]		April 1, 1980[b]	
	Male	Female	Male	Female
Under 1	1027	993	1806	1727
1–4	4328	4193	6556	6259
5–9	5419	5266	8539	8161
10–14	5952	5794	9316	8926
15–19	6180	6153	10 755	10 413
20–24	5692	5895	10 663	10 655
25–29	5451	5646	9705	9816
30–34	5070	5172	8677	8884
35–39	4746	4800	6862	7104
40–44	4419	4369	5708	5961
45–49	4209	4046	5388	5702
50–54	3753	3504	5621	6089
55–59	3022	2845	5482	6133
60–64	2412	2345	4670	5418
65–69	1871	1884	3903	4880
70–74	1271	1299	2854	3945
75–79	724	780	1848	2946
80–84	359	415	1019	1916
85 and over	156	208	682	1559
All ages	66 062	65 608	110 053	116 493

[a] R Grove and Hetzel A, *Vital Statistics Rates in the U.S. 1940–1960,* U.S. Department of HEW, Public Health Service Publication No. 1677, Washington, 1968.
[b] U.S. Bureau of the Census, Current Population Reports, Series P-25, No. 929, U.S. Government Printing Office, Washington 1983.

NUMERIC ANSWERS TO EXERCISES

Chapter 2

2-6a. 382
b. 739

2-7a. 31
b. 38

2-8. Using Equation 2-6, $n = 126$
Using Equation 2-7, $n = 152$
Using Equation 2-6 with $2\bar{P}\bar{Q}$ substituted for $2P_cQ_c$ (see page 32), $n = 150$

Chapter 3

3-1a. 1.30
b. 1.01, 1.68
c. 1.04, 1.63

3-2"a." .87
 "b." .45, 1.71
 "c." .44, 1.72

3-3a. $\geq 260/<220$ $\hat{OR} = 1.12$, $\hat{RR} = 1.09$
 $220–259/<220$ $\hat{OR} = .47$, $\hat{RR} = .55$
 b. $\geq 260/<220$ .54, 2.32
 $220–259/<220$ .24, .92

3-4a. FRW ≥ 120/FRW < 120 $\hat{OR} = 2.27$, $\hat{RR} = 1.70$
 b. Smokers/nonsmokers $\hat{OR} = 1.06$, $\hat{RR} = 1.04$
 c. DBP ≥ 90/DBP < 90 $\hat{OR} = 1.40$, $\hat{RR} = 1.29$

Chapter 4

4-1a. .0234
 b. 47%
 c. 28%

4-2a. $\hat{RR}$ for CHD = 1.17, $\hat{RR}$ for lung cancer = 3.79
 b. Excess mortality rate: for CHD = .00133, for lung cancer = .00117
 Population attributable risk: for CHD = .07, for lung cancer = .53
 c. Excess deaths: from CHD = 929, from lung cancer = 822

4-3a. $\hat{RR}$ for current cigarette smokers: CHD = 1.54, lung cancer = 9.37
 b. CHD = .48, lung cancer = .95
 c.

	Annual excess deaths	
Smoking category	CHD	Lung cancer
≥ 39/day	84	51
21–39/day	345	209
10–20/day	569*	230*
1–9/day	132	38

4-4.

SBP category	Excess risk	Excess risk (%)
≥ 180	.213	62
170–179	.187	59
160–169	.099	43
150–159	.086	40
140–149	.053	29

Chapter 5

	$\hat{RR}$	$\hat{OR}$
5-2a.	1.77	2.03
b.	1.93	2.27
c.	1.95	2.29
d.	1.90	2.23
e.	—	2.37
f.	—	2.36

	$\hat{RR}$	$\hat{OR}$
5-3a.	1.69	1.92
b.	1.55	1.73
c.	1.55	1.72
d.	1.53	1.70
e.	—	1.76
f.	—	1.75

5-4a. $\hat{OR} = 1.72$, $\chi^2_{M-H} = .66$, .95 CL $= .47, 6.35$
b. $\hat{OR} = 1.72$, .95 CL $= .64, 4.61$

Chapter 6

6-1a.	.197
b.	Men .265, women .136
ci.	2.29
cii.	2.40
ciii.	1.69
civ.	1.42
6-2ai.	.306
aii.	.080
bi.	.47
bii.	1.24
biii.	1.93
6-3ai.	.262
aii.	.077
bi.	.45
biii.	1.92

Chapter 7

7-1.

	$_{16}P_0$	SE $_{16}P_0$
≥ 165	.429	.084
< 165	.745	.037

7-2. $\chi^2_1 = 11.85$
7-3. $\hat{OR} = 2.97$, $\chi^2_1 = 11.76$
7-4. $\chi^2_1 = 11.78$

7-6.   Crude = .117
            Net   = .122
7-7. x $_{x+2}p_x$
            0   .947
            2   .921
            4   .929

Chapter 8

8-2. $_2\hat{d}_0 = 2$, $_2\hat{L}_0 = 405$, $_2\hat{m}_0 = .0099$; $_{10}\hat{d}_0 = 28$, $_{10}\hat{L}_0 = 1809$, $_{10}\hat{m}_0 = .155$
8-3. $_2\hat{d}_0 = 2$, $_2\hat{L}_0 = 392$, $_2\hat{m}_0 = .0102$; $_{10}\hat{d}_0 = 28$, $_{10}\hat{L}_0 = 1750$, $_{10}\hat{m}_0 = .160$
8-4. $_2\hat{d}_0 = 9$, $_2\hat{L}_0 = 335$, $_2\hat{m}_0 = .0537$; $_{10}\hat{d}_0 = 34$, $_{10}\hat{L}_0 = 1399$, $_{10}\hat{m}_0 = .243$
8-5.   45–54   20
            55–64   40
            65–74   30
            ≥75   10

Bibliography

Abbott RD, Y Yin, DM Reed and K Yano [1986], New Engl J Med **315**:717.

Abraham S [1986], Am J Clin Nutr **43**:839.

Abramson JH and E Peritz [1983], *Calculator Programs for the Health Sciences.* New York: Oxford University Press.

Armitage P [1971], *Statistical Methods in Medical Research.* New York: Wiley.

Axtell LM, AJ Asire and MH Meyers, eds. [1976], *Cancer Patient Survival,* Report No. 5, HEW NIH Publication 77–992. Washington, D.C.: U.S. Government Printing Office.

Bailar JC and F Ederer [1964], Biometrics **20**:639.

Breslow NE and NE Day [1980], *Statistical Methods in Cancer Research,* IARC Scientific Publications No. 32. Lyon: Int. Agency for Research on Cancer.

Chiang CL [1961a], in *Proceedings of the Fourth Berkeley Symposium on Mathematical Statistics and Probability* (J Neyman, ed). Berkeley: University of California Press.

Chiang CL [1961b], *Vital Statistics, Special Report 47 (no. 9).* Washington, D.C.: U.S. Government Printing Office.

Chiang CL [1968], *Introduction to Stochastic Processes in Biostatistics.* New York: Wiley.

Cochran WG [1963], *Sampling Techniques,* 2nd ed. New York: Wiley.

Cole P and B MacMahon [1971], Br J Prev Soc Med **25**:242.

Cook EF and L Goldman [1988], Am J Epidemiol **127**:626.

Cornfield J [1951], J Natl Cancer Inst **11**:1269.

Cornfield J [1959], Am J Mental Deficiency **64**:240.

Cornfield J, W Haenszel, EC Hammond, AM Lilienfeld, MB Shimkin and EL Wynder [1959], J Natl Cancer Inst **22**:173.

Cornfield J, T Gordon and WW Smith [1961], Bull Int Stat Inst **38** (Part II): 97.

Coronary Drug Project Research Group [1974], J Chron Dis **27**:267.

Cutler SJ and F Ederer [1958], J Chron Dis **8**:699.

Cox DR [1972], J Royal Stat Soc Series B **34**:187.

Dawber TR [1980], *The Framingham Study: The Epidemiology of Atherosclerotic Disease.* Boston: Harvard University Press.

Dawber TR, GF Meadors and FE Moore [1951], Am J Pub Health **41**:279.

Deming WE [1950], *Some Theory of Sampling.* New York: Wiley.

Diabetic Retinopathy Study Research Group [1976], Am J Ophthalmol **81**:383.

Documenta Geigy Scientific Tables, 7th edn. [1970], Basel: Ciba-Geigy.

Dorn HF [1950], Hum Biol **22**:238.

Draper NR and H Smith [1981], *Applied Regression Analysis,* 2nd ed. New York: Wiley.

Ederer F [1975], Am J Ophthalmol **79**:752.

Ederer F and N Mantel [1974], Am J Epidemiol **100**:165.

Feldstein MS [1966], J Royal Stat Soc Series **A 129**:61.

Fisher L and K Patil [1974], Am J Epidemiol **100**:347.

Fisher RA [1936], Ann Eugenics **7** (Part II):179.

Fisher RA and F Yates [1974], *Statistical Tables for Biological, Agricultural and Medical Research,* Table XXXIII. London: Longman Group.

Fleiss JL [1979], J Chron Dis **32**:69.

Fleiss JL [1981], *Statistical Methods for Rates and Proportions,* 2nd ed. New York: Wiley.

Fleiss JL [1984], Am J Epidemiol **120**:1.

Forthofer RN [1983], Am J Epidemiol **117**:507.

Gart JJ [1971], Rev Int Stat **39**:148.

Gart JJ [1982], Am J Epidemiol **115**:453.

Gordon T and WB Kannel [1968], *The Framingham Study, Section 1,* National Heart Institute.

Gordon T and D Shurtleff [1973], *The Framingham Study,* NIH Publication 74–478, Section 29. Department of Health, Education and Welfare.

Greenland S [1984], Am J Epidemiol **120**:4.

Greenland S, J Schlesselman and MH Criqui [1986], Am J Epidemiol **123**:203.

Greenwood M [1926], *Reports on Public Health and Medical Subjects,* No. 33, Appendix 1. London: H.M. Stationery Office.

Hadden WC and MI Harris [1987], Vital and Health Statistics Series 11, No. 237. Nat. Center Health Stat., DHHS Pub. No. (PHS) 87–1687. Public Health Service, Washington D.C.

Haldane JBS [1956], Ann Hum Genet **20**:309.

Halperin M [1977], Am J Epidemiol **105**:496.

Halperin M, E Rogot, J Gurian and F Ederer [1958], J Chron Dis **21**:13.

Halperin M, WC Blackwelder and JJ Verter [1971], J Chron Dis **24**:125.

Hill AB [1953], New Engl J Med **248**:995.

Hiller RA and HA Kahn [1976], Br J Ophthalmol **60**:283.

Holford TR, C White and JL Kelsey [1978], Am J Epidemiol **107**:245.

Hypertension Detection and Follow-up Program Cooperative Group [1976], Prev Med **5**:207.

Kahn HA [1966], National Cancer Institute Monograph 19.

Kahn HA, JH Medalie, HN Neufeld, E. Riss, M Balogh and JJ Groen [1969], Isr J Med Sci **5**:1117.

Kahn HA, JB Herman, JH Medalie, HN Neufeld, E Riss and U Goldbourt [1971], J Chron Dis **23**:617.

Kahn HA, H Leibowitz, JP Ganley, M Kini, T Colton, R Nickerson and TR Dawber [1975], Am J Ophthalmol **79**:768.

Kahn HA, RL Phillips, DA Snowdon and W Choi [1984], Am J Epidemiol **119**:775.

Kaplan EL and P Meier [1958], J Am Stat Assoc **53**:457.

Katz D, J Baptista, SP Azen and MC Pike [1978], Biometrics **34**:469.

Kelsey JL, WD Thompson and AS Evans [1986], *Methods in Observational Epidemiology*. New York: Oxford University Press.

Kleinbaum DG, LL Kupper and H Morgenstern [1982], *Epidemiologic Research*. Belmont, Calif.: Lifetime Learning Publications.

Kornberg A [1976], New Engl J Med **294**:1211.

Kupper LL and MD Hogan [1978], Am J Epidemiol **108**:447.

Kuzma JW [1967], Biometrics **23**:51.

Landis J, J Lepkowski, S Eklund and S Stehouwer [1982], Vital and Health Statistics. Series 2, No. 92. Nat. Center Health Stat., DHHS Pub. No. 82–1366. Public Health Service, Washington D.C.

Lee ET [1980], *Statistical Methods for Survival Data Analysis*. Belmont, Calif.: Lifetime Learning Publications.

Leibowitz HM, DE Krueger, LR Maunder, RC Milton, MM Kini, HA Kahn, RJ Nickerson, J Pool, TL Colton, JP Ganley, JI Lowenstein and TR Dawber [1980], Survey Ophthalmol **24** (suppl):517.

Lemeshow S and DW Hosmer [1982], Am J Epidemiol **115**:92.

Levin ML [1953], Acta Unio Int Contra Cancrum **9**:531.

Leviton A [1973], Am J Epidemiol **98**:231.

Lilienfeld AM and DE Lilienfeld [1980], *Foundations of Epidemiology*, 2nd ed. New York: Oxford University Press.

Liu K, J Stamler, A Dyer, J McKeever and P McKeever [1978], J Chron Dis **31**:399.

MacMahon B and TF Pugh [1970], *Epidemiology: Principles and Methods*. Boston: Little Brown.

Madow WG and LH Madow [1944], Ann Math Stat **15**:1.

Mantel N [1966], Cancer Chem Rep **50**:163.

Mantel N [1969], Am Stat **23**:32.

Mantel N [1977], Am J Epidemiol **106**:125.

Mantel N [1986], J Chron Dis **39**:154.

Mantel N [1988], The Confounder Crisis. Submitted for publication.

Mantel N and Haenszel W [1959], J Natl Cancer Inst **22**:719.

Mantel N and JL Fleiss [1980], Am J Epidemiol **112**:129.

Matanoski GM, R Seltser, PE Sartwell, EL Diamond and EA Elliott [1975], Am J Epidemiol **101**:188.

Miettinen OS [1969], Biometrics **25**:339.

Miettinen OS [1970], Am J Epidemiol **91**:111.

Miettinen OS [1974a], Am J Epidemiol **99**:325.

Miettinen OS [1974b], Am J Epidemiol **100**:350.

Miettinen OS [1976a], Am J Epidemiol **103**:226.

Miettinen OS [1976b], Am J Epidemiol **104**:609.

Miettinen OS [1979], J Chron Dis **32**:80.

Murphy EA [1982], *Biostatistics in Medicine*. Baltimore: Johns Hopkins University Press.

National Center for Health Statistics [1970], *Vital Statistics of the U.S.*, Vol. II, Part B. Washington, D.C.: U.S. Government Printing Office.

National Center for Health Statistics [1987], *Monthly Vital Statistics Report*, Vol. 36, No. 5.

National Diet-Heart Study Research Group [1968], Circulation **37** (suppl 1):1.

Oleinick A and N Mantel [1970], J Chron Dis **22**:617.

Pasquini P, HA Kahn, D Pileggi, A. Pana, J Terzi and E Guzzanti [1983], Am J Epidemiol **118**:699.

Peto R, MC Pike, P Armitage, NE Breslow, DR Cox, SV Howard, N Mantel, K McPherson, J Peto and PG Smith [1977], Br J Cancer **35**:1.

Pigou AC [1947], Proc Br Acad **32**:13.

Prentice R [1975], Biometrics **32**:599.

Remington RD and MA Schork [1970], *Statistics with Applications to the Biological and Health Sciences*. Englewood Cliffs, N.J.: Prentice-Hall.

Rogot E [1974], J Chron Dis **27**:189.

Rothman KJ [1974], Am J Epidemiol **99**:385.

Rothman KJ [1976], Am J Epidemiol **103**:506.

Rothman KJ and Boice JD [1979], *Epidemiologic Analysis with a Programmable Calculator*, NIH Publication 79–1649. Washington D.C.: U.S. Government Printing Office.

Schlesselman J [1974], Am J Epidemiol **99**:381.

Schlesselman JJ [1982], *Case-Control Studies*. New York: Oxford University Press.

Schlesselman J [unpublished tables available from the author].

Schoenberg BS [1983], Neuroepidemiology **2**:257.

Schwartzbaum JA, BS Hulka, WC Fowler, DG Kaufman and D Hoberman [1987], Am J Epidemiol **126**:851.

Seigel DG and SW Greenhouse [1973], Am J Epidemiol **97**:324.

Shryock HS and JS Siegel [1975], *Methods and Materials of Demography*, Vol. 2. Washington D.C.: U.S. Government Printing Office.

Shurtleff D [1970], *The Framingham Study: An Epidemiologic Investigation of Cardiovascular Disease*, Section 26. Washington D.C.: U.S. Government Printing Office.

Shurtleff D [1974], *The Framingham Study*, NIH Publication 74–599, Section 30. Department of Health, Education and Welfare.

Snedecor GW and WG Cochran [1980], *Statistical Methods*, 7th ed. Ames: Iowa State University Press.

The Rand Corporation [1954], *A Million Random Digits*. Glencoe, Ill. Free Press.

Truett J, J Cornfield and WB Kannel [1967], J Chron Dis **25**:11.

Tsiatis AA [1980], Biometrika **67**:250.

U.S. Bureau of the Census [1970], *Characteristics of the Population*, Volume 1, Part 1, U.S. Summary Section 1. Washington D.C.: U.S. Government Printing Office.

Walker SH and DB Duncan [1967], Biometrika **54**:167.

Walter SD [1976], Biometrics **32**:830.

Walter SD [1977], Am J Epidemiol **105**:387.

Walter SD [1978], Int J Epidemiol **7**:175.

Woolf B [1955], Ann Hum Genet **19**:251.

Yates F [1934], J Royal Stat Soc Suppl **1**:217.

Index